Trauma-Informed Research in Sport, Exercise, and Health

This is the first book to examine trauma research in the context of sport, exercise, and health. It outlines evidence-based, trauma-informed research practices, which qualitative researchers can use when conducting trauma research to prevent causing further harm to participants while maintaining a strengths-based approach.

Featuring the trauma research of leading qualitative sport, exercise, and health researchers from around the world, each chapter showcases the contributors' trauma research and participant context, followed by the 'what, why, and how' of trauma-informed research practices that were implemented. This book includes work from a wide range of contexts, including gender-based violence in sport and coaching, abuse in sport, the aftermath of abuse and violence, physical activity after spinal cord injury, trauma and limb amputation, trauma and homelessness, trauma and autistic adults, and sport for care-experienced youth. It provides researchers interested in working with populations affected by trauma with a qualitative research resource to build on, and highlights new directions in conducting trauma-informed research.

This is important reading for any researcher with an interest in trauma not only in sport, exercise, and health research but also in qualitative research contexts more broadly. It is a valuable resource for anyone working in athlete welfare, sport and exercise psychology, youth sport, sport development, physical activity and health, disability, gender, safeguarding, or social work.

Jenny McMahon is an Associate Professor in Education at the University of Tasmania, Australia. Before moving into academia, she was an elite swimmer who represented Australia at an international level, winning numerous medals. Her research centres on using qualitative methodologies such as creative analytical practices, visual methods, and narrative inquiry to explore trauma, athlete abuse, and education interventions in sport to bring about social change.

Kerry R. McGannon is a Professor in Kinesiology and Health Sciences at Laurentian University, Canada. Her research program centres qualitative methodologies (e.g., narrative inquiry, discourse analysis) to understand sport and exercise participation. Specific streams of this work explore cultural influences on identity and critical interpretations of sport and exercise. She is also Co-Editor of the journal *Qualitative Research in Sport, Exercise and Health*.

Qualitative Research in Sport and Physical Activity

Series Editors:
Michael D. Giardina
Florida State University, USA
Brett Smith
Durham University, UK

From ethnography and narrative inquiry to participatory action research and digital methods, feminist and poststructural theory to new materialism and onto-epistemologies, serious conversations about the practices, politics and philosophies of qualitative inquiry have never been stronger or more abundant in the field of sport, exercise and health. At the same time, the growth of new critical methodologies has opened up interdisciplinary space for sustained engagement with provocative questions over evidence, knowledge, and research practices. The *Qualitative Research in Sport and Physical Activity* series is the first of its kind within the field that has as its mandate the necessary advancement of qualitative methodologies and their intersection with theory and practice. Books in the series will develop new and innovative methodologies, serve as 'how-to' guides for conducting research, and present empirical research findings. It will serve the growing number of students and academics who promote and utilize qualitative inquiry in university courses, research, and applied practice.

Also available in this series:

For more information about this series, please visit: https://www.routledge.com/Qualitative-Research-in-Sport-and-Physical-Activity/book-series/QRSPA

Trauma-Informed Research in Sport, Exercise, and Health

Qualitative Methods

Edited by Jenny McMahon
and Kerry R. McGannon

Routledge
Taylor & Francis Group
LONDON AND NEW YORK

First published 2024
by Routledge
4 Park Square, Milton Park, Abingdon, Oxon OX14 4RN

and by Routledge
605 Third Avenue, New York, NY 10158

Routledge is an imprint of the Taylor & Francis Group, an informa business

British Library Cataloguing-in-Publication Data
A catalogue record for this book is available from the British Library

ISBN: 978-1-032-36610-4 (hbk)
ISBN: 978-1-032-36613-5 (pbk)
ISBN: 978-1-003-33290-9 (ebk)

DOI: 10.4324/9781003332909

Typeset in Optima
by KnowledgeWorks Global Ltd.

Contents

Foreword

At the heart of this Foreword is a story of trauma. Commencing in the early 1980s, it highlights the complexity of trauma experiences, and re-traumatising events, yet it would be familiar to scholars of sport, exercise, and health as in these environments such narratives are pervasive. Unlike the authors who comprise this collection, who emphasise language and practices that are trauma-informed, the setting for the story pre-dates the widespread use of trauma-informed approaches. Today, as the chapters in this collection attest, being trauma-informed enhances safety for those affected by trauma, by limiting the risk of re-traumatisation with the potential to encourage subsequent healing and growth. But these chapters also succeed in more meaningful, academic, and evidence-based ways. They engage critically with the way symptoms of trauma have been pathologised and illuminate how trauma touches wider networks of people. They highlight too how stories of trauma, so often upsetting to hear, are equally disturbing for researchers, who must be sensitive to the ways in which trauma is so often linked to systems of power. The story that follows offers a graphic illustration of my personal experience.

A Short Story of Trauma

I targeted initially friends as pilot interviewees when I commenced fieldwork for my PhD on professional football: individuals who I could be more re-laxed with, who would bear with me as I handled my research inexperience. With the few individuals I approached – all former professional football teammates – my only request was that we undertook the interview immediately. I had not spoken to some of these players/friends for some years, but all engaged fully in the research interview process. On one occasion, with a friend I had played with for four years as a young professional footballer in the 1980s, someone with whom I shared fateful turning points in our careers (his much more successful than mine), we settled in post-interview to reconnect. My friend listened aghast as I detailed my experience of treatment for Stage 4 Hodgkin's Lymphoma, the tribulations of chemotherapy, my parents, and infertility. He was annoyed he didn't know: he would have helped.

Keen to divert the conversation from a focus on me, I asked about him, his football career, and his family. He was both unguarded and caring with answers about his children. But then, unprompted, he started to talk about a former youth coach, well-known in the South of England and to both of us, and his experiences of what I recognised as appalling abuses of power. Little-by-little my friend talked of 'stripping' games, touching and, eventually, he talked of molestation. My friend had been a victim of sexual abuse by an individual who operated as an important gatekeeper for aspiring professionals. It happened in his teenage years, still a child, week-by-week, in and around *our* friends, he was not alone in these experiences, and over a drawn-out period, some of those affected had been able to find a supportive bond. Many years later legal action was triggered, and the coach was found guilty.

As he referenced the abuse to which he was subjected, simultaneously he spoke of the all-encompassing scale of the professional football industry vis-à-vis the inconsequentiality of an irrelevant would-be player. Who would care about him and his lost sense of humanity as an individual feeling silenced and isolated inside his profession. In our conversation he emphasised the point that, while suffering such a profound form of emotional shock and trauma, he was still required to bend and blend in ways that fit to powerful discourses of vocation, privilege, and economic capital both in and outside his workplaces.

From initially planning to meet over lunch, he asked if I would stay to meet his wife and children. And from that moment he directed our conversation, and we interlaced my experiences of being in remission for cancer with episodes and events in his professional playing career as well as youth football. Simply put, however, I was totally unprepared as either a friend or researcher for what he said. I was too inexperienced to know how to do anything more than listen. I remember distinctly that his words were not laced with the same dismay I recall feeling. He disclosed that other affected players had contacted him, and these connections were meaningful and had helped. Consequently, he was now receiving help, although this came only years after the abuse.

He shared his experiences with me then, but the trauma remains still. As an outcome of remaining silent – through shame and fear – and the compounding, re-traumatising impacts of protracted legal proceedings, my friend only now benefits from evidenced-based trauma-informed approaches to support that are the subject matter of this new collection.

This Book

It is unsurprising that people affected by trauma can be re-traumatised at any time, and in any context, but practices and situations can make it more likely to occur, such as the recalling of painful or traumatic memories which has become central to qualitative researchers' work. Such memories may impact researchers as well, through recalling their own lived experiences and/or by listening to others' stories. Given the recalling of lived experiences commonly occurs in research settings, it underscores the crucial need for qualitative researchers to be aware and responsive to the needs of participants by being trauma-informed and adopting evidence-based trauma-informed principles. When such practices are done, the potential risk of causing further harm can be reduced.

And so, in this book, an academic focus on the use of trauma-informed approaches in research contexts and researcher practice is foregrounded, as epitomised by the carefully curated chapters in this collection. Trauma is now recognised as a global health epidemic; thus, this is not just required, but paramount. As well as implementing evidence-based trauma-informed practices, recognising the significance of communities of care is fundamental, particularly in circumstances in which people can find themselves emotionally overwhelmed.

In the chapters in this edited volume, international researchers will showcase their trauma work, highlighting first-hand experiences of trauma and its lasting effects. They also provide strategies to reduce causing participants' further harm in their research and discuss some of these impacts on themselves. There is an expectation now for all people, at all levels of the organisation of sport, exercise, and health to understand this responsibility by understanding trauma and integrating trauma-informed practices. The chapters in this collection make therefore not just an original contribution to qualitative trauma research in the field of sport, exercise, and health, but foreground trauma-informed practices as an essential theme.

Professor Martin Roderick
Department of Sport and Exercise Sciences
Durham University, England
May 7, 2023

Acknowledgements

We would like to extend our sincerest thanks to each of the wonderful authors who contributed to this book. We are grateful to you for sharing your trauma research, insights, and experiences as part of our book. We also acknowledge that each of you have had experience with trauma, whether it be personally, or vicariously, from the trauma work that you have undertaken. Given that trauma is now acknowledged as a global health issue, your expertise relating to carrying out research with people affected by trauma is greatly appreciated and needed. We are certain that other researchers will benefit from your contributions and experiences within this topic of research. With that said, we hope that you are all proud to be part of this final product.

Thank you also to Simon Whitmore from Routledge, and to the Qualitative Research in Sport and Physical Activity series editors Professors Michael D. Giardina and Brett Smith for their support and guidance in developing this edited collection. We also thank the reviewers who offered their support and guidance from the early outset of our book's development.

Jenny's Acknowledgements

I would like to thank my partner Chris for his tireless support through our relationship and my career. I acknowledge that my 'history' of abuse and trauma does not make me an easy person to live with. I remember you saying when I first met you over two decades ago, that you were going to be my rock, and that the only way you could show me was through your unwavering support and by never giving up on me. Thank you, Chris, for being all that you said you would be. Thanks to my co-editor Kerry for mentoring and collaborating with me for the past ten years. I know I would not be the writer and researcher that I have become without you. Researching abuse and trauma is not easy. Acknowledging this along with having an insight into my background, you always tread carefully and are unwavering in your support of me. We know each other's boundaries, when to press each other and when to back off. I could not think of anybody else that I would rather do this work with.

Kerry's Acknowledgements

I would like to thank my partner, Ted Butryn, for his love, humour, and patience. You always support me without question, especially during difficult times. Witnessing your ongoing journey through sport and identity transformation is an inspiration. Thanks to co-editor Jenny for a cherished friendship and academic partnership. I had the privilege of first meeting you at the *International Conference for Qualitative Research in Sport and Exercise,* in 2014. My most vivid memory remains your talk on elite athlete self-presentation on social media, where you used footage of yourself as a 16-year-old swimmer in the Commonwealth Games. You engaged the audience on how problematic 'slim to win' cultural ideals result in insidious effects, and how for some athletes (including yourself) there is lost potential, compromised mental health, and trauma. Your work as a cultural insider on maltreatment and trauma in sport is vulnerable and evocative. When you approached me to co-edit this book I was – and remain – honoured, to be part of the vision and final product. I am grateful to you, and all trauma survivors, who share their stories.

Contributors

Natalie Barker-Ruchti is an Associate Professor in Sport Science (Sport Management) at Örebro University, Sweden. She is also currently employed as Expert Pedagogy/Science in the project Ethics in Sport at Swiss Olympic, Switzerland.

James Brighton is a Senior Lecturer in the Sociology of Sport and Exercise at Canterbury Christ Church University, UK.

Daryl T. Cowan is a Lecturer and Programme Leader in Sport Coaching in the Division of Sport, Exercise and Health at the University of the West of Scotland, UK.

Melissa Day is a Reader in qualitative sport psychology at the University of Chichester, UK.

Jordan A. Donnelly is a Lecturer in Sport Coaching and Development at the University of the West of Scotland's Division of Sport, Exercise & Health in the United Kingdom.

Kirsty Forsdike is an Associate Professor and Principal Research Fellow at La Trobe Rural Health School, La Trobe University in Australia. She specialises in the prevention of and response to gender-based violence in sport.

Fiona Giles is a Postdoctoral Research Fellow at La Trobe Rural Health School, La Trobe University and Department of General Practice, The University of Melbourne, Australia. Her research focuses on prevention and response to gender-based violence in health settings and health equity.

Oliver Hooper is a Lecturer in Physical Education and Sport Coaching at Loughborough University, UK.

Patrick Jachyra is an Assistant Professor in the Department of Sport & Exercise Sciences, at Durham University, UK. Patrick is appointed as an Affiliate Scientist at the Centre for Addiction and Mental Health, in Toronto, Canada, in Clinical Research, Adult Neurodevelopment and Geriatric Psychiatry.

Alixandra N. Krahn is a Postdoctoral visitor in the School of Kinesiology at York University, UK. She is also a part-time sessional instructor in the Faculty of Kinesiology at St. Francis Xavier University Canada.

William V. Massey is an Associate Professor for the College of Public Health and Human Sciences at Oregon State University, USA.

Sara McLaughlin is a Program Manager of Strategic Initiatives at the Laureus Sport for Good Foundation USA and worked with Dr Whitley as her Graduate Assistant for Adelphi University's Sport-Based Youth Development Specialization in the United States.

James McLeod is a PhD student in the Department of Psychology at Durham University in the United Kingdom.

Fiona J. Moola is an Associate Professor in the School of Early Childhood Studies at Toronto Metropolitan University, Canada. She is also Associate Professor in the Dalla Lana School of Public Health and Rehabilitation Sciences Institute at the University of Toronto Research Associate, Grandview Kids Hospital.

Anthony Papathomas is a Senior Lecturer in Sport and Exercise Psychology at Loughborough University, UK.

Erin Prior is a Doctoral Researcher and University Teacher at Loughborough University in the United Kingdom.

Thomas Quarmby is a Reader in Physical Education and Sport Pedagogy at Leeds Beckett University, UK.

Simon Rosenbaum is a Scientia Associate Professor in the Discipline of Psychiatry and Mental Health at the University of New South Wales, Australia.

Rachel Sandford is a Reader in Physical Education, Youth and Social Justice at Loughborough University, UK.

Andy Smith is a Professor of Sport, Physical Activity and Mental Health at Edge Hill University, UK, where he is also Director of the Centre for Mental Health, Sport, and Physical Activity Research.

Maria Luisa Pereira Vargas is a former Doctoral Researcher at Loughborough University, currently working as a Researcher at Durham University, UK.

Ross Wadey is a Professor of Sport Psychology at St Mary's University, Twickenham, UK.

Meredith A. Whitley is a Professor at Adelphi University, USA. She is also a Research Fellow at the Centre for Sport Leadership at Stellenbosch University, South Africa.

Toni L. Williams is an Associate Professor in the Department of Sport and Exercise Sciences at Durham University, UK.

Chris Zehntner is a Senior Lecturer with research interests in sport coaching; coach education; coach development pathways and coach/athlete wellbeing. He currently works at University of Southern Queensland, Australia.

Chapter 1

Introduction

Trauma-Informed Research Communities in Sport, Exercise, and Health

Jenny McMahon and Kerry R. McGannon

Researching the lived experiences of marginalised and oppressed groups in sport, exercise, and health contexts, including people who have suffered from or continue to suffer from trauma, has become central to qualitative researchers' work (Alessi & Kahn, 2023; Darroch et al., 2020; McMahon et al., 2023; van Ingen, 2016; Whitley et al., 2022). This is unsurprising, given that trauma is a global health epidemic with most adults experiencing a traumatic event at some point throughout their lives (Benjet et al., 2016; Magruder et al., 2017; SAMHSA, 2014, 2017, 2023). With high global trauma statistics such as these, it is likely that a person participating in sport, exercise, and health qualitative research projects, either as a participant or as part of the research team, will have experienced trauma in their lives.

Due to the prevalence of trauma and its subsequent effects, an awareness of trauma-informed practices is very much needed (SAMHSA, 2014, 2023) so that the risk of re-traumatisation for those affected is minimised and a strength-based approach is promoted. Such an awareness is important because the impact of trauma on a person is complex and can be subtle, insidious, or outright destructive impacting their health and well-being (McMahon et al., 2023). Trauma and vicarious trauma do not only occur through direct exposure (i.e., something that happens directly to an individual) but also by witnessing of an adverse event, or indirect exposure such as hearing about an adverse event can have trauma consequences (Acosta, 2017). While, experiencing or witnessing adverse events does not lead to trauma in every instance, when it does, it can impact a person developmentally in three ways: neurologically, physiologically, and psychologically (Dye, 2018; McMahon et al., Under Review; SAMHSA, 2014, 2023). Several other factors also increase the risk of trauma such as a cumulative exposure to adverse experiences (Gu et al., 2022) or when adverse experiences occur in a person's childhood and/or adolescence (Magruder et al., 2017; Massey & Williams, 2020; Mountjoy et al., 2016; SAMHSA, 2014, 2023). The effects of trauma may occur immediately following exposure to an adverse traumatic event or have a delayed onset, referred to as the "silent period" (McMahon et al., 2023; Teicher & Samson, 2016, p. 257).

DOI: 10.4324/9781003332909-1

Unsurprisingly, qualitative studies conducted in sport, exercise, and health contexts are responding to the global health epidemic status of trauma and as such, it has become an increasingly investigated theme with researchers reporting serious trauma consequences (e.g., Darroch et al., 2020; Massey & Williams, 2020; McMahon et al., 2023; van Ingen, 2016). Trauma consequences such as eating disorders, sexual addiction, abuse of prescription medication, alcohol use disorder, self-harm such as cutting, depression, and suicidal ideation have been reported in these related studies conducted in these contexts (McMahon & McGannon, 2021; Papathomas & Lavallee, 2014; Roderick et al., 2017; Smith, 2019). Consequently, those who have experienced or are experiencing, trauma have had their internal and external coping resources affected, requiring them to need ongoing, varied, and considered support (Dye, 2018; McMahon et al., Under Review; McMahon et al., 2023; SAMHSA, 2014, 2023).

Ongoing, varied, and considered support is important because the risk of re-traumatisation is high (SAMHSA, 2014, 2023). Re-traumatisation can occur in any situation or environment that resembles aspects of a person's original trauma literally or symbolically, and consequently difficult feelings and reactions can be triggered (BrightQuest, 2023; SAMHSA, 2017). When comparing re-traumatisation risks highlighted by general trauma researchers (i.e., outside of sport, exercise, and health) to commonly taken up qualitative research practices, there are many concerning alignments. For example, when a person (i.e., participant) is required to recall a lived experience of trauma (e.g., remembering and/or discussing specifics of their traumatic encounter), re-traumatisation may result (Butler et al., 2011; Hira et al., 2023; SAMHSA, 2014, 2017, 2023). Other potential triggers listed by trauma experts and researchers include environmental triggers where the space, place, or environment may remind the person of the adverse event they experienced (e.g., sport environment) (Butler et al., 2011; Hira et al., 2023; SAMHSA, 2014, 2017, 2023). Spatial triggers (i.e., physical distance between researcher and participant, small rooms, and restricted access to exit), physical triggers (e.g., touch and sounds), and interpersonal triggers (e.g., gender differentials between researcher and participant) were also listed as situations which may exacerbate the risk of re-traumatisation (Butler et al., 2011; Hira et al., 2023; SAMHSA, 2014, 2017, 2023). Further, the use of specific imagery such as memory prompts (e.g., photographs, movies, and news/media stories), a commonly taken up research method, may cause participants to have visual flashbacks relating to their adverse experiences, leading to further harm (Butler et al., 2011; Hira et al., 2023; SAMHSA, 2014, 2017, 2023). Hierarchical power relationships, where others hold power over those affected by trauma, can also be problematic (Butler et al., 2011; Hira et al., 2023; Sweeney et al., 2018). When applied to research settings, researcher-led investigations reduce participants' agency and control.

Without consideration of evidence-based trauma-informed guidelines, the adoption of commonly used or 'standard' research practices may cause research participants further harm, exacerbating their risk of re-traumatisation (Hira et al., 2023). If re-traumatisation occurs, the person (i.e., research participant) will experience a period of heightened sensibility and renewed vulnerability to traumatic memories (SAMHSA, 2014, 2017, 2023). Other re-traumatisation symptoms may include loss of trust, stress and anxiety, feelings of pessimism and fatalism, intense flashbacks/nightmares, paranoia, agoraphobic behaviour (e.g., fear of leaving the house), increase in vulnerability to triggers, greater reaction to stress, and higher incidence of self-harm (BrightQuest, 2023; Menschner & Maul, 2016; SAMHSA, 2014, 2023).

Re-traumatisation risks have been recognised and responded to through the implementation of trauma-informed practices in service-based contexts (i.e., outside of research). These contexts include social work, education, counselling, criminal and juvenile justice, health, mental, and behaviour health settings (McMahon et al., 2023). This recognition has resulted in the incorporation of evidence-based practices into areas such as programme design, facilitation of programmes, systems, care plans, and service providers/individual practices. While not related to research practices specifically, some qualitative researchers in sport, exercise, and health are drawing on trauma-informed practices to develop and deliver physical activity and/or sport services to mitigate the consequences of trauma (e.g., Darroch et al., 2020; van Ingen, 2016; Whitley et al., 2022). While this work continues to grow, the implementation and consideration of such practices into qualitative research contexts and researcher practices are less prevalent. Researchers in the social sciences have recently began making recommendations for trauma-informed practices in qualitative research contexts (Alessi & Kahn, 2023; Golden, 2022), with such consideration in sport, exercise, and health also beginning to emerge (McMahon et al., Under Review; McMahon et al., 2023; Palladino et al., 2023).

Although some researchers have reported that trauma survivors may find the research process beneficial (e.g., enhanced clarity and potential catharsis) (Jaffe et al., 2015; Rosetto, 2014), due to the above points and the unpredictability of trauma reactions (e.g., re-traumatisation can occur sometime after the research event which is not reported), the potential risk of causing re-traumatisation in research settings is likely high. When coupled with the effects of re-traumatisation, these points highlight the need for qualitative researchers to be trauma responsive to the needs of participants with whom they work alongside. Indeed, researchers' failure to implement evidence-based trauma-informed guidelines may result in them implementing unintended 'unsafe' practices. These consequences may compound the effects of adverse lived experience (e.g., athlete maltreatment) or trauma for participants (Bath, 2008; Filson, 2011; SAMHSA, 2023; Sweeney et al., 2018).

Ethical Issues and Considerations: Trauma-Informed Research

Implementing trauma-informed guidelines into research settings is a form of aspirational ethics (Lahman et al., 2011) (i.e., goes beyond the minimum ethical requirement). Yet surprisingly, many university research ethics boards have not made it a compulsory requirement when gaining ethical approval. Instead, ethical approval often involves researchers' adherence to a rigid procedural process (i.e., step-by-step method) as well as attending to the "more traditional considerations for trauma research (i.e., types of questions being asked, participant recruitment protocols, etc.)" (Hira et al., 2023, p. 9; McMahon et al., Under Review).

Further, many research ethics departments often view trauma as a potential vulnerability for people and in turn, stigmatise trauma as a debilitating condition (Hira et al., 2023). While trauma can be debilitating for some, not all people who have been exposed to an adverse event will experience it (Dye, 2018), and as noted some may experience benefits (e.g., clarity) from their involvement in the research process (Jaffe et al., 2015; Rosetto, 2014). People may also be at varying stages of their trauma recovery process and want to openly discuss their adverse experiences. Importantly, the assumption that trauma is a vulnerability, and the rigidity of guidelines imposed on researchers to gain the 'tick' of ethical approval, risks silencing stories that need to come forward to expose historical, cultural, and systemic harms and traumas, in sport, exercise, and health contexts.

Subsequently, many guidelines associated with gaining institutional ethical research approval sit at odds with a trauma-informed approach (SAMHSA, 2023), failing to acknowledge the complex, variable, and unpredictable nature of victims' histories and reactions to trauma (McMahon et al., Under Review; SAMHSA, 2014, 2023). Without providing safe spaces grounded in evidence-based trauma-informed practices to hear these stories, trauma may remain hidden and stigmatised (McMahon et al., 2023; van Ingen, 2016). This understanding is particularly important for qualitative researchers and Ethics Review Boards to acknowledge because the reactions of people who have experienced trauma cannot be predicted. Therefore, qualitative researchers need to be informed and equipped with a toolbox of evidence-based trauma-informed strategies to provide individualised, safe spaces for conducting trauma research as well as carrying out their research more broadly.

Adopting Evidence-Based Trauma-Informed Guidelines

One evidence-based trauma-informed framework that can be adapted and applied to research contexts and research practices to better protect participants from re-traumatisation is 'The practical guide for implementing a trauma-informed approach' (2023) which was first developed by the Substance Abuse and Mental Health Services Administration [SAMHSA] in 2014 and updated in 2023. This trauma-informed framework was developed by a working group of specialists who not only investigated the impact of trauma but also examined the body of work on trauma (e.g., research, professional practice knowledge, and survivor/victim knowledge) and the practices undertaken by experts who work with those affected by trauma (Baird, 2018; SAMHSA, 2014, 2023).

SAMHSA's (2023) trauma-informed framework is grounded in four assumptions and six key principles informed by a strength-based approach. These four assumptions are referred to as the 'four Rs' and require those (e.g., researchers) who work with people affected by trauma (e.g., participants) to 'realise' how pervasive trauma is as well as 'recognising' the signs and symptoms of trauma. They then need to 'respond' by putting theory into practice and, in turn, 'resist' doing further harm (SAMHSA, 2014, 2023). Coinciding with these points are six key principles underpinning the framework which include *safety*; *trustworthiness and transparency*; *peer-support*; *collaboration and mutuality*; *empowerment, voice, and choice*; and *cultural, historical, and gender issues* (SAMHSA, 2014, 2023). SAMHSA (2023) explains how these six evidence-based principles have been adapted and applied successfully to other (service-based) sectors (as detailed above) to offer better protection to people affected by trauma. In so doing, SAMHSA's (2014, 2023) framework can also be applied to researcher practice, and research settings more broadly, to minimise the risk of causing further harm.

When applied to the research process, being trauma-informed involves researchers adopting a holistic and fluid way of working, whereby they understand and adapt their practices to the specific trauma history and needs of each individual participant. In contrast, if researchers' practices do not stem from being trauma-informed, with their practices inflexible, not individualised, nor choice-based for participants, they may unintentionally cause re-traumatisation and further harm (Bath, 2008; Hira et al., 2023; McMahon et al., 2022; McMahon et al., Under Review; SAMHSA, 2014, 2023). SAMHSA's (2014, 2023) framework is just one evidence-based approach that qualitative researchers can adopt into their practice, with other strategies adapted and implemented into non-research settings. Another prominent approach is the guidelines outlined in the current trauma- and violence-informed care (TVIC) literature (Hira et al., 2023). Like SAMHSA (2014, 2023), TVIC relies on four key principles: understanding trauma, violence, and its impacts on people's lives and behaviours; creating emotionally and physically safe environments; fostering opportunity for authentic choice, collaboration, and connection; and providing a strengths-based and capacity-building approach to support coping and resilience (Arthur et al., 2023; Ponic et al., 2016; Wathen & Varcoe, 2021). TVIC's four principles along with the six evidence-based principles outlined by SAMHSA (2014, 2023) have many alignments, with their core focus to 'prevent further harm' while affirming strength and coping, underpinning their frameworks.

While the adoption of these evidence-based principles is essential, so too is ensuring that people with lived experience of trauma are integral to co-designing and co-implementing trauma-informed approaches into research settings. As explained by SAMHSA (2023), any re-design where trauma-informed practices is incorporated "should begin with a needs assessment and involve people with lived experience, their families, and communities, as part of the design, delivery, and ongoing evaluation of the services" (p. 9). By involving people with lived experiences of trauma when embedding trauma-informed guidelines into research settings and researcher practice, it may ensure the 'take-up' of such practices is authentic rather than being less informed, tokenistic, or a tick box checking exercise.

A superficial or tick box checking example could be researchers saying they have been *trustworthy and transparent* (one of SAMHSA's principles) in their research by providing participants with a study information sheet (i.e., informed consent). While this is a standard ethical practice in qualitative research, trauma-informed research goes further with a critically informed approach. Given that people who have experienced trauma often perceive the world as unsafe, which in turn causes them to be hypersensitive to their safety (Menschner & Maul, 2016; SAMHSA, 2014, 2023), providing a study information sheet is not enough to enhance safety and build trust between participants and researchers (SAMHSA, 2023). Moreover, such activities may (unintentionally) reinforce power divides between researchers and participants as well as communicate a lack of time and care investment. This practice also fails to fully capture the trustworthiness and transparency needed when working with those affected by trauma in this space (SAMHSA, 2023).

Likewise, it would be tokenistic or less informed, for qualitative researchers to say they have cared for the mental health of participants impacted by trauma by referring them to free mental health providers if needed. Having a mental health provider on the research team (e.g., psychologist and social worker) could be useful to mitigate issues; however, such inclusion should always be underpinned by trauma-informed guidelines. While provision of resources may again be standard ethical practice in qualitative research, trauma-informed researchers understand and consider that support needs are varied and different, depending on participants' trauma backgrounds (SAMHSA, 2014). Particularly, as some participants may hold a mistrust of health providers and services, due to historical and cultural traumas, and may need different support such as through peer-support and community-based resources (Darroch et al., 2020; McMahon & McGannon, 2020; van Ingen, 2016). An awareness of these potential impacts and addressing them in the research process necessitate researchers' reflexivity of their positioning (e.g., identities and institutional membership) and research practices (e.g., interpersonal triggers and research design in power over participants). Simply referring participants to psychologists or counselling services, without knowledge of trauma histories, coupled with researchers' lack of reflection on their own practices, risks doing further harm. SAMHSA (2023) reinforces these points by explaining, "creating a safe environment, for both physical and emotional safety, requires intentionally and comprehensively incorporating trauma-informed principles and practices into an organisation's structure, delivery, and culture" (p. 1).

While much of the emphasis in this opening chapter is centred on the research participants, attention and care should also be directed to the researchers themselves. Given trauma may occur as a result of adverse events such as exposure to various types of abuse or witnessing of abuse, having a family member with a mental health or substance use disorder, systemic discrimination, acquiring a traumatic injury, cancer, sexual assault, domestic violence, war, and incarceration of a family member among other things (Pinderhughes et al., 2016; SAMHSA, 2014, 2023), participants' stories or information relating to these events can undoubtedly be harrowing to witness. This is particularly the case when researchers bring their own personal trauma histories to qualitative research projects. Therefore, the beam of consciousness of potential harm that can be caused to participants when undertaking trauma research should also extend to researchers. This consideration is important because researchers may be at risk of experiencing vicarious trauma due to indirect exposure to the participants' sharing of their adverse experiences (e.g., telling/hearing their trauma stories), and as noted due to their own trauma histories as survivor-researchers (McMahon et al., Under Review).

Compassion fatigue is another risk to researchers resulting from their empathetic engagement (British Medical Association, 2023) with participants' trauma experiences and stories (SAMHSA, 2014, 2023). As such, trauma researchers should remain vigilant to their own health and well-being in and through trauma research, as should the research team to support one another's different needs (Clift et al., 2023; McMahon et al., 2023). One example of this vigilance related to a trauma research context in sport is the self-management framework designed by Brackenridge (1999) in response to her qualitative research work with sexual abuse survivors. The self-management framework used by Brackenridge ensured that she considered her own health and well-being at the forefront of her sexual abuse research work. The British Medical Association (2023) also offers some strategies for people at risk of experiencing vicarious trauma, such as maintaining a healthy work-life balance, utilising peer support to debrief, exercise, seeking social support from colleagues, and increasing self-awareness of well-being. Other strategies which could assist researchers experiencing vicarious trauma could be achieved through support provided from their work institutions (i.e., universities). By researchers' universities being trauma-informed in their approach to staff who are undertaking such research, risks of vicarious trauma can be mitigated. Finally, although a less studied area, the needs of researchers who are 'cultural insiders' with trauma histories and intersecting effects need to be considered so that they are also not (re)harmed in the research process (Alessi & Kahn, 2023; McMahon et al., Under Review).

About the Book: Scope and Organisation

The following book was produced in response to the growing body of trauma research being conducted with populations in sport, exercise, and health contexts (e.g., Darroch et al., 2020; McMahon et al., 2023; van Ingen, 2016; Whitley et al., 2022. This research growth along with the need for researchers to adopt trauma-informed practices in the research process to minimise the risk of doing further harm, while promoting a strength-based approach, was also central to the impetus of this book. As such, the book draws on the expertise of a collection of international qualitative researchers who have studied populations affected by trauma in sport, exercise, and health contexts. Of interest is the type of trauma research they conducted, the qualitative methodologies and methods they adopted, and the trauma-informed practices they implemented and/or recommend. With trauma-informed qualitative research practices is an emerging area in the social sciences and sport and exercise sciences; this book is the first of its kind which brings together a collection of work that centralises qualitative research on trauma in sport, exercise, and health as well as outlining evidence-based trauma-informed practices which can be used in research as its core theme. The book is organised into four key sections relating to different trauma events which include the following:

Part I: Trauma and Gender-Based Violence
Part II: Trauma In, and From Sport
Part III: Trauma and Disability, Injury, Chronic, and Life-Threatening Diagnosis
Part IV: Developmental Trauma and Youth Trauma

While each of these trauma events are presented in distinct sections, readers are encouraged to view them as overlapping since trauma origins and their effects are intersectional (SAMHSA, 2023). This point is underscored by our review of literature that frames this introduction and the chapters that follow, which further show that trauma events and the impacts are not easily categorised. Indeed, the chapters in this edited volume cross over into multiple terrains and open dialogues about tensions in the research process. We hope that readers will see such intersecting connections and the need for additional trauma-informed qualitative research in this complex and burgeoning field.

Excluding the introduction and closing chapters, the book features 13 chapters written by scholars from different research backgrounds and geographic regions. Within each chapter, authors will:

- Showcase their qualitative trauma research which they conducted in a sport, exercise, and health context.

- Outline any adverse reactions/effects experienced (if at all) by them as the researcher/research team when conducting their trauma research.
- Outline how their chosen methodology/ method(s) was most suitable for conducting trauma research. Focus will be placed on how their chosen methodology/method not only benefited the participants affected by trauma but also the audience to learn more about trauma.
- Outline which evidence-based trauma-informed practices they either implemented into their trauma research or alternatively recommend because of conducting their trauma work.
- Make three recommendations for other qualitative researchers wishing to undertake trauma research in sport, exercise, and health contexts. These recommendations can also apply to qualitative research more broadly.

Our intention with the above chapter structure and content was to address a significant gap in the market by providing a qualitative research resource that outlines the 'what', 'why', and 'how' of trauma-informed practices, in turn suggesting ways forward for those interested in conducting trauma research. Despite the application and embedding of trauma-informed practices into research practices and research settings being urgently needed, trauma-informed practices in qualitative research remains *emerging* in comparison to other contexts (e.g., social work, counselling, and judicial systems) that have embedded these principles for some time. Furthermore, with trauma research being central to qualitative researchers' work, the 'take up' and implementation of evidence-based trauma-informed practices in relation to the research process and qualitative methods and methodologies are in its infancy.

Ultimately, given that trauma is a global health issue and there are ongoing public conversations on trauma in health, sport, and exercise contexts, we predict that the 'take up' of trauma-informed principles into research practice and settings will continue to grow and evolve quickly in the coming years. In the meantime, this book provides qualitative researchers with a rich foundation and platform to inform their thinking and practices that they may wish to adopt, or use to spark new questions and directions, in trauma-informed qualitative research methods and methodologies. In this way, the book is a practical resource for those scholars interested in conducting qualitative research with populations affected by trauma by providing evidence-based practices, strategies, methods, and methodologies to better protect themselves as researchers as well as participants. Further, in the closing chapter, we reflect more on the research outlined in this introductory chapter, relating it to the other chapters, to suggest future considerations for trauma-informed qualitative research methods and methodologies. Our modest reflections are intended to continue the dialogue and expansion of trauma-informed practices and work in sport, exercise, and health contexts.

References

Acosta, M. (2017). Trauma-informed care and the aging population. *Geriatric Symposium: Texas health and human services.* https://www.hhs.texas.gov/sites/default/files/documents/doing-business-with-hhs/providers/resources/trauma-inform-care-holocaust-survivor.pdf

Alessi, E. J., & Kahn, S. (2023). Toward a trauma-informed qualitative research approach: Guidelines for ensuring the safety and promoting the resilience of research participants. *Qualitative Research in Psychology, 20*(1), 121–154. https://doi.org/10.1080/14780887.2022.2107967

Arthur, E., Seymour, A., Dartnall, M., Beltgens, P., Poole, N.,Smylie, D., North, N., & Schmidt, R. (2023). *Trauma-informed practice guide.* BC Provincial Mental Health and Substance Use Planning Council. https://bccewh.bc.ca/wp-content/uploads/2012/05/2013_TIP-Guide.pdf

Bath, H. (2008). The three-pillars of trauma informed care. *Reclaiming Children and Youth, 17*(3), 17–21.

Baird, C. (2018). A trauma-informed approach to substance abuse treatment. *Journal of Addictions Nursing, 29*(4), 262–263. https://doi.org/10.1097/JAN.0000000000000251

Benjet, C., Bromet, E., Karam, E. G., Kessler, R. C., McLaughlin, K. A., Ruscio, A. M., Shahly, V., Stein, D. J.,Petukhova, M.,Hill, E.,Alonso, J.,Atwoli, L.,Bunting, B.,Bruffaerts, R., Caldas-de-Almeida, J. M., Girolamo, G.,Florescu, S.,Gureje, O.,Huang, Y., Lepine, J. … Koenen, K. C. (2016). The epidemiology of traumatic event exposure worldwide: Results from the World Mental Health Survey Consortium. *Psychological Medicine, 46*(2), 1–9. https://doi.org/10.1017/S0033291715001981

Berger, R. (2020). Studying trauma: Indirect effects on researchers and self – And strategies for addressing them. *Dissociation, 5*(1), 100149. https://doi.org/10.1016/j.ejtd.2020.100149

Brackenridge, C. (1999). Managing myself: Investigator survival in sensitive research. *International Review for the Sociology of Sport, 34*(4), 399–410. https://doi.org/10.1177/101269099034004007

BrightQuest. (2023). *PTSD re-traumatisation.* https://www.brightquest.com/post-traumatic-stress-disorder/

British Medical Association. (2023). *Vicarious trauma: Signs and strategies for coping.* https://www.bma.org.uk/advice-and-support/your-wellbeing/vicarious-trauma/vicarious-trauma-signs-and-strategies-for-coping

Butler, L. D., Critelli, F. M., & Rinfrette, E. S. (2011). Trauma-informed care and mental health. *Directions in Psychiatry, 31*, 197–210.

Clift, B. C., Costas Batlle, I., Bekker, S., & Chudzikowski, K. (Eds.). (2023). *Qualitative researcher vulnerability: Negotiating, experiencing and embracing.* Routledge.

Darroch, F. E., Roett, C., Varcoe, C., Oliffe, J. L., & Montaner, G. G. (2020). Trauma-informed approaches to physical activity: A scoping study. *Complementary Therapies in Clinical Practice, 41*(3), 101224. https://doi.org/10.1016/j.ctcp.2020.101224

Dye, H. (2018). The impact and long-term effects of childhood trauma. *Journal of Human Behaviour in the Social Environment, 28*(3), 381–392. https://doi.org/10.1080/10911359.2018.1435328

Filson, B. (2011). Is anyone really listening? *National Council Magazine. Special Issue: Breaking the Silence: Trauma-informed Behavioral Healthcare, 2*(15), 15.

Golden, T. L. (2022). Innovating health research methods, part II: Arts-based methods improve research data, trauma-responsiveness, and reciprocity. *Fam Community Health*, *45*(3), 150–159. https://doi.org/10.1097/FCH.0000000000000337

Gu, W., Zhao, Q., Yuan, C., Yi, Z., Zhao, M., & Wang, Z. (2022). Impact of adverse childhood experiences on the symptom severity of different mental disorders: A cross-diagnostic study. *General Psychiatry*, *35*(2). https://doi.org/10.1136/gpsych-2021-100741

Hira, S., Sheppard-Perkins, M., & Darroch, F. (2023). The facilitator is not a bystander: Exploring the perspectives of interdisciplinary experts on trauma research. *Frontiers in Psychology*, *14*, 1225789. https://doi.org/10.3389/fpsyg.2023.1225789

Jaffe, A. E., DiLillo, D., Hoffman, L., Haikalis, M., & Dykstra, R. E. (2015). Does it hurt to ask? A meta-analysis of participant reactions to trauma research, *Clinical Psychology Review*, *40*, 40–56. https://doi.org/10.1016/j.cpr.2015.05.004

Lahman, M. K., Geist, M. R., Rodriguez, K. L., Graglia, P., & DeRoche, K. K. (2011). Culturally responsive relational reflexive ethics in research: The three rs. *Quality and Quantity*, *45*(6), 1397–1414. https://doi.org/10.1007/s11135-010-9347-3

Magruder, K. M., McLaughlin, K. A., & Elmore-Borbon, D. L. (2017). Trauma is a public health issue. *European Journal of Psychotraumatology*, *8*(1), 1375338. https://doi.org/10.1080/20008198.2017.1375338

Massey, W. V., & Williams, T. L. (2020). Sporting activities for individuals who experienced trauma during their youth: A meta-study. *Qualitative Health Research*, *30*(1), 73–87. https://doi.org/10.1177/1049732319849563

McMahon, J., & McGannon, K. R. (2020). The athlete-doctor relationship: Power, complicity, resistance and accomplices in recycling dominant sport ideologies. *Sport, Education and Society*, *25*(1), 57–69. https://doi.org/10.1080/13573322.2018.1561434

McMahon, J., & McGannon, K. R. (2021). 'I hurt myself because it sometimes helps': Former athletes' embodied emotion responses to abuse using self-injury. *Sport, Education and Society*, *26*(2), 161–174. https://doi.org/10.1080/13573322.2019.1702940

McMahon, J., McGannon, & Zehntner, C. (under review). Arts-based methods as a trauma informed approach to research: Enabling survivors and victims' experiences to become visible. *Methods in Psychology*.

McMahon, J., McGannon, K. R., Zehntner, C., Werbicki, L., Stephenson, E., & Martin, K. (2023). Trauma-informed abuse education in sport: Engaging athlete abuse survivors as educators and facilitating a community of care. *Sport, Education and Society*, *28*(8), 958–971. https://doi.org/10.1080/13573322.2022.2096586

Menschner, C., & Maul, A. (2016). *Key ingredients for successful trauma-informed care implementation*. https://www.samhsa.gov/sites/default/files/programs_campaigns/childrens_mental_health/atc-whitepaper-040616.pdf

Mountjoy, M., Brackenridge, C., Arrington, M., Blauwet, C., Carska-Sheppard, A., Fasting, K., Kirby, S., Leahy, T., Marks, S., Martin, K., Starr, K., Tiivas, A., & Budgett, R. (2016). International Olympic Committee consensus statement: Harassment and abuse (non-accidental violence) in sport. *British Journal of Sports Medicine*, *50*(17), 1019–1029. https://doi.org/10.1136/bjsports-2016-096121

Palladino, E., Darroch, F., Jean-Pierre, L., Kelly, M., Roberts, C., & Hayhurst, L. (2023). Landscape of practice: A participatory approach to creating a trauma- and violence-informed physical activity social learning space. *Qualitative Research in*

Sport, Exercise and Health, 15(2), 297–312. https://doi.org/10.1080/2159676X. 2022.2146163

Papathomas, A., & Lavallee, D. (2014). Self-starvation and the performance narrative in competitive sport. *Psychology of Sport and Exercise, 15*(6), 688–695. https://doi.org/10.1016/j.psychsport.2013.10.014

Pinderhughes, H., Davis, R., & Williams, M. (2016). *Adverse community experiences and resilience: A framework for addressing and preventing community trauma.* Prevention Institute. https://www.preventioninstitute.org/publications/adverse-community-experiences-and-resilience-frameworkaddressing-and-preventing

Ponic, P., Varcoe, C., & Smutylo, T. (2016). Trauma- (and violence-) informed approaches to supporting victims of violence: Policy and practice considerations. *Vic. Crime. Res. Dig, 9,* 3–15.

Roderick, M., Smith, A., & Potrac, P. (2017). The sociology of sports work, emotions, and mental health: Scoping the field and future directions. *Sociology of Sport Journal, 34*(2), 99–107. https://doi.org/10.1123/ssj.2017-0082

Rosetto, K. (2014). Qualitative research interviews: Assessing the therapeutic value and challenges. *Journal of Social and Personal Relationships, 31*(4), 482–489. https://doi.org/10.1177/0265407514522892

Smith, A. (2019). Depression and suicide in professional sport. In M. Atkinson (Ed.), *Sport, mental illness, and sociology* (pp. 9–96). Emerald.

Substance Abuse and Mental Health Services Administration (SAMHSA). (2014). *SAMHSA's concept of trauma and guidance for a trauma-informed approach.* https://ncsacw.samhsa.gov/userfiles/files/SAMHSA_Trauma.pdf

Substance Abuse and Mental Health Services Administration (SAMHSA). (2017). *Tips for survivors of disaster or other traumatic event: Coping with re-traumatisation.* https://store.samhsa.gov/sites/default/files/d7/priv/sma17-5047.pdf

Substance Abuse and Mental Health Services Administration (SAMHSA). (2023). *Practical guide for implementing a trauma-informed approach.* https://store.samhsa.gov/sites/default/files/pep23-06-05-005.pdf

Sweeney, A., Filson, B., Kennedy, A., Collinson, L., & Gillard, S. (2018). A paradigm shift: Relationships in trauma-informed mental health services. *BJPsych Advances, 24*(5), 319–333. https://doi.org/10.1192/bja.2018.29

Teicher, M., & Samson, J. (2016). Annual research review: Enduring neurobiological effects of childhood abuse and neglect. *Journal of Child Psychology and Psychiatry, 57*(3), 241–266. https://doi.org/10.1111/jcpp.12507

van Ingen, C. (2016). Getting lost as a way of knowing: The art of boxing within shape your life. *Qualitative Research in Sport, Exercise and Health, 8*(5), 472–486. https://doi.org/10.1080/2159676X.2016.1211170

Wathen, C. N., & Varcoe, C. (2021). Trauma- and violence-informed care (TVIC): A tool for health and social service organizations and providers. https://equiphealthcare.ca/files/2021/05/GTV-EQUIP-Tool-TVIC-Spring2021.pdf

Whitley, M. A., Donnelly, J. A., Cowan, D. T., & McLaughlin, S. (2022). Narratives of trauma and resilience from Street Soccer players. *Qualitative Research in Sport, Exercise and Health, 14*(1), 101–118. https://doi.org/10.1080/21596 76X.2021.1879919

Part I

Trauma and Gender-Based Violence

Chapter 2

Using a Trauma-Informed Lens in Ballet

A Case Study of One Professional Female Dancer

Fiona J. Moola and Alixandra Krahn

Introduction

Scholars suggest that trauma ruptures time and space and shatters the ground on which trauma survivors live. Trauma leaves a lasting effect on the individual, and, in this way, always carries a residue. It is often caused by factors that are external to the individual (Pedovic & Hedrih, 2019). In this chapter, we use a case study approach to understand a former professional ballerina's experiences in Canada whom we have called "Ava." Our research draws on a larger phenomenological investigation on the psychosocial experiences of ballet dancers in Canada. We utilized Martin Heidegger's phenomenology for our research. Unlike Husserl, who believed that phenomena could be divorced from context, Heidegger sought to explore the meaning of phenomena and the nature of being in the context of interpretation. We foreground the gender-based abuses that Ava was subjected to during her time as a dancer. In particular, we seek to understand the emotional, physical, and sexual trauma she experienced at the hands of dance teachers of all genders during the peak of her training and performance years. Whether sexual and emotional abuse was and/or is a deeper collective trauma that left an "indelible mark on the group consciousness" (Pedovic & Hedrih, 2019, p. 27) of ballerinas as a group deserves research attention.

Although it can be controversial, some scholars suggest that high-quality qualitative scholarship should be marked by a commitment to self-reflexivity (Olmos-Vega et al., 2023). Reflexivity should be emblematic of philosophical orientations and marked by a conscious process of thinking about how the subjectivity of the researchers has influenced the research process (Olmos-Vega et al., 2023). Although neither of us (authors) has experienced trauma in the context of professional ballet, both of us have lived experiences marked by the residue of trauma. As a woman of colour with ancestral roots from apartheid South Africa who is navigating Euro-centric society, Fiona (author 1) has lived experience of both ancestral and contemporary racial trauma (Saleem et al., 2020). Having spent several years in the hospital during late childhood and youth, Fiona experienced ableism and hospital-based medical trauma.

DOI: 10.4324/9781003332909-3

She is also a practicing Registered Psychotherapist (Qualifying), which has sensitized her to the ways in which trauma ruptures time, space, and ground. Alix (author 2) – who identifies as a White, cis-gender, able-bodied woman – is a former high-performance athlete with experiences of mental and emotional abuse from within the elite sporting realm. These experiences ultimately led Alix to pursue research that closely examined the power relationships operating within the high-performance sport context and how these relations may contribute to experiences of abuse and maltreatment among athletes. Although we can never understand the standpoint of the storyteller or the magnitude of the trauma Ava experienced, our own lived experiences of trauma have sensitized us to its profound impact on the body and self in society.

Review of the Literature

Since there is scant evidence on the topic of trauma in professional ballet, we turned to existing evidence on other adverse experiences that dancers have encountered in this art form more broadly (e.g., Abraham, 1996; Kelman, 2000; Novack, 1993; Papaefstathiou et al., 2013). These include the experience of eating disorders as well as the normalization of pain and injury. Cumulatively, both the normalization of pain and the experience of food and body image disorders are thought to worsen the psychosocial well-being of dancers (Abraham, 1996; Moola & Krahn, 2016). Turner and Wainwright (2003) and McEwen and Young (2011) have furthered understanding of the normalization of pain and injury in the context of professional ballet. Professional dancers are forced to deny their pain and injuries or else risk losing long-sought-after positions in ballet companies. Sometimes, this process entails enduring chronic pain as well as suffering from life-long pain in the future. Scholars (e.g., Alexias & Dimitropoulou, 2011) have also examined the experience of food and body disorders in ballet and the use of the body as a tool. While these militaristic bodily standards are thought to be improving over time, female dancers are still expected to be long and lean, almost ethereal, and ghost-like, an ideology/bodily standard born a few centuries ago. To achieve these aesthetic norms, many dancers forcibly restrict their nutritional intakes, limiting themselves to only a few hundred calories per day (Gvion, 2008).

Pirkko Markula's (2011) gender-based scholarship explored how dance and ballet cultures may perpetuate oppressive male gazes and reproduce gender binaries. Historically, dominant ballet plot lines (i.e., damsel in distress to be rescued by the prince) have reinforced gender stereotypes (Aalten, 1997) and the emergence of narratives that are deeply imbued in power relationships (Karthas, 2012). Although women were altogether absent from ballet during the 1600s, their debut into ballet (during the 1800s) was originally seen as downgrading this art form. As ballet became an institutionalized form of art, however, female dancers were used to portray dominant and/or acceptable forms of femininity (i.e., weak, fragile, and in need of rescue) (Karthas, 2012).

Methodological Reflections

In our original study entitled "a dance with many secrets" (see Moola & Krahn, 2016), we drew on a qualitative research tradition known broadly as phenomenology. This methodological framework underpinned our research with 20 former professional ballet dancers across the provinces of Canada as well as Canadian dancers who were working and performing in Europe. Phenomenology is a research tradition that purports to speak back to the "tyranny" of textual and cognitive approaches that are often over-used in the academy (Gunn & Rosberg, 2022). Instead, it is a deeply embodied approach that utilizes the body in the production of knowledge (Gunn & Rosberg, 2022). Given that dance is an embodied art form, and that so many of the dancers in our study experienced deeply embodied encounters like injury and eating disorders, we felt that phenomenology was the appropriate methodological choice for this particular study. Here, we understand embodiment to mean the essence of the body in contemporary society, including having a body, being a body, or even rejecting the body (Smith, 2017). We also recognize that materialist accounts of the body in Western academy challenge a long history of somatophobia of the body in modern, Euro-western thought. We aim to challenge the notion that the body is inferior that has characterized Western thought and instead (Smith, 2017), we value the wisdom of the body and the ways in which trauma may be housed in the body.

In this chapter, however, we used a case study methodological tradition so we could focus on one life – Ava's – in the context of a personal history, environment (i.e., ballet), and biography (Flyvbjerg, 2011). While case studies do have some methodological weaknesses (e.g., difficult to replicate), a strength is that they afford researchers the opportunity to capture detail, depth, and description (Flyvbjerg, 2011) that could be lost through a focus on a larger group of participants. We chose the intrinsic and exploratory case study which focuses on the investigation of a unique and understudied phenomenon. This case study approach affords the opportunity to carefully detail the nuances of the traumatic experiences that Ava was subjected to in her dance context, with attention to the details of her experiences. Indeed, for those unfamiliar with trauma, the case study approach utilized in conjunction with phenomenology may facilitate listening, hearing, and witnessing, which is so critical to breaking secrecy and silence around trauma (Bath, 2008).

In addition to the audience benefiting from the intrinsic and exploratory case study approach and phenomenology, arguably, participants like Ava may also benefit. Benefits can include being able to tap into embodied experiences and emotions, such as shame and humiliation or pride and joy as well as enabling an in-depth exploration of one life in the context of its history (Baxter & Jack, 2008). For these reasons, we believe that both of these methodologies may advance the field of trauma-informed research in sport and exercise contexts, giving attentiveness to the body, emotions, embodied experiences (Van Rhyn et al., 2021).

During our study, measures to protect the participant were put in place before, during, and after data collection. Long before the study began, we spent time forging a relationship with Ava, discussing and dialoguing about the purpose and rationale for the study. During the interview, we constantly reassured Ava that we valued her experiences and expertise. We also acknowledged the tremendous amount of gratitude that we felt towards her for her willingness to share with us. As researchers, we shared the emotional impact of the study on us and stepped into a place of shared vulnerability with the participant. These considerations are trauma-informed according to SAMHSA (2014), which we will expand on further below. Given the vulnerability that the participant courageously demonstrated with us, we feel that our shared mirroring of vulnerability back to the participants allowed for the development of an emotionally safe space (Bhattacharya, 2015). Emotional safety involves validation of participants' experiences and providing sources of support. In some cases, this entailed the appropriate sharing of some of our own experiences in a demonstration of vulnerability. When Ava became emotional or distressed during the interview, we let her know that it was OK to stop participating or to skip over questions that she did not feel comfortable with. Thus, prioritizing Ava's needs was more important than the execution of our research agenda. Upon completion of the interview, Ava was provided with a list of psychosocial resources via email in case she had unmet psychosocial needs. While this practice is standard in research, it is also important from a trauma-informed perspective.

Future researchers may also wish to consider the use of arts-based research (ABR) as a methodological framework in which to investigate the experience of trauma in professional ballet. ABR, such as self-portraits or body maps, refers to the production and/or dissemination of knowledge through the arts (Moola et al., 2022). Further, due to the fact that ABR considers the body and emotions – and the role of social inequity and power relationships – ABR may be particularly well suited for the study of trauma in dance (Moola et al., 2020). Drawing on the scholarship of dancer academic Pirkko Markula, researchers may also wish to consider employing performance ethnography, which is a type of research that works towards the development of a final artistic product through the collection of field notes and interviews (Bhattacharya, 2009). Markula (2011) suggests that performance ethnography might be a way in which to de-territorialize the molar category of femininity in dance while undoing the binary between theory and dance, academia, and movement. Markula used this approach to explore the experience of injury among modern dancers (2011). This approach may also be a useful embodied methodological platform in which to better consider trauma in the context of professional ballet, given that dance is an embodied art form.

Contextual Qualitative Data

Below, we present Ava's voice and experiences via verbatim narratives that exemplify the trauma she experienced at the hands of her ballet masters during the time of her training and performance years. During this time period, Ava moved away from home to live in the dormitory of the city ballet school. At the time when Ava was a member of the city Ballet school, which acts as a feeder programme for a professional ballet career, she was a minor/youth.

From Safety to Cruelty

Many abuse survivors describe the co-existence of love and safety with cruelty and abuse. Indeed, this coexistence makes the abusive cycle particularly toxic and difficult to eject oneself from. As is common in many abuse narratives, Ava explained that at the start of her ballet career, her dance masters (both male and female) made her feel safe and protected by "taking her under their wing" or "putting in a good word for her at a staff meeting."

> She put her arm around and said we take care of our students here and I felt very safe and loved in that moment that oh she's gonna take care of me.

Ava was so desperate for her dancer masters' approval that she often ignored her gut instincts and intuition, alerting her that something was wrong with their behaviour.

> I know even Aaron did that quite often of I'll put in good word for you in the staff meeting and even if your heart was saying this probably isn't right, you were so willing to do anything for acceptance and you weren't along with things that your gut said don't do it.

However, over time, her dance master's behaviour shifted from love and safety, to cruelty and abuse, which led her to terminate her involvement with the ballet company. Ava stated … "She was really the mainstay of cruelty and then in my final meeting in leaving the ballet she was just relentlessly and ridiculously cruel."

Villainizing the Female Body

Ava's body was frequently the brunt of abuse and she faced criticism from her coaches/masters as they expected her to be thin and svelte. Asexual female bodies were the expected aesthetic norm at the time of her ballet training. The dominant character roles that women play in traditional ballet often exemplify asexuality, such as dead virgins or animals. Ava stated … "especially with women in dance that you are asexual, you are supposed to play the role of a swan or a dead virgin." In contrast, Ava's body did not adhere to these aesthetic norms (e.g., no breasts and no bottom). Rather, Ava was frequently criticized for possessing a "female body", characterized by her curves, flesh, and breasts. Ava was also body shamed for "not having control" over her monthly menstruation cycles. The dance masters discouraged the female dancers from having a period/menstruating as this meant they were deemed overweight.

> So, if you are woman or have that womanly nature you are shunned upon or shamed about your breasts. I mean you tie them down or strap them in. I got kicked out of class for having my period and was completely shamed for being disgusting and that I didn't have control of my body and that something was wrong with me.

Ava's breasts were frequently regarded as being *"too big"* for ballet and her body antithetical contrasted that of the "12-year-old boy aesthetic" that her ballet masters demanded.

> … because I was on the pill my breasts increased by a cup size and we couldn't have that … you are these set of rules and not womanly. You are not supposed to have breasts or hips. When I was in the program, they really emulated the whole looking like a 12-year-old boy.

Additionally, she was often called "ugly" by her ballet masters and compared to other thinner dancers.

> … trying to be a professional dancer, that's all based on aesthetics and constantly being compared to girls in my class that somehow again I wasn't making the effort and trying hard enough to fix everything in my life to be a dancer, and I wasn't taking it seriously and that I was ugly … being called in about why I wasn't taking things seriously and that my face was ugly and did I not take my career seriously because I wasn't making the effort to get it corrected … and being told flat out that well you don't look like the other dancers and you can afford to lose five pounds because if you gain any weight you won't fit your costume or thing too of being too womanly, like having breasts or curves.

Physically Harmful Teaching

Ava's dance masters frequently engaged in physically harmful instructional practices. These physically dangerous teaching methods were also laced with sexual connotations, such as the touching of breasts in class while simultaneously biting a student. These physically harmful teaching methods were overlooked by the higher administration in the organization, but due to the belief that the teacher was "staff", their instructional methods were justified. For instance, as a form of punishment for poor dance performance and practice, a few of the male teachers often bit students in class, which included the biting of someone's breasts or buttocks. Ava reflects on these physically harmful practices and how they were ignored by the administration. Although she did not know it at the time, in retrospect, Ava regarded such behaviours as abusive in nature.

> ... that was always excused. And he did things in class, that even I went to staff and said "this needs to be dealt with" and they said "he is an instructor with the school and on contract" and they defend him if you raised it. So, it is okay for him to grab breasts or bite someone.

Ava also recalled that her dance master bit another student so hard that it led to bleeding... "He bit a friend of mine in class, he bit her bum so hard he made her bleed."

Other dance masters over stretched dancers' legs to the point of great pain or forced them to dance with broken bones,

> I remember a girl in my class that broke her wrist and she was told if she wasn't in class she would be out and she danced for six weeks with a cast on her wrist ... there were some instructors that went a little too far in demonstration with your body like pushing your leg to the point that you overstrained a muscle and being told that you couldn't seek treatment during class time because it took away from your rehearsals.

Blurring of Sexual Lines with Minors

Another normalized and unquestioned component of the ballet culture was that much older teachers often engaged in sexual relationships with minors. According to Ava, sexual relationships with minors were undertaken by male identifying dance teachers and not female identifying dance teachers. Given that the dancers were all minors at the time of these sexual transgressions, these behaviours were illegal. We engage in a discussion about this below. Sexual relationships were also laden with contradiction and paradox. Even though an "asexual, child-like body" was valued, as discussed above, sexual transgressions were permitted and/or ignored. Ava remarks on the normalization of sexual activity with minors by dance masters below.

> I mean even the instructors or directors who have affairs with extremely young students and it's perfectly normal for a 40-year-old man to have an affair with a 16-year-old girl.

Further, she also shares the story of another instructor who acted like a "paedophile" in class and circulated sexually explicit photography of dancers from the company, many of whom were minors:

> *He was pretty much the paedophile in the way he touched girls and demonstrated in class. He'd physically hit or hurt you to demonstrate ... he took a lot of us under his wing with the friendly nice guy but I'm sure you know about the whole photographs that he'd send.*

Ava also alluded to the entire sexualized culture with minors, commenting on the fact that female dance masters also engaged in such sexual transgressions.

> *There were female directors who had relationships with female students in the program as well. And there's this other whole sexual nature which is part in part with the whole thing with the photographs and the abuse of power in that you are taught in a studio.*

Carrying the Trauma Forward

In their article, McMahon and colleagues (2022) discuss the ways in which exposure to trauma significantly increases the risk of further re-traumatization and adverse psychosocial experiences in the future. Our findings clearly support McMahon's (2022) assertion. Although Ava eventually left this physically and emotionally abusive dance context, she acknowledges that she struggled with self-esteem issues for a long time and had to seek a great deal of psychological counselling after her career as a dancer. She compares ballet to the military and the church, acknowledging that the cruel way her dance teachers saw her came to invariably shape how she sees herself post her involvement with ballet. Ava acknowledges that the institution of ballet continued to have control over her mind for a long time:

> *It was after years that I'd felt like I never was gonna go anywhere or feel that acceptance to have that kind of window- then have it all taken away in one fell swoop. That was – to be honest and fair, I did a lot of counselling to fold that up. When I went to dance in another program, I had a lot of self-esteem issues and you felt like to carry it forward and it's that sort of part that – do they not realize the influence that have on people? It is just like well that's what was said to me and that's how I was treated – therefore, that's how you should be treated. Again, it perpetuates this sick cycle of "it's okay." I think that's because similarly with the military – as it is with the pro ballet world, you will find that the exact same stuff has been going on and it's continuing. Like we still have this dialogue or this framework of language that we use that keeps control over people because the longer that you can control them, you can make them do anything kind of thing.*

Trauma-Informed Practices Applied to Research

Since our research was carried out in 2015, we became aware that the experience of trauma can result in extremely distressing psychosocial impacts. As exemplified by Ava above in professional ballet, these impacts include shame, disgust, being and feeling silenced, and fear to name a few. In order to raise reflection and awareness, SAMHSA (2014) identifies six principles central to their trauma-informed approach which include *(a) safety in organizations; (b) trust and transparency; (c) peer support for those with lived experience of trauma by using survivor stories to heal; (d) collaboration; (e) empowerment, choice, and voice; and (f) being aware of the role of culture, history, and gender.* For the purpose of this chapter, we focus on how we addressed *Cultural, Historical, and Gender Issues* and *Peer Support* in our research to ensure re-traumatization was limited.

Cultural, Historical, and Gender Issues

To ensure gender considerations were addressed in our research, we did not engage in individualizing and/or pathologizing discourses and instead, tried to adopt a social and political way of thinking about abuse as born out of gender relationships that are deeply rooted in patriarchal power structures in society (Pemberton & Loeb, 2020). We did this specifically by constantly reassuring and reaffirming the participants experience as a victim in an institution, ballet, that historically has been embedded in patriarchal power relationships (Alterowitz, 2014). For instance, during the interview, to reaffirm the participants' experience as a victim in a male dominated institution, we used words such as "I imagine that it must have been so hard to be away from your parents and attending ballet school with ballet masters who hurt and betrayed you." Moreover, a section of our interview guide was dedicated to asking participants specific questions on gender and the gendered dynamics of power in their respective ballet worlds. For example, we asked participants to reflect on the differences between the female and male dancer experience with particular attention paid to those experiences of power and social support. Although we did not ask our participants to self-identify, the insights we obtained on gendered dynamics were attended to much more clearly in our earlier publication (Moola & Krahn, 2016), and we maintain that much more scholarship is required in this area in order to better understand the nuances of gender in the dance experience.

Additionally, we do not feel that our attentiveness to culture, history, and gender went far enough in unpacking the power relationships that contribute towards traumatic fields. Even though the SAMHSA (2014) principles call attention to the importance of intersectionality – and recognize that Black, Native, and Latina women consistently experience higher rates of trauma in comparison to White women (Pemberton & Loeb, 2020) – the field of post-colonial trauma studies might help to enrich this conversation. Indeed, it is important to de-centre Whiteness from trauma studies or the implicit Euro-centricity of the field and its continued focus on the West (Traverso & Broderick, 2010). This entails making sure that research teams reflect a diverse composition of intersectional identities, including equity-seeking and historically marginalized people. This also entails making sure that research teams engage in ongoing and reflective equity, diversity, and inclusion training. Finally, engaging directly with theoretical and methodological frameworks that de-centre Whiteness, such as decolonizing, arts-based, and post-colonial research, are some strategies that scholars can use. Although few of our dancers discussed race and culture, post-colonial trauma studies may help open a space to consider those traumas that have been laced with the atrocities of colonization, such as forced immigration, migration, racism, and slavery (Ward, 2013).

Further, more and more racialized dancers, such as US dancer Misty Copeland, are beginning to narrate stories about the complexities and challenges of being a Black dancer in a historically White, Euro-centric ballet profession. We encourage future trauma-informed dance researchers to enhance their understanding of gender, culture, and history in the SAMHSA framework with other post-colonial trauma principles that are sensitive and attuned to the ongoing impact of colonization and neo-colonization. For example, readers may wish to engage with the work of Tsibolane and Brown (2016). By drawing on the work of Said, Spivak, and Bhabha, these authors outline critical concepts in post-colonial informed research studies. For example, these authors suggest that the West (the Occident) has a historical fascination with what they imagine the East (Orient) to be (Tsibolane & Brown, 2016). Unfortunately, some of these imagined images and narratives about the Oriental Other are deeply problematic and colonial, such as imagining the other as a savage. Further, these constructions often serve the colonial interests of the Occident. Post-colonial scholars also suggest that racialized post-colonial identities are increasingly fractured and hybrid in post-colonial and post-modern times (Tsibolane & Brown, 2016).

Peer Support

The SAMHSA framework also outlines the importance of peer support when engaging in trauma work. Through the incorporation of lived trauma experiences, it may be possible to enhance trust and collaboration (2014). At the time of our study, we did not disclose to participants that both of us have experienced trauma outside of professional ballet. In retrospect, doing so may have allowed us to establish rapport, trust, and collegiality with the participant through the establishment of shared vulnerability. For example, in their paper, McMahon et al. (2022) discuss the inclusion of abuse survivors in sport as well as current athletes in the development of anti-abuse strate-gies in sport organization. Drawing on McMahon's professional and lived experience expertise as both a scholar and an abuse survivor and advocate, similar approaches could be taken to the establishing of research projects on abuse in ballet by inviting abuse survivors and current dancers onto re-search teams to co-design studies. Indeed, the inclusion of abuse survivors and current dancers, according to McMahon et al. (2022), may have several benefits, such as allowing victims to be heard in judgement-free spaces that make room for fear and other emotions to be shared. The inclusion of lived experience can also promote and facilitate recovery for victims and current athletes. Furthermore, the inclusion of abuse survivors can also facilitate nar-rative agency and ownership, or control over their own stories of abuse. Thus, the inclusion of peers on research teams may also enable narrative capital for victims and facilitate important shifts from "victim" to "advocate on behalf of abuse survivors." However, McMahon et al. (2022) warn that the inclusion of peers through lived experience must always be employed thoughtfully and carefully. If trauma-informed principles are not utilized when including lived experience peers, there is great potential for an escalation in trauma symp-toms, or even the risk of re-traumatizing. In the future, if we undertake work like this, we will make deliberate attempts to recruit "survivors" and current athletes onto our research team in a trauma-informed manner.

Additionally, one potential consequence and risk of trauma or abuse survivors facilitating such trauma research is the potential to experience vicarious trauma (Kadambi & Ennis, 2004). Despite our own experiences of trauma and abuse, and our best efforts to normalize trauma narratives with participants, it was nevertheless disturbing to listen to the experi-ences of abuse that participants encountered. Many of the normalized abusive practices that participants experienced, like biting, have not been reported in the literature and were bizarre and cruel. Research indicates that exposure to trauma through listening can have a very negative impact on the witness (e.g., vicarious trauma) (Kadambi & Ennis, 2004). In the future, we hope to better prepare and equip ourselves for any vicarious-trauma risks.

Ethical Reflections

During this study, past abuse was disclosed to us as researchers. We dis-cussed this with our research ethics board (REB) and since the participant was no longer a minor at the time and that the abuse was reported decades later in a research study, we did not have a duty to report. However, this was difficult for us as researchers. The fact that participants were minors at the time of the abusive experiences made listening to these narratives all the more disturbing and heart-breaking to hear. This is because the participants lacked both social and political power at the time to intervene in their own lives. At times, we found the material to be extremely emotional. As two equity-minded people, the grave injustices in the case were particularly striking. We did spend several months reflecting on the ethics of retrospective abuse reporting. Our thoughtful reflections were undertaken through engaging in deep dialogue, watching YouTube videos about ethical dilemmas, having discussions with the REB and journaling in research journals. Although we did not do so at the time, future researchers might also consider participating in therapy to help process the emotional experience of listening to abuse. Most importantly, future researchers engaging in abuse-based studies may need to seek adequate support from other trainees, mentors and supervisors, community agencies, and mental health networks. Trauma-informed research should never be taken lightly and requires adequate support.

Conclusions

To advance ethical and empathic trauma-informed scholarship in sport, exercise, health, sport, and dance, we propose three central future theoretical and methodological directions. First, we suggest that future researchers consider phenomenology, case study approaches, and arts-informed scholarship to methodological ground trauma-informed studies because all three of these methodologies provide an opportunity to centre the body and emotions – indeed, the place where trauma invades, harbours, and lives (Van der Kolk, 2014). Arguably, overly cognitive therapy and research approaches do little, if anything, to tap into trauma which, by definition, is locked in the body and profoundly scars the nervous system. To properly engage trauma-informed research, we need, therefore, to engage the body which houses it (Van der Kolk, 2014) through engagement with body-based approaches in research, including ABR and phenomenological research (Moola et al., 2022; Van Rhyn et al., 2021). Indeed, these are research approaches that engage the body through an exploration of sensory and emotional experiences. Second, researchers seeking to undertake investigations on sexual and emotional abuse should engage the rich field of traumatology (Thompson & Walsh, 2010) as well as the SAMHSA trauma-informed framework because they provide detailed theoretical perspectives on trauma as well as a set of evidence-based principles to use when working with traumatized people.

Third, we suggest that trauma-informed scholars draw from the vast theoretical richness of post-colonial trauma studies that better consider how power relationships contribute towards trauma and trauma-informed research practices. We must disrupt and de-centre the inherent Eurocentricity of trauma-based scholarship and open ourselves up to a polyphony of new trauma-informed theories outside of the West (Traverso & Broderick, 2010). Readers who are specifically interested in the disruption of power in research might consider reading heavily from participatory action research, decolonizing research (Thambinathan & Kinsella, 2021), and ABR (Moola et al., 2022).

All of these, in turn, are oriented towards de-centring traditional power relationships and listening to the other. Such approaches cultivate a "power-with" relationship with partners and participants rather than a "power-over" traditional academic research hierarchy (Ponic et al., 2010). Specific examples of how to de-centre Whiteness and power in sport, dance, and abuse research might include purposively engaging intersectional identities on research teams and among research participants, undertaking equity, diversity, and inclusion training, and engaging a diverse range of post-colonial epistemologies and theoretical frameworks. Engaging with polyphony of post-colonial and epistemological frameworks is important to sidestep the dominance of Euro-Western philosophy in current academic research. Further, in research settings, researchers and practitioners often possess instrumental power in that they define the research questions and decide what research agenda to pursue (Fritz & Binder, 2020). A less power-laden approach to knowledge production might entail having members of the racialized sexual abuse survivorship community co-design research questions with research teams, including all aspects of research design, such as ideation, execution, and dissemination. Funding agendas also dictate what research is deemed worthy at a particular cultural moment (Fritz & Binder, 2020). Decolonizing funding might look like having specific funding calls just for intersectionality in abuse in sport and dance research.

Finally, we encourage academic researchers to actively engage in the practice of vulnerability with participants in trauma-informed research contexts. Indeed, although shared vulnerability is extensively discussed in therapy writings (Aron, 2016), there has been very little engagement with the concept of vulnerability in academia and research. We actually began to discuss academic vulnerability about seven years ago when we noticed the failure of academics to ever discuss their feelings. As a young professor and master's student at the time, this was deeply frustrating for us. The practice of vulnerability (Råheim et al., 2016) is critical to the cultivation of emotional intimacy and is a practice that some academics have long since avoided due to the assumption that the academy is a place that values reason and cognition over emotion and embodiment. Demonstrating academic vulnerability entails researchers sharing their emotional experience with participants in a way that does not destabilize or upset them (Aron, 2016). For example, in response to hearing a trauma narrative such as Ava's, researchers might consider supportive, vulnerable, and empathic statements, such as "when you share this experience with me, it makes me feel very sad and also angry." Further, where relevant, researchers could consider safely sharing events from their own life that resonate or mirror participants own. Of note, the practice of vulnerability is not a "dangerous oversharing" by the researcher. Rather, it is a thoughtful and careful attempt to diminish the binary and the boundary between the researcher and the participant and to show the participant the humanity and relationality of the interviewer (Aron, 2016). In so doing, we show the participant that we are also subject to the same frailties and precarities of the human condition. We show them that we do not live behind a pretentious veiled curtain of knowledge or power, and, instead, humbly occupy a similar relational space as them. For communities that have been shamed, like sexual abuse survivors (MacGinley et al., 2019), seeing the fragilities and struggles of the Other can also help to diminish shame.

As our previous scholarship has shown (Moola & Krahn, 2016), the centuries-old institution of ballet is one that has guarded many secrets. Ethical, vulnerable, and empathic trauma-informed scholarship that is attentive to power and difference may help to shed light, transparency, and truth on the institution of ballet and the breaches of power it has engaged in over bodies like Avas.

References

Aalten, A. (1997). Performing the body, creating culture. *The European Journal of Women's Studies, 4*(2), 197–215. https://doi.org/10.1177/135050689700400205

Abraham, S. (1996). Eating and weight controlling behaviours of young ballet dancers. *Psychopathology, 29*(4), 218–222. https://doi.org/10.1159/000284996

Alexias, G., & Dimitropoulou, E. (2011). The body as a tool: Professional classical ballet dancers' embodiment. *Research in Dance Education, 12*(2), 87–104.

Alterowitz, G. (2014). Toward a feminist ballet pedagogy: Teaching strategies for ballet technique classes in the twenty-first century. *Journal of Dance Education, 14*(1), 8–17. https://doi.org/10.1080/15290824.2013.824579

Aron, L. (2016). Mutual vulnerability. An ethic of clinical practice. In D. Goodman & E. Severson (Eds.), *The ethical turn: Otherness and subjectivity in contemporary psychoanalysis*. Routledge.

Bath, H. (2008). The three pillars of trauma-informed care. *Reclaiming Children and Youth, 17*(3) 17–21. https://elevhalsan.uppsala.se/globalassets/elevhalsan/dokument/psykologhandlingar/trauma-informed-care.pdf

Baxter, P., & Jack, S. (2008). Qualitative case study methodology: Study design and implementation for novice researchers. *The Qualitative Report, 13*(4), 544–599. https://doi.org/10.46743/2160-3715/2008.1573

Bhattacharya, K. (2015). The vulnerable academic: Personal narratives and strategic de/colonizing of academic structures. *Qualitative Inquiry, 22*(5), 1–13. https://doi.org/10.1177/1077800415615619

Bhattacharya, K. (2009). Negotiating shuttling between transnational experiences: A de/colonizing approach to performance ethnography. *Qualitative Inquiry, 15*(6), 1061–1083. https://doi.org/10.1177/1077800409332746

Flyvbjerg, B. (2011). Case study. In N. Denzin & Y. Lincoln (Eds.), *The sage handbook of qualitative research* (pp. 301–316). Sage.

Fritz, L., & Binder, C. R.. (2020). Whose knowledge, whose values? An empirical analysis of power in transdisciplinary sustainability research. *European Journal of Futures Research, 8*(3). https://doi.org/10.1186/s40309-020-0161-4

Gunn, E., & Rosberg, S. (2022). Theorizing bodily dialogs – Reflection on knowledge production in phenomenological research. *Physiotherapy Theory and Practice, 38*(12), 1833–1842. https://doi.org/10.1080/09593985.2021.1923098

Gvion, L. (2008). Dancing bodies, decaying bodies: The interpretation of anorexia among Israeli dancers. *Nordic Journal of Youth Research, 16*(1), 67–87. https://doi.org/10.1177/110330880701600105

Kadambi, M., & Ennis, L. (2004). Reconsidering vicarious trauma. *Journal of Trauma Practice, 3*(2), 1–21. https://doi.org/10.1300/J189v03n02_01

Karthas, I. (2012). The politics of gender in the revival of ballet in early 20th century France. *Journal of Social History, 45*(4), 960–989. https://doi.org/10.1093/jsh/shr102

Kelman, B. (2000). Occupational hazards in female ballet dancers: Advocate for a forgotten population. *Workplace Health &Safety, 28*(9), 430–434. https://doi.org/10.1177/216507990004800904

MacGinley, M., Breckenridge, J., & Mowll, J. (2019). A scoping review of adult survivors' experiences of shame following sexual abuse in childhood. *Health and Social Care in the Community, 27*(5), 1135–1146. https://doi.org/10.1111/hsc.12771

Markula, P. (2011). Dancing the "data": (Im)Mobile bodies. *International Review of Qualitative Research, 4*(1), 35–50. https://doi.org/10.1525/irqr.2011.4.1.35

McEwen, K., & Young, K. (2011). Ballet and pain: Reflections on a risk-dance culture. *Qualitative Research in Sport, Exercise and Health, 3*(2), 152–173. https://doi.org/10.1080/2159676X.2011.572181

McMahon, J., McGannon, K., Zehntner, C., Webicki, L., Stephenson, E., & Martin, K. (2022). Trauma-informed abuse education in sport: Engaging athlete abuse survivors as educations and facilitators: A community of care. *Sport, Education & Society, 28*(8)1–15. https://doi.org/10.1080/13573322.2022.2096586

Moola, F. J., Buliung, R., Posa, S., Moothathamby, N., Woodgate, R., Hansen, N., & Ross, T. (2022). Understanding the impact of visual arts-based research (ABR) in the lives of disabled children and youth as well as methodological insights in ABR application. Canadian *Journal of Disability Studies, 11*(2), 119–160. https://doi.org/10.15353/cjds.v11i2.891

Moola, F., & Krahn, A. (2016). A dance of many secrets: The experiences of emotional harm from the perspective of past professional female ballet dancers in Canada. *Journal of Aggression, Maltreatment & Trauma, 27*(3), 256–274. https://doi.org/10.1080/10926771.2017.1410747

Moola, F. J., Moothathamby, N., McAdam, L., Solomon, M., Varadi, R., Tullis, D. E., & Reisman, J. (2020). Telling my tale: Reflections on the process of visual storytelling for children and youth living with cystic fibrosis and muscular dystrophy in Canada. *International Journal of Qualitative Methods, 19*, 1–8. https://doi.org/10.1177/1609406919898917

Novack, J. (1993). Ballet, gender and cultural power. In H. Thomas (Ed.), *Dance, gender and culture* (pp. 34–48). Palgrave MacMillan. https://doi.org/10.1007/978-1-349-22747-1_3

Olmos-Vega, F., Stalmeijer, R., Varpio, L., & Kahlkem, R. (2023). A practical guide to reflexivity in qualitative research: AMEE guide no. 149. *Medical Teacher, 45*(3), 241–251. https://doi.org/10.1080/0142159X.2022.2057287

Papaefstathiou, M., Rhind, D., & Brackenridge, C. (2013). Child protection in ballet: Experiences and views of teachers, administrators and ballet students. *Child Abuse Review, 22*(2), 127–141. https://doi.org/10.1002/car.2228

Pedovic, I., & Hedrih, V. (2019). Social trauma and emotional attachment. *Facta Universitais, 18*(1), 27–37. https://doi.org/10.22190/FUPSPH1901027P

Pemberton, J., & Loeb, T. (2020). Impact of sexual and interpersonal violence and trauma on women: Trauma-informed practice and feminist theory. *Journal of Feminist Family Therapy, 32*(1–2), 115–131. https://doi.org/10.1080/08952833.2020.1793564

Ponic, P., Reid, C., & Frisby, W. (2010). Cultivating the power of partnerships in feminist participatory action research in women's health. *Nursing Inquiry, 17*(4), 324–335. https://doi.org/10.1111/j.1440-1800.2010.00506.x

Råheim, M., Magnussen, L. H., Tveit Sekse, R. J., Lunde, Å, Jacobsen, T., & Blystad, A. (2016). Researcher–researched relationship in qualitative research: Shifts in positions and researcher vulnerability. *International Journal of Qualitative Studies on Health and Well-Being, 11*(1), 1–12. https://doi.org/10.3402/qhw.v11.30996

Saleem, F., Anderson, R., & Williams, M. (2020). Addressing the myth of racial trauma: Developmental and ecological considerations for youth of colour. *Clinical Child and Family Psychology Review, 23*(1), 1–14. https://doi.org/10.1007/s10567-019-00304-1

SAMHSA. (2014). *SAMHSA's concept of trauma and guidance for a trauma-informed approach.* Scholar Works. https://scholarworks.boisestate.edu/cgi/viewcontent.cgi?article=1006&context=covid

Smith, J. (2017). *Embodiment: A history.* Oxford University Press.

Thambinathan, V., & Kinsella, E. A. (2021). Decolonizing methodologies in qualitative research: Creating spaces for transformative praxis. *International Journal of Qualitative Methods, 20.* https://doi.org/10.1177/16094069211014766

Thompson, N., & Walsh, M. (2010). The existential basis of trauma. *Journal of Social Work Practice, 24,* 377–389. https://doi.org/10.1080/02650531003638163

Traverso, A., & Broderick, M. (2010). Interrogating trauma: Towards a critical trauma studies. *Continuum: Journal of Media and Cultural Studies, 24*(1), 3–15. https://doi.org/10.1080/10304310903461270

Tsibolane, P., & Brown, I. (2016). Principles for conducting critical research using postcolonial theory in ICT4D studies. *Global Development 2016, 3.* http://aisel.aisnet.org/globdev201

Turner, B., & Wainwright, S. (2003). Corps de ballet: The case of the injured ballet dancer, *Sociology of Health and Illness, 25,* 269–288. https://doi.org/10.1111/1467-9566.00347

Van der Kolk, B. (2014). *The body keeps the score: Brain, mind, and body in the healing of trauma.* Penguin Books.

Van Rhyn, B., Barwick, A., & Donelly, M. (2021). The phenomenology of the body after 85 years. *Qualitative Health Research, 31*(12), 12, 2317–2327. https://doi.org/10.1177/10497323211026911

Ward, A. (2013). Understanding postcolonial traumas. *Journal of Theoretical and Philosophical Psychology, 33*(3), 170–184. https://doi.org/10.1037/a0033576

Chapter 3

Investigating Gender-Based Violence Experienced by Female Coaches and How Trauma-Informed Research Approaches Were Used to Prevent Further Harm

Chris Zehntner, Jenny McMahon, and Kerry R. McGannon

Introduction

The population central to this trauma research was female swim coaches within the context of Swimming Australia (SA). An independent review recently conducted on SA occurred and was circulated in the media. This review revealed SA's treatment of female athletes was the result of a toxic culture where women were at the receiving end of groping, sexual innuendo, body shaming, and physical and mental abuse. Governance issues were also found, along with the President of Swimming Australia criticised for discouraging victims from testifying about their abuse (Linden, 2023). Similar to the findings of this independent review of the toxic culture, this research found that female coaches working within this swimming culture were subjected to gender-based violence through literal and ideological force to (re)create a gendered order. This finding is unsurprising, given that research outside of sport contexts has shown that women experience higher rates of assault or abuse, with sexual abuse being the most common type to be reported (The Substance Abuse and Mental Health Services Administration [SAMHSA], 2023; U.S. Department of Veterans Affairs, 2023).

SA is the peak body for the sport of swimming in Australia and coordinates or oversees coach education by setting coach accreditation standards and making selection choices in relation to representative teams for both swimmers and coaches. Ultimately, SA is the decision maker regarding coach education, employment of high-performance coaches, and selection of athletes in their funded high-performance programmes, among other things. Given this consolidation of decision making, SA holds power over its coaches and athletes.

Within SA, male coaches dominate the coaching workplace, with a minority of female coaches holding the higher levels of coaching accreditation. Recent figures show that only 8% of females achieve 'Platinum' accreditation (i.e., the highest level of coach accreditation) (ASCTA, 2015). In contrast,

DOI: 10.4324/9781003332909-4

the percentage of female coach representation holding lower levels of coach accreditation is significantly higher (ASCTA, 2015). These figures show how female coaches are failing to progress through the levels, and alarmingly, are leaving the profession/industry.

The reasons why female swimming coaches are failing to progress (i.e., hold higher levels of accreditation) or leaving the profession all together remains an underexplored area and is central to the research presented in this chapter. One possible reason for female coaches' inability to progress in coaching pathways was reported by Norman (2008), who explained that as a group, females have endured what can only be described as a difficult progression beset with bottlenecks and barriers. This complex cultural phenomenon, which favours and advantages male coaches, also shows how coaches are evaluated through filters such as 'gender' (Holmes, 2018). Another potential reason for the lack of female coaches in senior roles in SA could be due to their poor treatment as witnessed by Author 1 during his time as a fulltime practising coach. Together, these points provided the impetus for our research, which explored the central question: *what barriers do female coaches' face within the profession regarding their progression and treatment, and what are the consequences?*

At the completion of this qualitative study, it became known that female coaches were subjected to non-accidental violence, gender-based violence, and psychological abuse from male coaches (Zehntner et al., 2023). Their adverse experiences in their workplace (i.e., sports coaching) led to trauma in many instances, which profoundly affected their ongoing health and well-being. Indeed, some of the ongoing challenges experienced by the female coaches who took part in this research not only profoundly shaped their practice (e.g., they were scared to deviate from the accepted practice promoted by their male coach counterparts) but had an ongoing legacy of this trauma on their lives outside of work (e.g., depression, anxiety, panic attacks, trouble sleeping, becoming withdrawn from family and friends, etc.). This ongoing legacy resulting from their treatment sat at the forefront of our conversations throughout the research process. Visceral and emotional evidence of their trauma was also evident. For instance, one female coach burst into tears during the interview when she began explaining how speaking out against the male coaches' toxic practices (with SA leadership) resurrected all the feelings she had experienced during the traumatic event itself. This traumatisation through engagement with the organisational structures of SA, designed to resolve issues, aligns with SAMHSA's (2014, 2023) suggestion that systemic factors (e.g., in the organisation) can interfere with desired outcomes (i.e., resolution of an incident).

Long-lasting adverse effects that manifest as traumatic reactions such as de-motivation or avoidance can be so deeply embedded or normalised that the connection between the adverse event/s and resulting effect(s) might be mis-recognised (Treloar et al., 2023). This was exemplified by one female coach whose coaching practice was commanding and polished in real life, but she revealed a very different side during her interview. She explained how she had to manage ongoing intense anxiety and was on the verge of tears for extended periods (i.e., months) while working on pool deck. To navigate her workplace, she was in a state of constant arousal, vigilant to practices that might have a negative impact (e.g., male coaches' judgement and condemnation of her). Nonetheless, she was locked into the process, seemingly unaware of the wearing down effect it was having on her mental health.

Another female coach, in response to trivialisation and control, modified her practice within the organisation to align with powerful male coach characters, as a way of avoiding potential conflict situations with them (Zehntner et al., 2023). This misrecognition of powerful social actions to control her behaviour was first consented to by the participant and was done (in her words) to "survive in this workplace," therefore characterising this change in practice as an act of self-determination rather than coercive control through persuasion and enforcement (Walker & Sartore-Baldwin, 2013). Soon after this, devastated and disillusioned, she quit coaching altogether.

The objectification of female coaches by male coaches was another common occurrence in the workplace, which female coaches had to constantly negotiate but remained silent about. Coach 'C' describes this,

> Not long after I successful won a job, I had to go in for surgery. I was telling one of the senior male coaches about it and he just looks at me and says, 'Elective?' He motions with his hands clutched around imaginary breasts – inferring a breast implant procedure. I was like, 'No, I'm having abdominal surgery, I'm really unwell.
>
> (Zehntner et al., 2023)

This male coach in the above example not only attempted to subordinate Coach 'C,' asserting his dominance and control over her (Bryson, 1987), but also enacted sexual harassment, the most common form of gender-based violence to occur in the workplace (Australian Human Rights Commission, 2022). Moreover, while sexual harassment can take many forms, Coach 'C' was subjected to verbal sexual harassment from a senior male coach "through his sexually suggestive, offensive, comment or joke" (Australian Human Rights Commission, 2022.). Connell (1987, 1995) explains how these practices become normalised by other male coaches and shows how an idealised hegemonic masculinity is perpetuated (Aboim et al., 2016).

The female coaches also expressed how the constant control of them by male coaches, along with their criticism, objectification, critique of their physical appearance (e.g., *Coach C was chastised by a male coach for wearing lipstick to a finals session*) and exclusion, affected their health and well-being. Some of the effects experienced by the female coaches included anxiety, migraines, depression, sleeping disorders, disordered eating, and withdrawal from their family and friends. These none-too-subtle interplays were Coach C's cultural reality and contributed to a broader impact on her and those close to her.

> My family tries to help me fight the fight, but it's too big; there are too many levels of resistance. And it crushes me, it has impacted me as a person, it has changed the way that I interact with people, and that is not good. It's like being in an abusive relationship where you are getting hammered and thinking, just shut up and take it, and it will be OK, just close your eyes, put your mind somewhere else and you will be ok. And that is how I feel sometimes when I am on deck particularly when I am around some personalities. I just close my eyes and think of some place nice. That is a pretty bad workplace, and you can see that I must really love coaching to stay.
> (Zehntner et al., 2023, p. 112)

What is evident here for Coach C is how multiple victimisation experiences compound and result in trauma symptoms such as depression and anxiety (Wall et al., 2016). While there is a great deal of speculation by coach researchers (e.g., Fielding-Lloyd & Mean, 2011; Norman, 2008, 2010a, 2010b) and pundits (Carney, 2018) around the reasons for female coaches leaving the profession, it is only through the examination of their stories that understanding of the mechanisms at play within this SA social system became known.

Methodology

Given that gender-based violence and the subordination of female swim coaches were central to this investigation, the chosen methodology needed to provide opportunities for their voices of experience relating to their treatment to be foregrounded. Foregrounding the female coaches' voices and experiences was imperative because researchers have shown how female victims of abuse and violence have had their voices silenced or suppressed, including control taken from them (Delker et al., 2020; McMahon et al., 2023). We also wanted the opportunity for their lived experiences to be accessible to others in a format that could be more easily understood so they could potentially be used for coach learning (McMahon, 2013) with the hope that social action may result (e.g., change to practices and policy).

Narrative inquiry was therefore purposely chosen as a methodology, as it centralises the female coaches' stories and narratives that frame them as the primary data set. Indeed, the stories of experience told by the female coach participants become the object of the investigation (Polkinghorne, 1988). By employing narrative inquiry, female coach participants have agency and autonomy over their stories, including what they tell and the way they tell it, which is important in trauma research (McMahon et al., Under Review). Riessman (2008) further states how narrative/life story interviewing places a great emphasis on participants' autonomy, choice, and voice to tell it in their own words.

As Polkinghorne (1988) explains, narrative inquiry entails not only the collection of stories but also their analysis, which is considered the primary way in which life is made meaningful. By appropriately engaging the audience with stories of gender-based violence that result from this project, it may lead to social change, increased empathy, and the opportunity for others to resonate (McMahon & McGannon, 2020). Therefore, the use of accessible data forms is imperative, which in the case of our research was stories, to enable 'witnessing' to occur (Ropers-Huilman, 1999). As Ropers-Huilman (1999, p. 23) explains, witnessing occurs through the act of "reading, feeling, and experiencing the lived experiences of others, therefore accessibility to such information is imperative."

Deductive reflexive thematic analysis (Braun & Clarke, 2019) and a story analyst approach (Smith, 2016), expanded below in the method section, were used to address the aims of this research and enhance the audience's potential 'witnessing' (Ropers-Huilman, 1999) of gender-based violence and trauma. From a literature standpoint, the complexity of the female coaches' experiences within this sport culture required relevant theory to be applied, so a deeper insight and better understanding into their treatment (i.e., social and structural barriers) could be gained. While the more traditional researchers' interpretive voice was present, it was incumbent on us (i.e., the researchers) to provide the reader with relevant theoretical and interpretive tools so they could make [their own] critical judgements (Zehntner et al., 2023). Therefore, to provide potential connections between male coaches' 'pattern[s] of practice' (Connell & Messerschmidt, 2005, p. 832) and their actions that might have allowed 'men's dominance over women' (Connell & Messerschmidt, 2005, p. 832), we utilised the concept of hegemonic masculinity (Connell, 1987, 1995; Connell & Messerschmidt, 2005). Hegemonic masculinity can be characterised as practices that justify men's dominant position in a cultural setting (Connell, 1995; Connell & Messerschmidt, 2005) and illuminate how social practices (re)produce the 'dominant position of men and the subordination of women' (Connell, 1995, p. 77). In this way, and through the application of theory in the narrative inquiry process, a better understanding of the treatment of female coaches by their male counterparts, along with the subsequent effects (e.g., trauma and leaving the profession), can be made known.

While none of these methodological considerations and decisions can provide immediate tangible relief to participants who may experience trauma, it was hoped that aspects of the narrative inquiry may potentially benefit them by providing them with some clarity and understanding of their experiences. As McMahon and Penney (2011) state, catharsis may result from in-depth discussion and deep introspection, along with providing participants with the requisite tools to share and analyse their own stories.

Method

Ethical approval was gained from Author 1's institution; however, we were also mindful of Sparkes and Smith's (2014) call for researchers to strive for aspirational ethics beyond the minimum standard (Lahman et al., 2011). We realised that disclosure of traumatic experiences could likely cause discomfort, and so we sought to minimise the length of interviews and took great care to avoid pressing participants, instead enabling them to direct the topic and detail they wished to share (expanded on below). Participants also controlled the time of interviews and the direction of the conversations that ensued via the key points or barriers they had listed in their mind maps (see below). We were also mindful of the power imbalance between the male researcher (interviewer), who was a cultural insider (swim coach), and the female coach participants. As such, when undertaking interviews, Author 1 was responsive to instances that might compromise the dignity, psychological safety, and privacy of the participants and implemented trauma-informed strategies (see the trauma-informed strategies section below) to minimise the possibility of causing further harm.

The research method or process that was undertaken was partly designed in response to the scarcity of participants and the cultural insider status of two of the researchers (Zehntner and McMahon). McMahon (Author 2) is a past elite swimmer who was subjected to abuse and subsequent trauma in the SA culture, and Zehntner, a swim coach for over 20 years, meant that between them, they had access to many female coaches of varying experience. As a result of this, participants were recruited through purposive sampling (Sparkes & Smith, 2014). After consenting to be a part of the investigation, the female coaches were asked to produce a mind map. The instructions were simply to produce a graphic organiser like a mind map (visual exemplars were provided) in response to the prompt question, "can you describe some of the instances in your coach education journey that had a significant (positive or negative) impact on your progress as a coach?" Participants were encouraged to bring their mind map to their interview, which was held at a time of their choosing via an online format. An example of a mind map produced by one of the participants for their interview is presented directly below in Figure 3.1. The mind map and personal topics listed by each of the participants subsequently directed the focus of the interview/conversation rather than the researcher (Author 1) controlling or directing it.

Unstructured interviews were then conducted by Author 1, and open-ended questions stemming from the participant's mind map were asked. As an example of one of the open-ended questions included, *in terms of the challenges you faced in the coach education pathway, what incidents have you listed in your mind map had the biggest impact on your progression as a coach?* (Zehntner et al., 2023). Reference to examples from the mind map aided in the identification of critical information points and the general

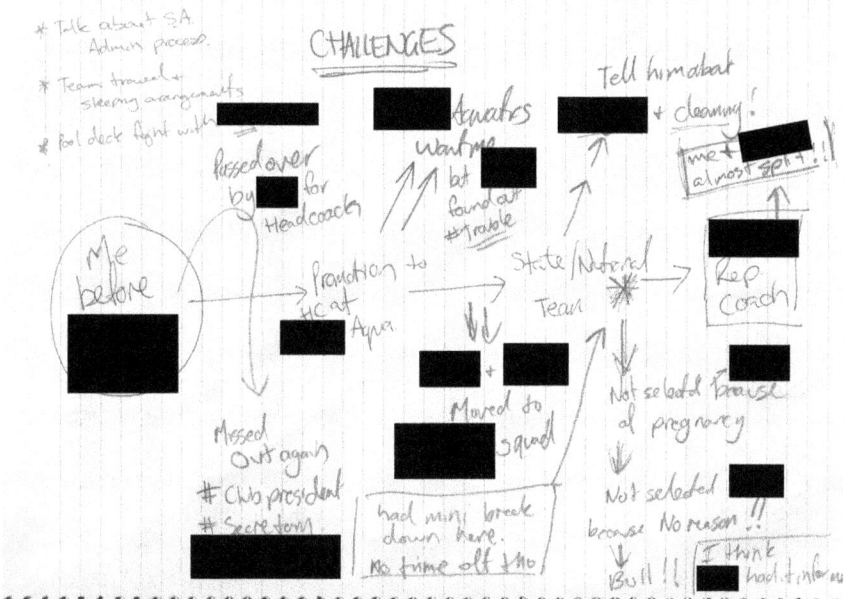

Figure 3.1 Mind map generated by participant. Redacted sections for anonymity.

flow of the interview. Doing this avoided narrative development becoming a "more sensitive version of the 'old' men's studies" (Messner, 1990, p. 137); instead the storyteller (i.e., participant) decided the context and content (Walk, 2000, p. 33) of the stories that followed. Story telling during the interview was a natural, rather than forced, preference for the participants to detail their experiences and practices they were subjected to within the SA culture (Messner, 1990; Tong, 2018). Towards the conclusion of the discussion, Author 1 revisited points within their stories that remained unclear before finalising the interview.

After the interview, Author 1 refined the participants' stories (i.e., removed ums and identifiable information) into discrete narratives. Some of the stories told by the participants were not sequential or told in a linear way, however still provided important details relating to their gender-based violence, subordination, and trauma. This is unsurprising, given that trauma may affect people's ability to tell a story with emplotment (i.e., detailing a comprehensive account) and sequence (Day & Wadey, 2023; Neimeyer & Levitt, 2001). Therefore, in some instances, and as a way of developing the female coaches' narratives a little further (Moon, 2010; Sparkes, 2009), a back-and-forth process between the interviewer (Author 1) and the participant occurred, allowing for additional information to be added (e.g., background or context specific information). The impetus of this back-and-forth process (between

Author 1 and participant) stemmed from the guide provided by SAMHSA's (2014, 2023) for relaying trauma information. Thus, when relaying trauma information, the three E's of trauma should be made known, including (1) the trauma Event[s], (2) Experience of the event[s], and (3) the Effect. By foregrounding the participants' experiences using this format, details around what occurred can be made known, along with their feelings of hurt, humiliation, embarrassment, or betrayal relating to the trauma event, so both the lay reader and academic audience might better understand trauma. In this way, narrative trauma representations can be used as a pedagogical tool for learning and shared understanding (Douglas & Carless, 2009; McMahon, 2013; McMahon et al., 2018).

Following narrative development, deductive reflexive thematic analysis (Braun & Clarke, 2006, 2019) was performed, and themes relating to hegemonic masculinity and gender-based violence were identified. The first stage in this process involved familiarisation with the narratives by the co-authors. This was achieved by engaging in multiple readings of the participants' accounts and collaborative discussions (between authors) that centred on analytical sensibility within and across the stories. This process aided in drawing out keywords and phrases that directly related to the core tenets of hegemony (i.e., practices representative of social manipulation, social censure, or social mechanisms) or gender-based violence. Using a collective critical approach between Author 1 and critical friends (Authors 2 and 3), the themes were refined and finalised. Finally, the analysis of the data corpus (i.e., series of individual narratives) occurred through illustration and analysis by using social theory (e.g., hegemonic masculinity) to interpret events in extracts from the narratives.

Pseudonyms were used to protect participants' identities; however, as the data related to events, including interactions with past and present employees of SA, the development of narratives relating to identifiable events could potentially compromise participants' safety. Therefore, the locations and timing of interaction/events required layers of confidentiality (Pittman & Maxwell, 1992). This was done in consultation with each of the participants, who were "central to decision making around their security and anonymity" (p. 109).

Evidence-based Trauma-Informed Practices Applied to Research

We were acutely aware from the outset of this research that the experiences of female coach participants could contain themes of trauma and gender-based violence, particularly as Author 1 had witnessed their poor treatment during his own immersion in the SA culture. What Author 1 (primary interviewer) was not fully prepared for was the sharing of personal trauma experiences and the ongoing legacy of it on the participants and their lives. Upon first hearing the stories, Author 1 found himself, at times, shocked and angry, and by the end of data collection, frustrated by what was found.

Given the ongoing legacy of trauma on these female coach participants, the importance of researchers needing to be trauma aware (SAMHSA, 2023; Wall et al., 2016) by implementing trauma-informed practices is very much needed, so potential further harm is minimised. SAMHSA (2014, 2023) outlines six key principles of a trauma-informed approach, of which two were largely influential in this research. While these two principles are expanded on below, there was indeed overlap across all six principles.

Physical and Psychological Safety

When undertaking a trauma-informed approach, the principle of safety is essential because people who have experienced gender-based violence or trauma often perceive the world as 'unsafe' (Menschner & Maul, 2016; SAMHSA, 2014, 2023). This means that if the female coach participants experiencing trauma were to feel physically, socially, or emotionally unsafe at any time in the research process, it could lead to them experiencing anxiety or even re-traumatisation (Menschner & Maul, 2016). Therefore, when designing and implementing this research, we realised that addressing the physical and psychological safety of the female coach participants needed to be prioritised to ensure that the risk of causing them further harm was limited.

Before we even commenced the research design, Author 2's experiences as an abuse victim, abuse survivor, and trauma survivor within the SA context were drawn upon. As SAMHSA (2014, 2023) highlights, it is important to utilise an individual with lived experience of trauma (i.e., Author 2) to help identify how "the physical and psychological experience can be more trauma-informed" (SAMHSA, 2014, p. 21). Therefore, much of the interview design was centred on Author 2's insider experiences of abuse and trauma, in conjunction with the trauma-informed guidelines outlined by SAMHSA (2014, 2023). The first primary concern outlined by Author 2 was the gender differentials between Author 1 (the interviewer), who is a male former swimming coach, and the female coach participants. This point was of particular concern as male coaches were primarily the perpetrators of the female coach participants' harm. As Hira et al. (2023) state, gender differentials can be an interpersonal trigger for women experiencing trauma that can lead to re-traumatisation; therefore the consideration of gender differences is very much needed. As a way of addressing gender differentials and this potential trigger in the interview process, the female coach participants were provided with the option of completing the interview process with Author 1 (former male coach) or Author 2 (former female swimmer who was subjected to abuse by male coaches in the SA culture). While the recommendation of Hira et al. (2023) relates to the application of trauma-informed practices in the medical field, they state the importance of providing women with access to and choices regarding the preferred gender they would like to engage with. While the female coach participants in this study were provided with options and choices, all the participants expressed that they were happy to undertake the interviews with Author 1. Nonetheless, as an additional precaution and option, Author 2 remained available during each scheduled interview, ready to dial in if needed.

As a cultural insider of SA, Author 1 (coach) had a particular history and knowledge within this 'coaching' subculture that proved beneficial. This meant that he had an intricate understanding of how power was and is deployed in and through the coaching sub-culture, which was integral to the subsequent conversations and shared understanding that ensued in interviews. This is not to suggest that as a male coach, Author 1 could fully recognise the social forces experienced by female coaches. Instead, as a past coach, cultural insider, and reflective researcher, he had an elevated understanding of the possible ways that ideological force or coercive power could be deployed in this hierarchical environment. As such, he could share, and validate, coaching stories with participants, enhancing the richness of the conversations (Goodson & Gill, 2011).

Another suggestion made by Author 2 relating to the participants' safety in the interview process was to implement online interviews rather than conducting them in a face-to-face mode, an approach that was incorporated by her in her research with athletes' survivors of abuse (McMahon et al., 2023). As Veletsianos and Houlden (2019) explain, the online environment is far more predictable; therefore unforeseen events can be limited, thus enhancing the physical safety of the participants (McMahon et al., 2023. This consideration is important because spatial triggers (e.g., distance between two people and small rooms) have been identified as a potential cause of re-traumatisation for women affected by trauma (Hira et al., 2023). Further, as explained by Marlowe (2019), in contexts where there are gender differentials, online approaches are preferred because in a face-to-face context, situations may prove more difficult for the person (i.e., participant) to control. Online settings therefore enable people with 'implied control' over the time (i.e., when the female coach participants chose to complete the interview) and location chosen by the participant (e.g., home, garden, or in a parked car) (McMahon et al., 2023; Veletsianos & Houlden, 2019). Moreover, through the implementation of online interviews, the maintaining of healthy interpersonal boundaries could also occur between Author 1 and the female coach participants, along with elevated levels of physical comfort (Veletsianos & Houlden, 2019).

Another benefit of the online format for interviews is that participants can make use of personal comfort or soothing devices, such as their pet or a favourite blanket, to soothe themselves if needed throughout the interview (Marlowe & Allen, 2023). By encouraging personal comforts (e.g., a pet in the room) (McMahon et al., 2023) and the ability to move (i.e., lie down in the room if needed), we hoped their comfort levels would be increased.

The participants' psychological safety was another important consideration, and as explained by SAMHSA, it centred on interpersonal interactions
(SAMHSA, 2014, 2023). As described in the method section above, we aimed
to promote a sense of psychological safety by limiting instances of 'power
over' the participant (i.e., power differentials occurring between the researcher and the researched). As explained by trauma researchers (e.g., Butler
et al., 2011; Sweeney et al., 2018), re-traumatisation can occur in the use of
'power-over' relationships and, when applied to research settings, may relate
to participants having a lack of agency and control. Therefore, the participants
had 'power over' the chosen time and date that the interview occurred. They
also had 'power over' the topics of discussion in the interview process, with
only points they had listed in their mind map (see example in Figure 3.1
above) being discussed. Moreover, through the employment of narrative inquiry, they maintained 'power over' what they did and did not share with the
audience in their storied representations. In this way, the research participants
expressed choice (SAMHSA, 2014, 2023) in relation to identifying the topic,
detail, and depth of stories and further, which narratives were selected for
inclusion in subsequent publications.

Cultural, Historical, and Gender Issues

SAMHSA's (2023) sixth TIP of *cultural, historical, and gender issues* outlined
in their *'Guidance for a Trauma-Informed Approach Framework'* centres on
the idea that within a trauma-informed approach, cultural stereotypes and
biases should be moved beyond, with gender responsive practices incorporated, along with providing authentic cultural connections. Given *'gender'*
underpinned the aim of this research, we felt it was non-negotiable to implement this principle into the research design and researcher practices, so
no unintended gender harms resulted. We achieved this in several discreet
ways. The first related to the overall aim of the research project, which was
gender responsiveness to a particular issue affecting women (i.e., female
coaches). Indeed, our overall aim centred on the need to find out more
about why female coaches are failing to progress in their professions in SA
and further why they are leaving the profession all together. In this respect,
the impetus of the research was based on attempting to reduce gender inequalities in the SA context and identify gender [mis]treatment within the SA
coaching workforce. With this noted, it could be assumed that this research
was therefore *gender-biased* due to the impetus and research aim; however,
it was hoped that the findings of this research may primarily benefit female
coaches, such as through policy change. We also felt that the male coaches
could also benefit in the education sense through their engagement with
the female coaches' stories, which may assist them to reflect and adapt
their mentoring practices (Douglas & Carless, 2009; McMahon, 2013). Likewise, SA, as a predominantly male dominated organisation, may respond by

implementing strategies and procedures to better support female coaches. Subsequently, this may assist them as an organisation in maintaining an equal ratio of gender within their coaching staff (particularly at the higher levels), equal work opportunities, and having power more equally distributed (United Nations, 2023).

The *gender representation* of the research team was another important consideration, given the topic of the research. While the team contained three researchers, equal gender representation was unable to be achieved. However, given the topic of gender-based violence against female coaches, we felt it was important to 'tip the scales' by including two female researchers to work with Author 1 (the primary researcher), who was a male. Like Author 1, Author 2 provided a unique 'insider' perspective to this project as a former female swimmer within the SA culture who was subjected to abuse by male coaches, which led to subsequent trauma. While Author 3, a sport psychology researcher who has extensively investigated gender equity and psychological safety in sport, was also integral to this *gender-responsive* research. Through the female representation on the research team, a *gendered lens* could be authentically applied to ensure communications were conveyed in a *gender-sensitive manner*. By doing this, we strove for a research process that was *gender transformative* by centralising the experiences of female coaches while also striving for their psychological and cultural safety from a gender equity perspective. Our hope was that this may potentially lead to progressive changes in power relationships between female and male coaches within SA (World Health Organisation, 2011).

Relating to the cultural component of this sixth TIP while it can also relate to race, ethnicity, and other intersecting identities (SAMHSA, 2014), we focused on cultural issues intersecting with gender occurring within the context of SA. SAMHSA (2014, 2023) explains the importance of having a good 'cultural fit' when being trauma-informed. This 'fit' can be achieved by using cultural 'insiders' when undertaking ethnographic research work to enhance better communication (Goodson & Gill, 2011) and more authentic engagement than what is possible with an outsider (SAMHSA, 2014). Author 1 and Author 2 functioned in multiple roles in the research process by providing much needed cultural insider positions. For example, Author 1, who is an accredited coach within SA with over 25 years of experience and possesses extensive 'insider' knowledge of this culture, undertook the roles of primary interviewer and research designer. While Author 2, as a former athlete within the SA culture, was able to provide a unique insider perspective of trauma, abuse, and maltreatment within the SA culture. The 'insider' knowledge of both Authors 1 and 2 was imperative because an 'outsider' would not be able to share the same cultural insight, knowledge, or expertise, limiting the potential research outcomes and experience for the recipients (McMahon et al., 2022). Goodson and Gill (2011) explain the importance of being a cultural 'insider' for collaboration and reciprocation so that rich and culturally relevant conversations occur (Goodson & Gill, 2011; McMahon et al., 2022). As such, in the interviews carried out, Author 1 adopted appropriate cultural language from SA (e.g., culturally specific terms were used such as mentor, sets, pbs, laps, taper, stroke rates, and information relating to specific camps or trips) to resonate with participants' own understandings (McMahon et al., 2023).

Conclusions

It is important to acknowledge that researchers are not trauma clinicians, but we are encouraged by Greenwald's (2015) assertion that some healing from trauma may potentially occur in non-clinical settings (i.e., research contexts). However, as Bath (2008) explains, potential healing is more likely to result in environments, which are trauma-informed. While we do not suggest that this research is a panacea for healing, we do assert that creating a safe environment for female coach participants through the implementation of evidence-based trauma-informed practices can facilitate meaningful sharing (SAMHSA, 2014, 2023). As such, some degree of the ethical loneliness (Stauffer, 2015) experienced by female coach participants can also be addressed.

As a result of our experience conducting this research and through reflection undertaken when compiling this chapter, we have identified three future directions for conducting research with sport, exercise, and health populations that have experienced trauma. These include (1) greater consideration of the cultural context prior to the study; (2) addressing gender differentials in the research process through evidence-based practices; and finally (3) drawing on the expertise and insight of an individual with lived experience of trauma.

1 Understanding the socio-political, cultural, and gender-based systems of privilege and oppression will impact researchers' ability to understand how "these dynamics promote or violate the assumptions of healing centered engagement" (Voith et al., 2020, p. 5). Thus, pre-study engagement with the population should inform trauma-informed research design to learn about their histories, lives, and how these intersect with sport cultures. So, to truly plumb the depths of the system, a deep understanding is first required to be trauma-informed. Such understanding can be achieved when grounded in a historical/intergenerational perspective to learn more about how gender-based violence practices are deeply embedded, recycled, and circulated in the everyday lives of coaches/participants.
2 Researchers should consider gender differentials in researcher and researched relationships. This consideration includes the researchers' reflexive recognition of their gendered identities in relation to power and privilege and how these impact co-participants and the research team during the process. This is urgently needed because, as Hira et al. (2023) highlight, gender differentials can be an interpersonal trigger for women

experiencing trauma that can lead to their re-traumatisation. Some strategies to address this are to ensure equal gender representation on research teams, along with a critical eye towards how the gender dynamics in the research team relate to participants, and to ensure research is gender-responsive, to name just a few.

3   Finally, we encourage researchers to draw on the expertise of a person with lived experience of trauma and/or work with cultural/contextual insiders, who can advise about the research design and researcher practices throughout a project. As SAMHSA (2014, 2023) explains in the principle of peer support, utilising the lived experience of trauma survivors to co-design research can help identify how "the physical and psychological experience can be more trauma-informed" (SAMHSA, 2014, p. 21). This practice may also facilitate understanding of trauma meanings and experiences throughout the research process to enhance safety and trust (SAMHSA, 2014).

References

Aboim, S., Hearn, J., & Howson, R. (2016). Hegemonic masculinity. In The Blackwell encyclopaedia of sociology. Blackwell. https://doi.org/10.1002/9781405165518. wbeosh022.pub2

Australian Human Rights Commission. (2022). *Sexual harassment.* https://humanrights. gov.au/quick-guide/12096

Australian Swim Coaches and Teachers Association (ASCTA). (2015). *2015 annual report from Australian Swim Coaches and Teachers Association.* https://ascta.com/about/governance/

Bath, H. (2008). The three pillars of trauma-informed care. *Reclaiming Children and Youth, 17*(3), 17–21.

Braun, V., & Clarke, V. (2006). Using thematic analysis in psychology. *Qualitative Research in Psychology, 3*(2), 77–101. https://doi.org/10.1191/1478088706qp0 63oa

Braun, V., & Clarke, V. (2019). Reflecting on reflexive thematic analysis. *Qualitative Research in Sport, Exercise and Health, 11*(4), 589–597. https://doi.org/10.1080/21 59676X.2019.1628806

Bryson, L. (1987). Sport and the maintenance of masculine hegemony. *Women's Studies International Forum, 10*(4), 349–360. https://doi.org/10.1016/0277-5395(87)90052-5

Butler, L. D., Critelli, F. M., & Rinfrette, E. S. (2011) Trauma-informed care and mental health. *Directions in Psychiatry, 31*(3), 197–210.

Carney, S. (2018). *Kate Palmer: Gross under-representation of women in high-performance coaching and executive positions.* https://ministryofsport.com.au/kate-palmer-gross-under-representation-of-women-in-highperformance-coaching-and-executive-positions/

Connell, R. W. (1987). *Gender and power.* Allen and Unwin.

Connell, R. W. (1995). *Masculinities.* University of California Press.

Connell, R. W., & Messerschmidt, J. W. (2005). Hegemonic masculinity: Rethinking the concept. *Gender & Society, 19*(6), 829–859. https://doi.org/10.1177/0891243205278639

Day, M., & Wadey, R. (2023). Learning to put on the brakes: Trauma-informed narrative interviewing after limb amputation. In. J. McMahon & K. R. McGannon (Eds.), *Trauma-informed research in sport, exercise, and health: Qualitative methods*. Routledge.

Delker, B., Salton, R., & McLean, K. (2020). Giving voice to silence: Empowerment and disempowerment in the developmental shift from trauma 'victim' to 'survivor-advocate. *Journal of Trauma and Dissociation, 21*(2), 242–263. https://doi.org/10.1080/15299732.2019.167821

Douglas, K., & Carless, D. (2009). Exploring taboo issues in professional sport through a fictional approach. *Reflective Practice, 10*(3), 311–323. https://doi.org/10.1080/14623940903034630

Fielding-Lloyd, B., & Mean L. J. (2011). "I don't think I can catch it": Women, confidence, and responsibility in football coach education. Soccer and Society, *12*, 344–363.

Goodson, I., & Gill, S. (2011). *Narrative pedagogy: Life history and learning*. Peter Lang.

Greenwald, R. (2015). *Child trauma handbook: A guide for helping trauma-exposed children and adolescents*. Routledge.

Hira, S., Sheppard-Perkins, M., & Darroch, F. (2023). The facilitator is not a bystander: Exploring the perspectives of interdisciplinary experts on trauma research. *Frontiers in Psychology, 14*, 1225789. https://doi.org/10.3389/fpsyg.2023.1225789

Holmes, T. (2018). *New sport Australia boss out to tackle gender inequality in sport governance and coaching*. https://www.abc.net.au/news/2018-11-09/sport-boss-gender-inequality-in-sport-governance-and-coaching/10479876

Lahman, M. K., Geist, M. R., Rodriguez, K. L., Graglia, P., & DeRoche, K. K. (2011). Culturally responsive relational reflexive ethics in research: The three Rs. *Quality and Quantity, 45*(6), 1397–1414. https://doi.org/10.1007/s11135-010-9347-3

Linden, J. (2023). Swimming legend Kieren Perkins secretly criticised by high-level investigators for comments they claim discouraged whistleblowers. *The Australian*. https://www.theaustralian.com.au/sport/olympics/swimming-legend-kieren-perkins-secretly-criticised-by-highlevel-investigators-for-comments-they-claim-discouraged-whistleblowers/news-story/9b1137ee0bc8cc9d7e114fae422a4597

Marlowe, J. (2019). Refugee resettlement, social media and the social organization of difference. *Global Networks, 20*(2), 274–291. https://doi.org/10.1111/glob.12233

Marlowe, J., & Allen, J. (2023). Relationality and online interpersonal research: Ethical, methodological and pragmatic extensions. *Qualitative Social Work, 22*(3), 484–501. https://doi.org/10.1177/1473325022108791

McMahon, J. (2013). The use of narrative in coach education: The effect on short- and long-term practice? *Sports Coaching Review*. https://doi.org/10.1080/21640629.2013.836922

McMahon, J., Knight, C. J., & McGannon, K. R. (2018). Educating parents of children in sport about abuse using narrative pedagogy. *Sociology of Sport Journal, 35*(4), 314–323. https://doi.org/10.1123/ssj.2017-0186

McMahon, J., & McGannon, K. R. (2020). Acting out what is inside of us: Self-management strategies of an abused ex-athlete. *Sport Management Review, 23*(1), https://doi.org/10.1016/j.smr.2019.03.008

McMahon, J., McGannon, K. R., & Zehntner, C. (Under Review). Arts-based methods as a trauma-informed approach to research: Enabling survivors and victims' experiences to be visible and limiting the risk of re-traumatisation. *Methods in Psychology*.

McMahon, J., McGannon, K. R., Zehntner, C., Werbicki, L., Stephenson, E., & Martin, K. (2023). Trauma-informed abuse education in sport: Engaging athlete abuse survivors as educators and facilitating a community of care. *Sport, Education and Society*, *28*(8), 958–971. https://doi.org/10.1080/13573322.2022.2096586

McMahon, J., & Penney, D. (2011). Empowering swimmers and their bodies in and through research. *Qualitative Research in Sport, Exercise and Health*, *3*(2), 130–151. https://doi.org/10.1080/2159676X.2011.572176

Menschner, C., & Maul, A. (2016). *Key ingredients for successful trauma-informed care implementation*. https://www.samhsa.gov/sites/default/files/programs_campaigns/childrens_mental_health/atc-whitepaper-040616.pdf

Messner, M. A. (1990). Men studying masculinity: Some epistemological issues in sport sociology. *Sociology of Sport Journal*, *7*(2), 136–153. https://doi.org/10.1123/ssj.7.2.136

Moon, J. (2010). *Using story: In higher education and professional development*. Routledge.

Neimeyer, R. A., & Levitt, H. (2001). Coping and coherence: A narrative perspective on resilience. In S. Snyder (Ed.), *Coping with stress* (pp. 47–67). Oxford University Press.

Norman, L. (2008). The UK coaching system is failing women coaches. *International Journal of Sports Science & Coaching*, *3*(4), 447–476. https://doi.org/10.1260/174795408787186431

Norman, L. (2010a). Bearing the burden of doubt: Female coaches' experiences of gender relations. *Research Quarterly for Exercise and Sport*, *81*(4), 506–517. https://doi.org/10.1080/02701367.2010.10599712

Norman, L. (2010b). Feeling second best: Elite women coaches' experiences. *Sociology of Sport Journal*, *27*(1), 89–104. https://doi.org/10.1123/ssj.27.1.89

Pittman, M. A., & Maxwell, J. A. (1992). Qualitative approaches to evaluation: Models and methods. In M. D. LeCompte, W. L. Millroy, & J. Preissle (Eds.), *The handbook of qualitative research in education* (pp. 729–770). Academic Press.

Polkinghorne, D. E. (1988). *Narrative knowing and the human sciences*. Suny Press.

Riessman, C. K. (2008). *Narrative methods for the human sciences*. Sage.

Ropers-Huilman, B. (1999). Witnessing: Critical inquiry in a post structural world. *Qualitative Studies in Education*, *12*(1), 21–35. https://doi.org/10.1080/095183999236312

Smith, B. (2016). Narrative analysis in sport and exercise: How can it be done? In B. Smith & C. Sparkes (Eds.), *Routledge handbook of qualitative research in sport and exercise* (pp. 260–274). Routledge.

Sparkes, A. (2009). Ethnography and the senses: Challenges and possibilities. *Qualitative Research in Sport and Exercise*, *1*(1), 21–35. https://doi.org/10.1080/19398440802567923

Sparkes, A., & Smith, B. (2014). *Qualitative research methods in sport, exercise, and health: From process to product*. Routledge.

Stauffer, J. (2015). *Ethical loneliness: The injustice of not being heard*. Columbia University Press.

Substance Abuse and Mental Health Services Administration (SAMHSA). (2014). *SAMHSA's concept of trauma and guidance for a trauma informed approach.* Substance Abuse and Mental Health Services Administration.

Substance Abuse and Mental Health Services Administration (SAMHSA). (2023). *Practical guide for implementing a trauma-informed approach.* https://store.samhsa.gov/sites/default/files/pep23-06-05-005.pdf

Sweeney, A., Filson, B., Kennedy, A., Collinson, L., & Gillard, S. (2018). A paradigm shift: Relationships in trauma-informed mental health services. *BJPsych Advances, 24*(5), 319–333. https://doi.org/10.1192/bja.2018.29.

Tong, R. (2018). *Feminist thought, student economy edition: A more comprehensive introduction.* Routledge.

Treloar, C., Idle, J., & Valentine, K. (2023). Child sexual abuse, alcohol and other drug use and the criminal justice system: The meanings of trauma in survivor narratives for a national royal commission. *Qualitative Health Research, 33*(1–2), 117–126. https://doi.org/10.1177/10497323221144923

United Nations. (2023). *Sustainable Development Goals: The world is failing girls and women, according to new UN report.* https://www.un.org/sustainabledevelopment/blog/2023/09/press-release-the-world-is-failing-girls-and-women-according-to-new-un-report/

U.S. Department of Veterans Affairs. (2023). *How common is PTSD in adults?* https://www.ptsd.va.gov/understand/common/common_adults.asp

Veletsianos, G., & Houlden, S. (2019). An analysis of flexible learning and flexibility over the last 40 years of distance education. *Distance Education, 40*(4), 454–468. https://doi.org/10.1080/01587919.2019.1681893

Voith, L. A., Hamler, T., Francis, M. W., Lee, H., & Korsch-Williams, A. (2020). Using a trauma-informed, socially just research framework with marginalized populations: Practices and barriers to implementation. *Social Work Research, 44*(3), 169–181. https://doi.org/10.1093/swr/svaa013

Wall, L., Higgins, D. J., & Hunter, C. (2016). *Trauma-informed care in child/family welfare services.* Australian Institute of Family Studies Melbourne.

Walk, S. R. (2000). Moms, sisters, and ladies; Women student trainers in men's intercollegiate sport. In J. McKay, M. A. Messner, & D. Sabo (Eds.), *Masculinity, gender relations and sport* (pp. 31–46). Sage.

Walker, N. A., & Sartore-Baldwin, M. L. (2013). Hegemonic masculinity and the institutionalized bias toward women in men's collegiate basketball: What do men think? *Journal of Sport Management, 27*(4), 303–315.

World Health Organisation. (2011). *Gender mainstreaming: A practical approach.* Participant's notes. Geneva. https://apps.who.int/iris/bitstream/handle/10665/44516/9789241501064_eng.pdf?sequence=2

Zehntner, C., McMahon, J., & McGannon, K. R. (2023). Gender order through social censure: An examination of social exclusion in sport coaching. *Sport, Education and Society, 28*(1), 105–116. https://doi.org/10.1080/13573322.2021.1979506

Chapter 4

Critical Reflection on Research into Women's Experiences of Gender-Based Violence in Sport

The Application of Trauma-Informed Research Practices

Kirsty Forsdike and Fiona Giles

Introduction

We embarked on this chapter with trepidation. Whilst our meta-synthesis was meant to guide us in our journey in exploring gender-based interpersonal violence in sport, we were not going out to speak with victim survivors. We were worried we would not have anything to provide of use to this edited book. On reflection, in the process of undertaking a meta-synthesis, we were surprised by the disparity across studies and how study authors approached this sensitive topic over time. We struggled with the application of standard "critical appraisal tools" throughout our review as we considered trauma-informed approaches in research.

As such, we focus the chapter on what authors discuss (or not) in their papers in terms of the process of undertaking research with populations who have experienced trauma, and how critical appraisal tools hinder or support such work for ensuring trauma-informed, and therefore ethical, research in this space. We also acknowledge the impact of potential vicarious trauma on the researchers themselves (including us, as we read the papers forming part of the meta-synthesis).

Positionality

We have both participated in sport since our early 20s, in different sports and across different levels albeit all at the grass roots community level. We have also both experienced gender-based violence, including intimate partner violence and sexual violence, either in sport or in other areas of our lives. These experiences shape our view of the world and the research we undertake.

DOI: 10.4324/9781003332909-5

Background

Gender-Based Interpersonal Violence

Gender-based interpersonal violence in sport, the focus of this chapter, is a somewhat broad umbrella term that can cover violence against women and some forms of family violence. The United Nation's definition of violence against women in Articles One and Two of the Declaration on the Elimination of Violence against Women (Proclaimed by General Assembly resolution 48/104 of 20 December 1993) is "any act of gender-based violence that results in, or is likely to result in, physical, sexual or psychological harm or suffering to women, including threats of such acts, coercion or arbitrary deprivation of liberty, whether occurring in public or in private life" (Article 1). This definition includes violence within the family or general community or violence that is perpetrated or condoned by the state. Given we use the term "interpersonal", we are not looking at violence perpetrated or condoned by the state. We are also focused on adult, rather than child, gender-based interpersonal violence. This focus can be challenging to define, given the age boundary between child and adult is not always clear, legally (in terms of age of consent for sex) or across social and cultural differences.

What is clear is that gender-based interpersonal violence can result in significant harm to victim survivors, including ongoing trauma. Such violence has been shown to significantly impact the physical and mental well-being of women and children (Lum On et al., 2016; Savopoulos et al., 2022). Yet, it was not until feminist movements brought "the tyranny of private life" (Herman, 2015, p. 31), sexual and domestic violence, out into the open through the political contexts of western democracies that the public became aware of such violence as trauma.

Trauma was gradually recognised through the first and second world wars but was really seen as a health condition after the Vietnam War (Herman, 2015). As Herman (2015) argues, those who are "devalued" (p. 16) such as women and children, can find that what they experience as trauma may not be socially validated. Women do not necessarily respond to trauma in the same way; they experience complex intersections across individual and environmental contexts (Harvey, 1996; Tseris, 2013). As such, "her experience becomes unspeakable" (Herman, 2015, p. 16). The context of trauma experience is key.

Given the need for trauma-informed approaches, we examine studies of adult women who have experienced gender-based interpersonal violence. We consider researcher positioning and reflexivity as well, and how researchers applied trauma-informed practices in and through their research. We then consider how these studies can be reviewed through a trauma-informed lens and the challenges faced with adhering to qualitative research method critical appraisal tools.

Methodology

Qualitative approaches provide avenues to explore, make sense of, critique, and challenge what happens and how it is experienced in the social and material world. The development of qualitative research literature exploring gender-based interpersonal violence mirrors growing political movements. At a societal level, growth in gender-based violence research in sport alongside political movements that support it can counteract the norm of "silencing and denial" (Herman, 2015, p. 16) of such violence. On an individual level, Lamb and colleagues (2020) argue that most women who speak about their experiences report finding it affirming and empowering, as the trauma they went through could be used to help others, giving meaning to their experience and pain. It can also aid their healing and recovery (Lamb et al., 2020). However, some participants may encounter negative experiences from participating in trauma focused research (Valpied et al., 2014). Not surprisingly, SAMHSA (2014) highlights the need for implementing evidence-based trauma-informed practices because those working with people experiencing trauma may be inadvertently contributing to their re-traumatisation (SAMHSA, 2014).

We undertook a qualitative meta-synthesis to examine published qualitative studies and construct an overarching interpretation of the collective that could answer the research question: "what are women's experiences of gender-based interpersonal violence in sport?". Our meta-synthesis was informed by Noblit and Hare's (1988) meta-ethnographic approach as used by Thomas and Harden (2008) and Williams and Shaw (2016). A meta-ethnographic approach interprets qualitative studies collectively, creating a new interpretation (third-order construct) beyond the individual studies reviewed (Noblit & Hare, 1988). We chose this methodology because it develops third-order constructs through the translation of concepts from one study into another and is therefore ideal when the topic under review is broad and engaged across very different studies (Noblit & Hare, 1988; Thomas & Harden, 2008). We are not reporting the full results from our meta-synthesis in this chapter; these will be reported elsewhere. Rather, we will reflect upon our findings on the methodologies and methods being used, and the implications for future studies with respect to trauma-informed practice.

Search Strategy

We searched five databases: CINAHL, Web of Science, SPORTDiscus, PsycINFO, and Sociological Abstracts; using four categories of search terms (1) Gender-based violence/abuse/harassment; (2) Sport/exercise; (3) Woman/Female; and (4) Qualitative. Keywords and MeSH terms were both used. We only included papers that were published in the English language. Included studies needed to use qualitative methods where women described their experiences of any gender-based violence at any point in the lifespan. We excluded studies where gender-based violence against women could not be distinguished from other types of abuse. Fiona carried out the title and abstract review, with Kirsty reviewing those that Fiona was unsure of whether to include. We both carried out full text screening. For one study we contacted the primary author as we were uncertain about the gendered nature of the violence. Following correspondence and clarification, we included the study in our meta-synthesis.

Quality Appraisal

As qualitative methods use has grown, so too has critique and confusion relating to its rigor or trustworthiness, a hangover from traditional positivist quantitative research. Long et al. (2020) argue that given the rising expectations of qualitative researchers to show rigor in their research (e.g., Excellence in Research in Australia and the research Excellence Framework (REF) in the United Kingdom) there is a "need to develop appropriate standards by which to judge quality" (p. 32). Qualitative research appraisal tools reflect this drive for quality.

We used the Critical Appraisal Skills Programme's (CASP) (CASP, 2022) qualitative studies checklist to appraise the quality of the studies we included in the meta-synthesis. The CASP is a generic tool that asks ten methodology focused questions. It is the most used qualitative research appraisal tool in Cochrane and the World Health Organisation guidelines (Noyes et al., 2018). The ten questions posed by the CASP tool are supported by guiding prompts.

We both undertook the appraisal independently and met to discuss if there were any areas where we disagreed. We did not exclude any papers based on quality appraisal, but merely recorded our assessment of the studies.

Box 1   The ten questions of the CASP qualitative checklist tool (CASP, 2022)

1 Was there a clear statement of the aims of the research?
2 Is a qualitative methodology appropriate?
3 Was the research design appropriate to address the aims of the research?
4 Was the recruitment strategy appropriate to the aims of the research?
5 Was the data collected in a way that addressed the research issue?
6 Has the relationship between researcher and participants been adequately considered?
7 Have ethical issues been taken into consideration?
8 Was the data analysis sufficiently rigorous?
9 Is there a clear statement of findings?
10 How valuable is the research?

Data Extraction and Analysis

We developed a form to extract descriptive information such as: research aim; study characteristics (e.g., population description, country in which the study was conducted); researcher positioning; method of recruitment and data collection; type of violence specified and definition used; ethical considerations; and evidence of trauma-informed practice (if any). We then imported all the included literature into NVivo qualitative software to assist with coding for first-order constructs (participant quotations as they appeared in the literature) and second-order constructs (findings/interpretations of those quotes).

We used reflexive thematic analysis as our method of analysis (Braun & Clarke, 2019). This aligns with the meta-ethnographic approach of establishing first- and second-order constructs across the included studies and constructing a third-order construct that translates and speaks to those first- and second-order constructs (Noblit & Hare, 1988). We immersed ourselves in the literature and generated initial descriptive themes across the first- and second-order constructs. We explored these further individually and then in discussion we created interpretive themes as we translated the concepts across the studies into one another. This evolved into our third-order constructs, new interpretations that went beyond the individual studies. This process occurred iteratively and flexibly over the course of two full days.

Throughout the search and our initial assessments, we regularly discussed how our own experiences impacted our approach to this work. We kept a reflective diary and established protocols to care for each other's well-being. This practice included limits on the amount of time spent on this work each day; discussing responses to individual studies; and ensuring we had access to appropriate psychological support. As the work progressed, we increasingly recognised the importance of care of ourselves and of each other, and the importance of the need to document this.

Findings

In what follows, we present our reflections. We first provide a brief overview of the studies we reviewed, to contextualise our reflections.

The Studies

Twenty-five records representing 24 studies were included in our meta-synthesis. Papers were published between 1997 and 2022. The majority (17) were published since 2010. Most of the studies were conducted in Western countries, particularly Canada (5) and Norway (4). The included studies reflected the breadth of methods found in qualitative research.

Whilst the majority used interviews, the range of methodologies across the studies included case study, narrative analysis, narrative inquiry, collaborative autoethnography, phenomenology, and interpretative phenomenological analysis. Eight studies did not specify a particular methodology, two studies were mixed methods surveys that included open-ended questions and one study was a qualitative meta-synthesis. In one study, victim impact statements were used as data, whilst for a small number of other studies, interview data were supplemented with supporting material such as media reports. Fifteen studies reported the application of a theoretical framework, many with a feminist lens.

Study participants were predominantly current or former athletes (22), with coaches (1), officials (1), and managers (2) making up the remainder. Perpetrators were predominantly coaches (17), followed by peers (6) and members of the public (6), other authority figures (4), and in one study, family members. A wide range of team and individual sports were represented. Participants in the included studies experienced many forms of gender-based violence, for example, sexual, physical, psychological, economic, drug, and technology facilitated. These often appeared as composite forms of abuse, intersecting, and overlapping. As was expected, following Forsdike and O'Sullivan's recent scoping review (2022), many studies focused on exploring experiences of sexual.

The impact of the violence women described included emotional responses such as feelings of shame and self-blame, and fear of recriminations and others finding out. This often resulted in long term mental health impacts. Many participants reported they changed coaches, moved to a different sport, or dropped out of sport entirely.

Quality Appraisal

Quality appraisal tools focus reviewers on the quality of the study being reported. As such, it is dependent upon what the researchers have reported and so does not necessarily assess how the study was conducted (Long et al., 2020). In our review of the studies using the CASP tool, we found the quality of studies to be mixed. Most of the studies included a clear statement of the aims, and demonstrated the appropriateness of the methodology, research design, and the value of the research. However, many studies either did not report researcher positioning or provided scant detail. Also, most studies provided little detail of any potential ethical issues nor how they were addressed. Ethical issues may well have been addressed during researchers' human ethics committee reviews but not reported in detail in publication, the inclusion of confirmation of ethics approval being considered sufficient by journal editors.

Researcher positioning has the potential to impact the research process and how data are analysed, pertaining to the quality of the study and its findings (Newton et al., 2012). Researchers bring their own experiences and biases to qualitative research, and the process of constant and critical self-examination of their stance in relation to the research being conducted (i.e., "reflexivity") is necessary and, we argue, crucial when conducting research with participants who have experienced trauma (Guillemin & Gillam, 2004). This improves the rigor of the research, and importantly, provides greater attentiveness to transparency so the reader can also reflect on researchers' construction of themes or interpretations of participants' reported experiences (Berger, 2015; Newton et al., 2012). Only ten items of literature clearly reported on the relationship between the researcher and the participants in their study. What was reported ranged between researchers reporting themselves to be insiders to the topic, usually former athletes themselves, to in-depth critical reflections on their potential bias, influences, and subsequent potential impact on their research from recruitment through to analysis. Aside from credibility of researcher interpretations of the data, such reflexivity on researcher relationship with participants also has ethical implications (Guillemin & Gillam, 2004). Two studies reflected at length on the relationship between the researcher and the participant, and then also provided much greater detail of ethical considerations in their research than the other studies (Owton, 2016; Owton & Sparkes, 2017; Rodriguez & Gill, 2011). These studies used a phenomenological interpretive framework and feminist ethics of care respectively which may explain the depth of reflections. We had expected recently published articles to be more attentive to researcher positioning and ethical issues; however, there was no clear relationship between these components and the year of publication.

An additional limitation we found in using the CASP quality appraisal tool was where a study had only one participant. These types of qualitative studies provide rich, in-depth insights into how gender-based interpersonal violence manifests in the sporting environment (e.g., the process of grooming by a coach), yet the CASP tool assumes that studies contain multiple participants, and that "thematic" style analysis is undertaken. There were five studies that reported on the experience of one or two athletes, providing rich insights to interpersonal violence experiences (Bisgaard & Stockel, 2019; Fasting & Sand, 2015; McMahon & McGannon, 2020; Owton, 2016; Owton & Sparkes, 2017; Van Ingen, 2020).

Trauma-Informed Approach in Practice

Very few of the studies reported using trauma-informed practices in their research, either explicitly or indirectly (Bisgaard & Stockel, 2019; McMahon & McGannon, 2020; McMahon et al., 2021; Owton, 2016; Owton & Sparkes, 2017; Stirling & Kerr, 2009; Van Ingen, 2020). These can be viewed through the lens of SAMHSA's (2014) six principles of trauma-informed approaches:

safety; trustworthiness and transparency; support provision; collaboration and mutuality between researchers and participants; ensuring participant empowerment, voice, and choice; and consideration of cultural, historical, and gender issues. Furthermore, these principles need to apply across all stages of the research process. For example, in studies using interviews, stages include research design, preparation for interview, during the interview, and after the interview (Isobel, 2021). Isobel (2021) provides useful insights on conducting qualitative research in a trauma-informed manner across these stages. For example, during the design phase research aims, where possible, should be co-designed with participants, aligning with collaboration and mutuality. In preparation for an interview, Isobel (2021) advises the development of a distress protocol and also raises the importance of the physical environment and adjusting it, accordingly, ensuring safety for the participants. She suggests to:

> scan the physical environment that you will be using, adjust furniture and layout to promote safety and where possible, provide choice. This may include considering cues of safety (e.g., visibility to exit, space for belongings, glass of water) and potential unexplained cues of power (e.g., internal doors or windows, posters on the wall, positioning of recording device).
>
> (p. 1460)

During the interview, Isobel highlights the importance of experience and knowledge of the researcher in trauma-informed practice and trauma more broadly. She advises looking for signs that the participant is uncomfortable, disengaged, or disassociating (for example, using a monotone voice or a fixed stare) and knowing when to provide grounding actions such as offering a glass of water.

The trauma-informed practices reported across the studies mostly aligned with four of SAMHSA's (2014) six principles including: safety; collaboration and mutuality between researchers and participants; ensuring participant empowerment, voice, and choice; and support provision.

Safety

Across those studies indicating a trauma-informed approach, safety involved understanding the sensitive nature of the topic, the potential for re-traumatisation of the participant, and addressing these through ethical practices (beyond the procedures required of human research ethics committees). Stirling and Kerr (2009) were explicit in acknowledging the sensitive nature of the topic, the vulnerability of the participants, and the potential for distress during interview. They report the interviews "were approached in a sensitive manner" and that "questions were communicated in a style that was best suited for the participant's emotional state at each stage of the interview" (p. 230).

Owton (2016) went a step further in detailing that she attended training on supporting those working with trauma. In comparison, Van Ingen (2020) reflected on the fact that whilst she had extensive experience interviewing survivors of violence, this study was the first in which she had explicitly asked about their experiences. She explained approaching "our conversation with much care" (p. 3). Owton and Van Ingen's awareness of their own limitations in experience and how they sought to address that is commendable.

Owton's (2016) use of "friendship as method" and its potential to minimise power imbalances is important in terms of safety. Minimising power imbalances in the researcher and participant relationship is an important safety consideration because in trauma-informed research, replicating similar power imbalances to what participants experienced when the violence occurred must be avoided (McMahon et al., 2022; SAMHSA, 2014).

Collaboration and Mutuality

Collaboration and mutuality are about working with participants and minimising potential power imbalances to the point of sharing power in research production. McMahon and McGannon (2020) explicitly referred to the need for trauma-informed practice across research design, and the need to protect the athlete "in and through the research process" (p. 31). Whilst they did not detail specific trauma-informed practices, their choice of methodology, narrative inquiry, and creative non-fiction can be viewed as working with the participant and providing a platform to tell their story and control over content (McMahon & McGannon, 2020). This balances power between researcher/s and participant. McMahon and McGannon's (2020) used a storyteller method, removing themselves from analysing the experience of the participant. They let the participants' stories stand alone with analysis being left to those who engage with them. This methodology has been shown to empower participants as it provides the opportunity to "gain new insight and/ or clarity into her experiences" (McMahon & McGannon, 2020, p. 31). Similarly, minimising power in the research process was also outlined in a later study by McMahon and colleagues (2021) where participants had the "power to decide what they wanted to share with the audience and how they wanted to share it" (p. 4).

As an example of collaboration and mutuality in the research process, data production, analysis, and presentation, Owton (2016) explains using "friendship as method" (p. 9). As a form of relational ethics (Ellis, 2007), it frames how researchers interact with participants over time, before during and after the research with an "ethic of friendship" (Tillmann-Healy, 2003, p. 729). In "friendship as method", the roles of researcher and friendship combine. As Owton (2016) described, they develop

> a shared sense of alliance and emotional affiliation with the subject matter and we built upon foundations of trust, honesty, safety, support, generosity, loyalty, understanding and acceptance towards each other and ourselves.
>
> (p. 9)

However, Owton (2016) acknowledged that such a method does not necessarily remove power imbalance. Ellis (2007) argues: "the problem comes not from being friends with participants but from acting as a friend yet not living up to the obligations of friendship" (p. 10). Choice of methodology can be a critical way of aligning with trauma-informed practice. However, trauma-informed practice does require ongoing reflexive consideration of ethical practice and relational ethics throughout the research process.

Ensuring Participant Empowerment, Voice, and Choice

Whilst no specific trauma-informed practice under this principle was directly apparent, some practices that researchers engaged in may align with it. Bisgaard and Stockel (2019) felt it important for participants to feel in control of an interview and so, rather than using an interview guide, researchers focused on listening to the participant and only seeking clarification when needed. Debriefing with participants afterwards also enabled participants to "address any new feelings that may have arisen" (p. 230). In Stirling and Kerr's (2009) study, participants chose to continue with an interview despite being offered to end it when they cried in the retelling of their story. Lamb et al. (2020) have raised the importance of participant choice to continue rather than have the interview stopped by the researcher (Orb et al., 2001).

Support Provision

Although relatively unreported, support provision was clear in three studies. Stirling and Kerr (2009) gave participants details of local counselling services if they needed additional support and McMahon and colleagues (2021), Owton (2016), and Owton and Sparkes (2017) detailed psychological support being available to participants. Through "friendship as method", narrative inquiry, and creative non-fiction methodologies, peer support between the researcher and the participant may also be considered in this principle (McMahon & McGannon, 2020; McMahon et al., 2021; Owton, 2016; Owton & Sparkes, 2017).

Structural Integration of a Trauma-Informed Approach

It is important for researchers to reflect upon their research practice to ensure they implement evidence-based trauma-informed approaches that avoid re-traumatising participants. A focus on procedural ethics rather than ethics in practice, including trauma-informed approaches across all stages of research, may run the risk of reported studies perpetuating harmful narratives. One of the studies, whilst detailing ethical procedures, did not appear to take a trauma-informed approach and concerned us. The authors seemed to "victim-blame" by appearing to admonish participants for ignoring or avoiding harassment instead of reporting it (Fasting et al., 2007). The authors reflection that "perhaps the most frustrating finding is that many of the athletes did nothing to stop the harassers. They reacted with either passivity or avoidance" (p. 428) did not sit well with us, nor that "her perpetrator will probably continue his harassing behaviour towards other female athletes" (p. 428) if she leaves the sport without actively addressing the harassment. We felt that this placed responsibility on the athlete to stop the perpetrator's behaviour and perpetuated a victim blaming attitude. It also runs the risk of harm to the participant should they read the researchers' reflections, a situation that Carolyn Ellis (1995) acknowledged occurred in her own ethnographic research.

Given this, we propose some changes to existing research structures to support, guide, and ultimately ensure such trauma-informed practice becomes embedded in this type of research. We consider the role of quality appraisal tools and relational ethics.

Reporting a Trauma-Informed Approach

Whilst ethics committees will oversee procedural ethics issues relating to risk of harm for participants, detail pertaining to trauma-informed practice should be standard practice when conducting research with people affected by trauma, particularly those who have experienced gender-based violence. Qualitative researchers can use SAMHSA's guidelines for a trauma-informed approach (2014) in and through their research practice. Aligning this with existing quality assessments, such as the CASP tool, would serve two purposes (1) inform journal editors and their reviewers as to the quality of the study being presented and (2) provide greater recognition of the need for and adherence to trauma-informed practice when conducting research on gender-based violence. The CASP tool would act as a reminder to researchers of appropriate practices in conducting qualitative research and that they will be held accountable in the reporting of those practices. Taking SAMHSA's (2014) six principles of trauma-informed approaches as our overarching framework, together with Isobel's (2021) considerations for trauma-informed practice in qualitative research, we propose the following adaptation to a tool such as CASP where the research engages with those who have experienced trauma through gender-based violence in sport.

Box 2   Suggested revision to the CASP

[CASP Question 7] Have Ethical Issues Been Taken into Consideration?

if the study addresses directly or indirectly trauma or populations that may have experienced trauma, the following question should also be considered.

Has the Research Been Designed with Trauma-Informed Practice in Mind?

When answering this question, consider each of the four stages of the research process (1) research design, (2) preparation for data collection, (3) data collection, and (4) post data collection.

The following sub-questions can be used as a guide:

- What evidence is there that the study has been designed and data collection process conducted to ensure safe settings, physically and psychologically, were being used?
- To what extent have researchers exhibited trustworthiness and transparency to potential participants before, during, and after the study?
- What supports for the participants, peer/s or otherwise have been incorporated into the research design and made available before, during, and after the study?
- To what extent have the researchers engaged collaboratively with participants, and in what ways does that enhances mutuality in the research process across all stages of research?
- How have the researchers ensured participant empowerment, voice, and choice at each stage of the research process?
- What cultural, historical, and gender issues have been explicitly considered by the researchers and how have these been addressed throughout the research process?

Trauma-Informed Approach: Care for the Researcher

As researchers, we also need to think of our own care and potential for re-traumatisation when conducting trauma research (e.g., vicarious trauma). Clearly missing from the studies in our meta-synthesis was the impact of the research on those engaging with it and acknowledgement of potential for vicarious trauma. Our weekly reflective discussions highlighted the impact that our research was having on us. Fiona expressed concerns over one text and its impact on her. She had interpreted the title of the paper she was reading as being potentially about self-care practices. She was shocked to then read a description of a rape. There was no trigger warning or preparation for the reader that the paper would include such content. Indeed, the authors(s) appeared to have purposely written the paper in such a way as to provoke a strong reaction. Fiona is an experienced researcher, but the paper surprised her, and despite her experience with sensitive topics, she had a distressing and traumatic reaction to it. She needed to step away from the work and debrief with Kirsty. We considered the ethics not only of research itself, but ethical practices in presenting such research. The impact of published studies, and the stories told therein, on the reader in trauma research is not considered by ethics committees or researchers alike because they are not included in guidelines for research conduct (The National Health and Medical Research Council et al., 2018; World Medical Association, 2022). As such, any potential for recognition and mitigation of the impacts of vicarious trauma or re-traumatisation is bypassed. Dickson-Swift (2022) explains that research has been so focused on the impact on participants, that the impact of our research on ourselves as researchers and our future publication audience is often forgotten. The impact of researching sensitive topics such as trauma can be physically and emotionally demanding and can extend to long after the study has completed, including the publication and presentation of research (Dickson-Swift, 2022; Kiyimba & O'Reilly, 2016; Woodby et al., 2011). Despite the potential impact on those other than research participants (i.e., researchers, professional transcribers, audience), such risks of harm are rarely considered by ethics review committees (Dickson-Swift, 2022; Dickson-Swift et al., 2008). Bedera (2021) offers some useful guidance. Whilst her focus is on the context of teaching sexual violence in universities, her suggestion to go beyond a "trigger-warning" is just as valid in the context of presenting gender-based violence research. Bedera (2021) argues that it is important to speak to survivors. For example, offer guidance and support to empower them to prepare for self-care ahead of hearing about gender-based violence, which may include their choice to step away. When writing up our studies, it is perhaps pertinent to consider who we are writing for, as well as who may read our work. One of Bedera's key questions in the preparation of, or choice of material to share with others, is the impact it would have on someone who has experienced sexual assault regardless of whether they are trying to make sense of the assault or healing from sexual trauma. Another strategy that Bedera (2021) suggests is providing space to consider and write down individual reactions to material on violence. Openly acknowledging and preparing the reader enables them to consider what they would like to do to prepare themselves for potential discomfort or being triggered (such as going to a quiet space, going for a walk outside, having a glass of water), and engaging them more directly as co-constructors of the research and its impact. As Bedera argues, "studying sexual violence is emotionally taxing. Making space for the feelings that surface not only makes them more manageable, but it also can teach us a lot about the nature of sexual violence" (2021, p. 272). In addition to Bedera's (2021) suggestions, we recommend researchers be proactive regarding professional and individual support for themselves and their team. This may include peer and independent support/debriefing for researchers, time limits on aspects of some work such as reading and reviewing literature, creating an environment where it's ok to say something was triggering and therefore step away to seek support (Sexual Violence Research Initiative, 2023). We undertook these things as experienced trauma researchers who have also experienced trauma ourselves. Such actions are not always automatic across researchers and their teams.

Conclusions

We have provided insights into the methodological challenges we came across when conducting a qualitative meta-synthesis on women's experiences of gender-based violence. We have three key messages for informing future research of this type. First, a trauma-informed approach must underpin research with women who have experienced gender-based violence in any context. Some women want to tell their stories to help others. However, we must be sensitive to their needs, of ourselves as researchers, and of the audiences to our work to ensure we do not inadvertently cause further harm. Therefore, when thinking about what a trauma-informed approach looks like, we must apply it across the whole spectrum of the research process, from study design, the ethical conduct of our work, and through to presentation and publication.

Second, the systems and structures that support research should encourage and promote research on sensitive topics to be conducted using a trauma-informed approach. Until there is system-wide change to research infrastructure, the onus will remain with individual researchers to ensure that women are not potentially re-traumatised from their participation in and through research participation.

Finally, research institutions have a responsibility to proactively care for the well-being of researchers conducting this type of research. It is not enough to inform researchers that support is available "if they need". Being proactive assumes that this type of work will impact researchers and that both formal and informal supports are in place before a study starts. This may include training by specialist services in how to recognise and manage vicarious trauma, services being alerted to the conduct of trauma research setting up regular engagement with the research teams, and peer support programmes being established.

We end this chapter on a personal reflection. Given the sensitive nature of this research and our own experiences with gender-based violence, we created an environment in which we both felt safe to share our past experiences, our emotional responses to what we were reading, and the need to temporarily step away and seek peer or external support as needed. It fostered a mutual trust and care for one another that enabled us to produce a body of work that we hope honours the voices of the women who have experienced gender-based violence in sport.

References

Bedera, N. (2021). Beyond trigger warnings: A survivor-centered approach to teaching on sexual violence and avoiding institutional betrayal. *Teaching Sociology, 49*(3), 267–277. https://doi.org/10.1177/0092055X211022471

Berger, R. (2015). Now I see it, now I don't: Researcher's position and reflexivity in qualitative research. *Qualitative Research, 15*(2), 219–234. https://doi.org/10.1177/1468794112468475

Bisgaard, K., & Stockel, J. T. (2019). Athlete narratives of sexual harassment and abuse in the field of sport. *Journal of Clinical Sport Psychology, 13*(2), 226–242. https://doi.org/10.1123/jcsp.2018-0036

Braun, V., & Clarke, V. (2019). Reflecting on reflexive thematic analysis. *Qualitative Research in Sport, Exercise and Health, 11*(4), 589–597. https://doi.org/10.1080/2159676X.2019.1628806

Critical Appraisal Skills Programme (CASP). (2022). *CASP qualitative studies checklist.* (online) https://casp-uk.net/images/checklist/documents/CASP-Qualitative-Studies-Checklist/CASP-Qualitative-Checklist-2018_fillable_form.pdf

Dickson-Swift, V. (2022). Undertaking qualitative research on trauma: Impacts on researchers and guidelines for risk management. *Qualitative Research in Organizations and Management, 17*(4), 469–486. https://doi.org/10.1108/QROM-11-2021-2248

Dickson-Swift, V., James, E. L., Kippen, S., & Liamputtong, P. (2008). Risk to researchers in qualitative research on sensitive topics: Issues and strategies. *Qualitative Health Research, 18*(1), 133–144. https://doi.org/10.1177/1049732307309007

Ellis, C. (1995). Emotional and ethical quagmires in returning to the field. *Journal of Contemporary Ethnography, 24*(1), 68–98. https://doi.org/10.1177/089124195024001003

Ellis, C. (2007). Telling secrets, revealing lives. *Qualitative Inquiry, 13*(1), 3–29. https://doi.org/10.1177/1077800406294947

Fasting, K., Brackenridge, C., & Walseth, K. (2007). Women athletes' personal responses to sexual harassment in sport. *Journal of Applied Sport Psychology, 19*(4), 419–433. https://doi.org/10.1080/10413200701599165

Fasting, K., & Sand, T. S. (2015). Narratives of sexual harassment experiences in sport. *Qualitative Research in Sport Exercise and Health, 7*(5), 573–588. https://doi.org/10.1080/2159676x.2015.1008028

Forsdike, K., & O'Sullivan, G. (2022). Interpersonal gendered violence against adult women participating in sport: A scoping review. *Managing Sport and Leisure,* 1–23. https://doi.org/10.1080/23750472.2022.2116089

Guillemin, M., & Gillam, L. (2004). Ethics, reflexivity, and "Ethically important moments" in research. *Qualitative Inquiry, 10*(2), 261–280. https://doi.org/10.1177/1077800403262360

Harvey, M. R. (1996). An ecological view of psychological trauma and trauma recovery. *Journal of Traumatic Stress, 9*(1), 3–23. https://doi.org/10.1007/BF02116830

Herman, J. L. (2015). *Trauma and recovery: The aftermath of violence – From domestic abuse to political terror.* Basic Books.

Isobel, S. (2021). Trauma-informed qualitative research: Some methodological and practical considerations. *International Journal of Mental Health Nursing, 30*(1), 1456–1469. https://doi.org/10.1111/inm.12914

Kiyimba, N., & O'Reilly, M. (2016). An exploration of the possibility for secondary traumatic stress among transcriptionists: A grounded theory approach. *Qualitative Research in Psychology, 13*(1), 92–108. https://doi.org/10.1080/14780887.2015.1106630

Lamb, K., Amanda, C., Fiona, Parker, R., Novy, K., & Hegarty, K. (2020). *The family violence experts by experience framework. Research report and framework 2020.* https://safeandequal.org.au/wp-content/uploads/DVV_EBE-Framework-Report.pdf

Long, H. A., French, D. P., & Brooks, J. M. (2020). Optimising the value of the critical appraisal skills programme (CASP) tool for quality appraisal in qualitative evidence synthesis. *Research Methods in Medicine & Health Sciences, 1*(1), 31–42. https://doi.org/10.1177/2632084320947559

Lum On, M., Ayre, J., Webster, K., Gourley, M., & Moon, L. (2016). *Examination of the burden of disease of intimate partner violence against women in 2011: Final report* (ANROWS Horizons, 06/2016). Australia's National Research Organisation for Women's Safety (ANROWS).

McMahon, J., & McGannon, K. R. (2020). Acting out what is inside of us: Self-management strategies of an abused ex-athlete. *Sport Management Review, 23*(1), 28–38. https://doi.org/10.1016/j.smr.2019.03.008

McMahon, J., McGannon, K. R., & Palmer, C. (2021). Body shaming and associated practices as abuse: Athlete entourage as perpetrators of abuse. *Sport, Education and Society, 27*(5), 1–14. https://doi.org/10.1080/13573322.2021.1890571

McMahon, J., McGannon, K. R., Zehntner, C., Werbicki, L., Stephenson, E., & Martin, K. (2022). Trauma-informed abuse education in sport: Engaging athlete abuse survivors as educators and facilitating a community of care, *Sport, Education and Society, 28*(8), https://doi.org/10.1080/13573322.2022.2096586

Newton, B. J., Rothlingova, Z., Gutteridge, R., LeMarchand, K., & Raphael, J. H. (2012). No room for reflexivity? Critical reflections following a systematic review of qualitative research. *Journal of Health Psychology, 17*(6), 866–885. https://doi.org/10.1177/1359105311427615

Noblit, G. W., & Hare, R. D. (1988). *Meta-ethnography: Synthesizing qualitative studies.* Sage Publications.

Noyes, J., Booth, A., Flemming, K., Garside, R., Harden, A., Lewin, S., Pantoja, T., Hannes, K., Cargo, M., & Thomas, J. (2018). Cochrane qualitative and implementation methods group guidance series—Paper 3: Methods for assessing methodological limitations, data extraction and synthesis, and confidence in synthesized qualitative findings. *Journal of Clinical Epidemiology, 97*, 49–58. https://doi.org/10.1016/j.jclinepi.2017.06.020

Orb, A., Eisenhauer, L., & Wynaden, D. (2001). Ethics in qualitative research. *Journal of Nursing Scholarship*, *33*(1), 93–96. https://doi.org/10.1111/j.1547-5069.2001.00093.x

Owton, H. (2016). *Sexual abuse in sport: A qualitative case study*. Palgrave Macmillan. https://doi.org/10.1007/978-3-319-46795-5

Owton, H., & Sparkes, A. C. (2017). Sexual abuse and the grooming process in sport: Learning from Bella's story. *Sport, Education & Society*, *22*(6), 732–743.

Rodriguez, E. A., & Gill, D. L. (2011). Sexual harassment perceptions among Puerto Rican female former athletes. *International Journal of Sport and Exercise Psychology*, *9*(4), 323–337. https://doi.org/10.1080/1612197x.2011.623461

Savopoulos, P., Bryant, C., Fogarty, A., Conway, L. J., Fitzpatrick, K. M., Condron, P., & Giallo, R. (2022). Intimate partner violence and child and adolescent cognitive development: A systematic review. *Trauma Violence & Abuse*. https://doi.org/10.1177/15248380221082081

Sexual Violence Research Initiative. (2023). *Researching with Hart: Promoting researcher wellbeing through self and collective care*. SVRI. https://www.svri.org/svrinterest/researching-hart-promoting-researcher-wellbeing-through-self-and-collective-care

Stirling, A. E., & Kerr, G. A. (2009). Abused athletes' perceptions of the coach-athlete relationship. *Sport in Society*, *12*(2), 227–239. https://doi.org/10.1080/17430430802591019

Substance Abuse and Mental Health Services Administration (SAMHSA). (2014). *SAMHSA's concept of trauma and guidance for a trauma-informed approach. HHS Publication No. (SMA) 14-4884*. Substance Abuse and Mental Health Services Administration.

Thomas, J., & Harden, A. (2008). Methods for the thematic synthesis of qualitative research in systematic reviews. *BMC Medical Research Methodology*, *8*(1), 45–45. https://doi.org/10.1186/1471-2288-8-45

Tillmann-Healy, L. M. (2003). Friendship as method. *Qualitative Inquiry*, *9*(5), 729–749. https://doi.org/10.1177/1077800403254894

Tseris, E. J. (2013). Trauma theory without feminism? Evaluating contemporary understandings of traumatized women. *Affilia: Journal of Women and Social Work*, *28*(2), 153–164. https://doi.org/10.1177/0886109913485707

The National Health and Medical Research Council, Australian Research Council, & Universities Australia. (2018). *National Statement on Ethical Conduct in Human Research*. The National Health and Medical Research Council. https://www.nhmrc.gov.au/file/9131/download?token=4Qw7LMvh

Valpied, J., Cini, A., O'Doherty, L., Taket, A., & Hegarty, K. (2014). "Sometimes cathartic. Sometimes quite raw": Benefit and harm in an intimate partner violence trial. *Aggression and Violent Behavior*, *19*(6), 673–685. https://doi.org/10.1016/j.avb.2014.09.005

Van Ingen, C. (2020). Stabbed, shot, left to die: Christy Martin and gender-based violence in boxing. *International Review for the Sociology of Sport*, *56*(8). https://doi.org/10.1177/1012690220979716

Williams, T., & Shaw, R. (2016). Synthesising qualitative research: Meta-synthesis in sport and exercise. In B. Smith & A. C. Sparkes (Eds.), *Routledge handbook of qualitative research in sport and exercise* (pp. 274–288). Taylor & Francis Group.

Woodby, L. L., Williams, B. R., Wittich, A. R., & Burgio, K. L. (2011). Expanding the notion of researcher distress: The cumulative effects of coding. *Qualitative Health Research, 21*(6), 830–838. https://doi.org/10.1177/1049732311402095

World Medical Association. (2022). *WMA declaration of Helsinki – Ethical principles for medical research involving human subjects*. World Medical Association. https://pdf-it.dev.acw.website/please-and-thank-you?url=https://www.wma.net/policies-post/wma-declaration-of-helsinki-ethical-principles-for-medical-research-involving-human-subjects/&pdfName=wma-declaration-of-helsinki-ethical-principles-for-medical-research-involving-human-subjects

Part II

Trauma In, and From Sport

Chapter 5

Abstracting the Legacy of Abuse in Post-Sport

Using Arts-Based Methods and Friendship as Method to Limit Re-Traumatisation in Abuse and Trauma Research

Jenny McMahon and Kerry R. McGannon

Introduction

Researchers have shown that sport contexts are distinctive socio-cultural environments where athlete abuse can occur (Kerr et al., 2019; Mountjoy et al., 2016). Two reasons identified for such abuse is the 'win at all costs' and 'meritocratic' nature of sport which encourages coaches, athletes, and other sport insiders to engage in toxic and damaging practices perceived to enhance competitive performance outcomes. Such damaging practices may include training while sick or injured, ignoring athletes for their lack of performance, severe calorie restriction diets, and screaming, hitting, ridiculing of athletes for performance failures (Kavanagh & Brady, 2014; Kerr et al., 2019; McMahon et al., 2012). Athlete abuse statistics are high, with emotional abuse (also known as psychological abuse) and neglect identified as the most predominant types (Alexander et al., 2011; Kerr et al., 2019). The extent of these types of abuse were revealed by researchers in a study conducted in Canada, where it was shown that 67% of current athletes experienced neglect, while 59% were subjected to psychological abuse (Kerr et al., 2019).

There are severe long-term consequences for those exposed to abuse (McMahon & McGannon, 2021). For instance, in abuse literature outside of sport, alarming medical issues have been reported including physical injury, headaches, depression, fear, low self-esteem, inability to trust, anger, sexual dysfunction, eating and sleeping disorders, post-traumatic stress disorder, and suicide (UNICEF, 2010). Researchers who contributed to the International Olympic Committee (IOC) consensus statement on harassment and abuse in sport also highlighted the consequences of athlete abuse saying that the "risk of non-suicidal self-injury/self-harm, suicide attempts, and completed suicide attempts increases with the number of harassment types that an adolescent experience[s]" (Mountjoy et al., 2016, p. 6). The consequences of my (Jenny) own experiences of abuse have impacted me well into adulthood, which led

DOI: 10.4324/9781003332909-7

to abusing prescription medication, and consuming excessive alcohol as a way of coping as detailed in the vignette below.

> I get home late. My anxiety is unbearable, and I am finding it hard to even cope doing the simplest daily activities. I know sleep will evade me again tonight, so I open the pantry door and remove a container of tablets. They are diazepam (anxiety medication). I remove the lid and tip the powdery textured tablets into my hand. Even though I have been prescribed one tablet in the evenings, I take seven tablets as I want to feel nothing. I want to be numb immediately, so I wash them down with half a bottle of red wine. My body gets more and more pent up as I wait for the effects to take hold. It is like my insides have been wound with a winch so tightly, that with just one more turn, I will snap. While I know that I will shortly succumb to the effects of diazepam and wine, waiting for that to happen is pure torture as my mind is swirling so fast, like I am in the midst of a hurricane.
>
> (McMahon & McGannon, 2021)

With consequences such as these, it is unsurprising that sport researchers (e.g., Kavanagh & Brady, 2014; McMahon & McGannon, 2021) have recommended sport scholars to undertake more studies regarding how athlete abuse victims cope once they leave sport, and whether there are long-term impacts. Investigating the legacy of abuse post-sport is important because it will lead to better informed interventions and support strategies (McMahon & McGannon, 2021).

Research Impetus and (My) Researcher Background

Exposure to abuse, or the witnessing of abuse is listed as an adverse experience that can lead to trauma by the Substance Abuse and Mental Health Services Administration [SAMHSA] (2014, 2023). The impact of trauma can be subtle, insidious, or outright destructive with survivors' reactions acknowledged as complicated and variable (McMahon et al., under review; SAMHSA, 2014, 2023). Not surprisingly, their internal and external coping resources can be affected, therefore their support needs differ (Dye, 2018; SAMHSA, 2014). Relating to (qualitative) research practice specifically, there is an urgent need for those working with populations affected by trauma to implement evidence-based trauma informed principles (TIPs) into their practice, so research spaces are safe and choice-based and the potential for re-traumatisation is limited (McMahon et al., Under Review; SAMHSA, 2014, 2023).

Given the high rates of trauma occurring from abuse in sport, in this chapter, we outline how arts-based methods align with certain principles listed in the evidence-based trauma-informed framework created by SAMHSA (2014, 2023). In so doing, we will show the potential application of these trauma-informed approaches to researcher practice and research contexts more broadly to highlight its benefits (i.e., value) for other researchers considering undertaking research with abuse victims/survivors in sport.

I (Jenny) am a former national representative athlete who experienced firsthand, a *'win at all costs'* culture where I was subjected to abusive practices in the sport of swimming. I was subjected to non-sexualised types of abuse (e.g., psychological abuse, non-contact physical abuse) during my time in the national team. This abuse affected me not only during my immersion in the sport at age 15, 16, and 17 years of age, but also in my post-sport life. While this chapter centres on detailing my post-sport experiences of "how my abuse and trauma from sport impact my post-sport adult life?" Co-author (Kerry) plays a key role at various points in the research process. Given our roles, the chapter will show an interchange between 'I' and 'we' to highlight when this research was conducted independently and/or collaboratively. Accordingly, the 'voice' in the chapter will shift to 'I' as my (i.e., Jenny's) experiences are brought to the fore and discuss the methodological approach and research.

Methodological Considerations When Conducting (My) Trauma Research

When considering the appropriate methodology to investigate my post-sport experiences of trauma, I wanted a methodology which would foreground my lived experiences in a way that I felt comfortable. Another consideration that was important was engaging the reader and wider field to my trauma information using accessible 'data' forms. As Ropers-Huilman (1999, p. 23) explains, 'witnessing' occurs through the act of reading, feeling, and experiencing the lived experiences of others, therefore accessibility to such information is imperative. Similarly, Sparkes (1999) highlights how "an emotional response in the reader, enhances their empathetic understanding of selected issues, and enable[s] them to reflect upon their actual worlds from different vantage points" (p. 24). However, a caveat is provided by Ropers-Huilman (1999) relating to the potential "dangers inherent in the process of witnessing others' lives and constructing meanings about those experiences" (p. 24) in that vicarious trauma may result. This point is pertinent for trauma and abuse research because when victims and survivors engage with data sets that centre on these topics, they may become triggered (Owton, 2016). Subsequently, researchers should be mindful of audience impact and provide potential trigger warnings. With that, we thus caution readers that the data that follows contains themes of trauma and self-injury, and may be distressing, or triggering, for some. A final consideration, related to my choice to use visual or alternate ways to present my lived experiences which could generate, interpret, and communicate new knowledge, thus broadening the ways that my trauma information is communicated.

Methodology: Arts-Based Autoethnography

Considering the above methodological points in conjunction with my research question, I decided that *arts-based autoethnography* (defined below) was the optimal methodological approach. This is because arts-based autoethnography foregrounds my post-sport lived experiences infused with emotional and socio-cultural layers, using a combination of visual-arts methods and literary arts-methods (e.g., poetry, vignettes, drawings) (Holman Jones & Adams, 2023; Leavy, 2018). Arts-based approaches *show* and *tell* of my lived experiences and render complex vulnerable moments and 'taboo' aspects of my experiences, so they can be accessible and understood (Holman Jones & Adams, 2023). Trauma researcher Davies (2018) explains how arts-based methods make trauma symptoms visible and broadens the communication and understanding of trauma information. In her research, visual art making processes made visible the biopsychosocial impact of trauma, the creative process looked at how trauma can be embodied from a first-person perspective, with the intention of evoking empathy from the audience while offering alternative ways to view one's life (Davies, 2018). For Moon (1999), the physical and emotional dimensions associated with the art, enabled individuals to express themselves, unblock emotions and circumvent the need for verbal representations.

Arts-based autoethnography combines autoethnography with arts-based practices. Autoethnography focuses on an author's personal experiences (i.e., 'auto') using writing techniques to convey theoretical, cultural, and sometimes political layers (Holman Jones & Adams, 2023). Autoethnographers expose meaningful vulnerabilities, epiphanies, and socio-cultural happenings, by joining thought and action in creative ways (Holman Jones & Adams, 2023). While autoethnographies often rely on the written word, the craft of personal storytelling need not be confined to one representation form or genre (Holman Jones & Adams, 2023). Indeed, arts-based methods use artistic forms such as, photography, creative writing, poetry, dance, theatre performances, collages, digital storytelling, murals, filmmaking, paintings, craft, drawings, and body mapping to generate, interpret, or communicate knowledge about lived experience (Knowles & Cole, 2008; Leavy, 2018). Arts-based forms in qualitative research can also serve as data collection methods and/or cultural sites of analysis (Leavy, 2018). For my trauma and abuse research, arts-based methods and autoethnography were combined to invite the audience to 'step into' my experience by providing alternative, visual and creative ways of presenting my lived experience, in contrast to 'realist tales' that present decontextualised textual interview excerpts (Barone & Eisner, 2012; Coemans & Hannes, 2017).

Method

After receiving ethical approval, I revisited artefacts of my life collected since retiring from elite sport which included video and audio diary recordings as well as photographs. While revisiting these artefacts, I conducted 'relational analysis' (Kirk, 1999) by exploring if any themes from my adolescent elite sport experiences were being played out, resisted, or continued in my post-sport life. I focused on dominant themes intertwined with ideologies relevant to my elite adolescent swimming experiences which included, 'slim to win' (i.e., engaging in damaging practices based on the belief that the leaner the body is, the better it performs), 'body hatred' (i.e., negative thoughts/beliefs about my body, actions used to check on, tend to, alter, or conceal my body), 'problematic eating behaviours' (e.g., extreme calorie restriction, binge eating, no eating, avoidant eating, repetitive eating, self-surveillance, body avoidance) and 'self-harm' (e.g., purposely using prescription medication and alcohol in excess, exercising as punishment to point of pain and injury, scratching/burning of skin) (McMahon & Barker-Ruchti, 2017; McMahon & McGannon, 2021; McMahon et al., 2012). This relational analysis (Kirk, 1999) enabled me to recognise which of my sport experiences were persisting in the present day (i.e., post-sport). This further enabled me to link the *exposure* of the abusive/toxic practices that I was subjected to by others, or in turn, engaged with myself, with their *effect* (McMahon, 2010). From there, I identified which arts-based methods would best represent my trauma experiences (e.g., drawing, sculpture, written or poetic prose) which I detail below.

Vignettes: Storying (My) Trauma

Vignettes were a natural choice for me in this trauma research because I had used diary writing previously as a teenager to detail my hurt and pain. Similar to my written diary excerpts in my adolescence, vignettes are short written storied forms (Sparkes & Smith, 2014) enabling me to detail my experiences or scenarios as an adult woman post-sport. Recognised as a literary arts method, I commenced the construction of my vignette by following a process that worked for me in the writing, transcribing, or detailing of my previous lived experiences relating to abuse and trauma. I jotted down points relating to how specific scenarios that I wished to share occurred. Next, I detailed who was present and the conversations (if applicable). I then filled in the blanks which included intricate details where other relevant information such as the weather on the day of the incident, clothes worn, body language of people present (if any), and the conversation tone (if relevant).

While intricate details of my trauma and abuse legacy are important to include, I acknowledged my relational ethical responsibilities regarding people who potentially feature in my lived experience (i.e., perpetrator/s of abuse) as their identity should be protected (Holman Jones & Adams, 2023). As such, where relevant, I used pseudonyms instead of actual names and omitted physical or contextual characteristics which could identify those who feature indirectly. While informed consent is not needed for those featuring indirectly in my data (Bochner & Ellis, 2016), care and consideration ensued using 'interpretive authority' (Bochner & Ellis, 2016, p. 148). This means that as the researcher, I became accountable for what I did and did not include, and how I interpreted the findings (Bochner & Ellis, 2016). As Bochner and Ellis (2016) summarise, we cannot always know or predict the effects of our words on another, or the offence it may cause, but we should be mindful in our writing to minimise any possible harm(s).

Detailing Pain through Poetry

During my elite athlete experiences, I was often constrained, silenced, and bound to rules and ideologies that were stifling and abusive. Therefore, in the research process, it was important for me not to be bound by similar constraints nor be restricted to one method or way of telling. I found the use of poetry enabled me freedom to detail my experiences without having to adhere to stylistic rules associated with academic writing conventions. Therefore, I made use of the free verse style of poetry which does not have rules (e.g., meter and rhythm) and lacks a consistent rhyme scheme, metrical pattern, or musical form (Kidder, 2019). I did, however, purposely use *stylistic punctuation* (e.g., to create short pauses, to accentuate something) to guide the reader on how I would like my poem to be read. I also used *capitalisation* to emphasise certain elements relating to (my) traumatic events, emotions, along with the (de-identified) perpetrators involved in my encounter. I pondered and searched for appropriate word/s to use to explain my feelings, with the hope that the audience could, in turn, reflect on, feel, or empathise with, my experiences of trauma and abuse. As I preferred a minimalist poem, I ensured every word included was essential to how my trauma story was told. As Hogue (2006) explains, the poet needs to 'show', rather than simply 'tell', by transporting readers to place, time, and experience, which, if the image is effective, affords understanding of emotions conveyed in the poem.

Drawing the Self: Inside-Out

Drawing was also a useful way to detail my pain and ongoing trauma associated with the abuse I experienced as an athlete, so my trauma experiences could be shown in a visual way. Phoenix (2010) highlights how "drawings can allow those who are the subjects of the research to shape how they see themselves and are potentially seen by others" (p. 99). For me, drawing was a device that assisted me to convey my trauma and abuse experiences, but also acted as a buffer, as it protected me from having to say, or detail my most hidden painful experiences into a written form (Mc-Mahon et al., Under Review). In this respect, I wanted to use drawing to detail my 'self-harm' rather than having to story it in a written form with a beginning, middle, and ending (McMahon et al., Under Review). As a neophyte drawer, I was apprehensive about detailing my self-harm, so I asked my son who is studying a creative arts degree at university, how I might approach such a drawing process. As explained by Leavy (2018), although 'special skills' are not needed to undertake arts-based research, to 'think like an artist' may entail working with, and learning from, people who have mastered an arts-based craft (e.g., drawing). My son and I initially spent time searching the internet looking at various drawings and techniques, to identify what drawing type would best show my feelings and trauma experiences. From there, he showed me different techniques (e.g., shading) which I needed to master to create specific mood(s) relating to communicating my emotions.

I began drawing light proportion lines of the object (i.e., my body, weight scales) which I later removed. Regarding the drawing of my body (shown in 'body disgust'), I drew rough shapes of my shoulder, arm, hand, hair, and stomach. Notably, the first version of my body drawing was a skinnier body than I have. To add the necessary and realistic fat rolls, the next step required refining the 'actual' shapes of my arm, hand, stomach, and shoulder. I then added shading with instruction and encouragement from my son (Leavy, 2018), which gave my body a three-dimensional look. Shading was an ongoing process which took hours to finalise. I finalised my body drawing by adding a red colour to emphasise the scratches made when I self-harmed. My intention through drawing is to bring my visual and visceral lived experience of self-harm and 'disgust' towards my body to life, with the hope of evoking empathy, and alternative ways of viewing my life (Barone & Eisner, 1997). Relating to my drawing of 'scales', after completing the feet and object outline, I purposely wrote the words and statements that coaches, and team managers said to me about my swimmer body. I used capitalisation for common words and repeated them multiple times for emphasis. Given that having a low weight number and a fatless body was perceived to enhance competitive performance by coaches, I purposely made the scales the starting blocks of a competition pool. In what follows, I present my drawings, vignette, and poem to *show* and *tell* of my post-sport difficulties of trauma, including how dominant ideologies and practices embodied during my elite swimming career, continue to play out in my post-sport life (Figures 5.1 and 5.2).

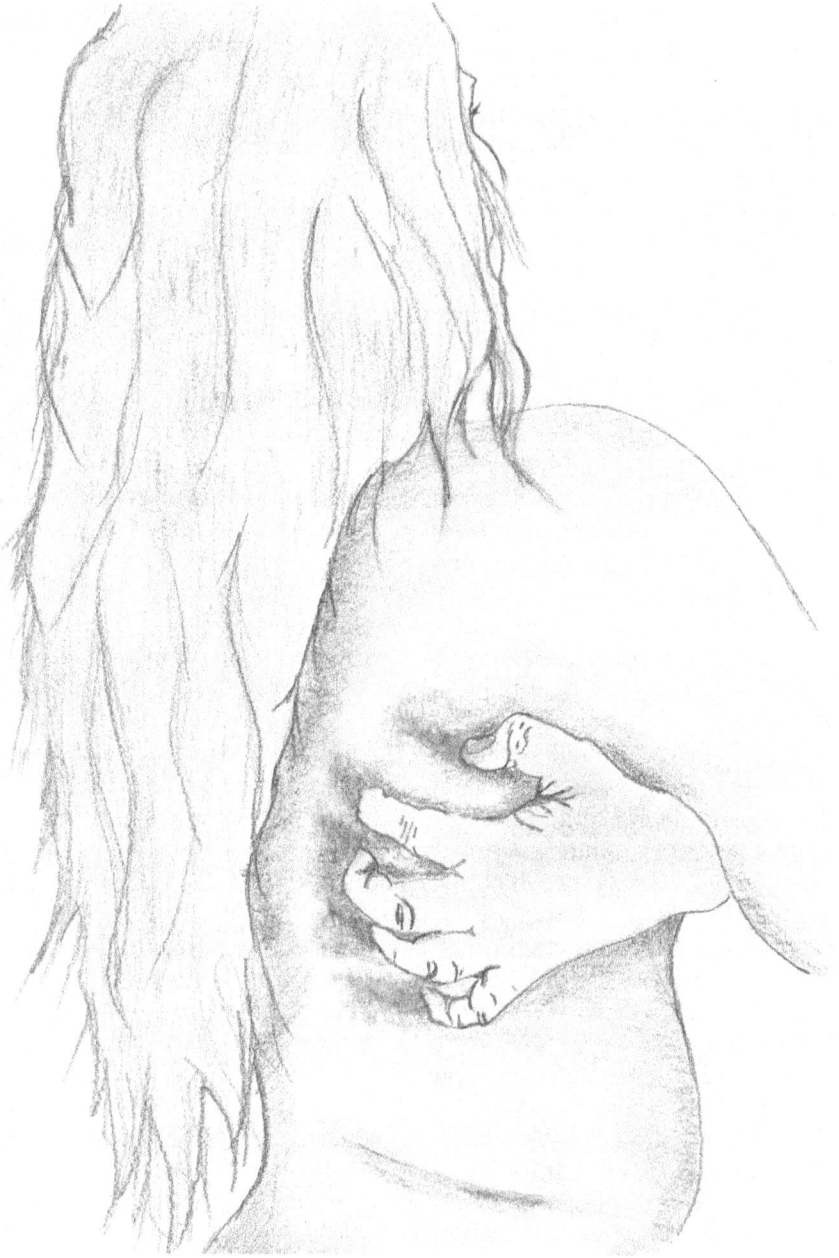

Figure 5.1 Body disgust (pencil on paper).

After succumbing to the food noise in my head and consuming a huge plate of spaghetti carbonara with garlic bread, I sit on my bed disgusted in myself. Eating the pasta felt good for a second, but the guilt now is unbearable. Then the self-hatred creeps in, and I fixate on the fat rolls of my stomach and back which are bigger and flabbier than ever before. Disgust overwhelms me, and the words of others who critiqued my body when I was swimming, re-emerge. The disgust becomes too much so I begin scratching my fat rolls, digging in with my fingernails so hard that my skin becomes red and inflamed. I begin to bleed and my skin stings. The stinging, a pain that I deserve for my disgusting failure body. I hop into the shower and turn the hot tap to the highest setting scorching my skin, purposely burning it, punishing it for looking as it does.

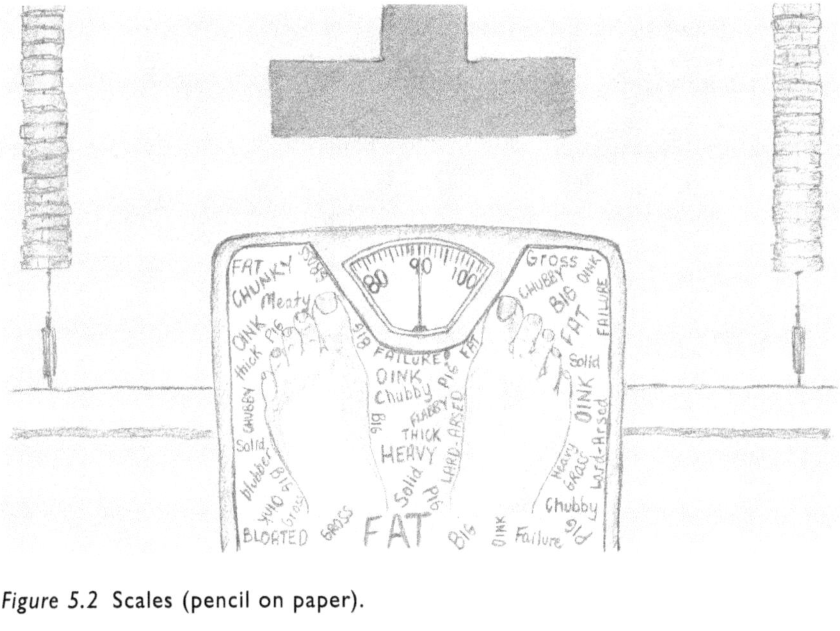

Figure 5.2 Scales (pencil on paper).

The door swings, I see something that terrifies ME
Body freezes
Hairs on arms stand
Lump in throat appears
Acid in stomach gurgles

I stare at THEM
WORDS reappear, that were once said to ME
WORDS, I try to supress
WORDS, I try to bury
WORDS, said by COACHES
WORDS, said by MANAGERS
WORDS said, when I was forced onto the SCALES

OINK OINK OINK, HE says
LARD ARSE, THEY say
TOO BIG, YOU are
Carrying a bit of BLOAT, HE says
BUM FAT, THEY say
A FAILURE, THEY say
TOO BIG, HE says
CHUNKY legs, HE says
MEATY, THEY say
OINK OINK OINK, HE says
SOLID legs, THEY say
CHUBBY, HE says
HEAVY, THEY say
BLOATED, THEY say
BLUBBER, HE says
HEAVY, THEY say
BIG, THEY say
SOLID, THEY say
OINK OINK OINK, HE says

WORDS, I wish I could escape
WORDS, I wish I could forget
WORDS, I wish wouldn't haunt

FAILURE, they said
FAILURE, I felt
FAILURE, I believe
FAILURE, I was
FAILURE, I am.

Applying Trauma-Informed Practices to Abuse and Trauma Research

Although this chapter features self-research whereby my decision making and choices were central, the implementation of evidence-based TIPs was still intertwined with this work, to ensure my safety and well-being was protected along with limiting the possibility of (my) re-traumatisation. As Owton (2016) warns, disclosing or recounting the experience of abuse or its ongoing effects can be traumatic and lead to a 'double trauma'. Even though the abuse I was subjected to during my adolescence occurred decades ago, and the resulting trauma is less prevalent today, an ethic of care was still needed. As SAMHSA (2014, 2023) highlights, the internal and external coping resources available to those exposed to adverse experiences can be affected, creating a sense of extreme threat that has lasting negative consequences for victims' functioning and well-being. Thus, it is no surprise that those affected by trauma differ in their support needs (Dye, 2018; SAMHSA, 2014), highlighting the need for trauma-informed approaches to be implemented by researchers.

Below, due to word restriction, we focus on two evidence-based trauma-informed principles (TIPs) (*peer support* and *empowerment, voice, and choice*) recommended by SAMHSA (2014, 2023) which were implemented into this self-research. These same principles should be considered by other researchers wishing to conduct research with those who have suffered or are suffering from trauma and an abuse legacy. This is not to say that the other principles outlined by SAMHSA (2014, 2023) were less important or not implemented by us.

Peer Support: Friendship as Method

When implementing the TIP of peer support, we found '*friendship as method*' an appropriate means to support my needs as the researcher/participant in and through the research process to limit re-traumatisation. 'Critical friends' (Smith & McGannon, 2018) could also fall under the banner of 'peer support' which involves a "process of critical dialogue between people, with researchers giving voice to their interpretations in relation to other people who listen and offer critical feedback" (Smith & McGannon, 2018, p. 13). While this approach in qualitative research has been conducted in sport/exercise/health contexts over the past decade, it did not resonate as appropriate for my emotional needs in this self-research. Other trauma researchers (e.g., Delker et al., 2020; SAMHSA, 2014, 2023) caution that people with reported histories of trauma and abuse may have fragile self-esteem and may suffer from extreme sensitivity to criticism. While the critical friend process opens constructive dialogue, I found the associated concepts and connotations of *criticism, scrutinising, scanning*, or *inspecting* (Smith & Caddick, 2012), profoundly confronting. This process could be problematic for those subjected to, or surviving, abuse and affected by trauma (Delker et al., 2020). As the National Association of State Mental Health Program Directors [NASMHPD] (2018) warn, if we are not alert to power differentials in peer support relationships, similar power dynamics may unintentionally be recreated to the original trauma/abuse experienced. Therefore, the role of the critical friend or the process itself could sit in contrast to a trauma-informed approach and should either be modified to support the well-being of trauma participants, or adopt an alternative, which was the case in this research.

'Friendship as method' involves the practices, pace, contexts, and the ethics of friendship when undertaking research (Tillmann, 2015). The 'friendship as method' is grounded in the interpretive turn, meaning that objectivity is not possible, and that collaboration through friendship is a resource that embraces multiple standpoints and truths in the research process. This meant, Kerry (friend/co-author) was "somebody to talk to, depend on, rely on for help and support and was caring" (Rawlins, 1992, p. 271) in the research process. Equally, I (friend/co-author) also held that role for Kerry, so the process became two-way. We engaged in 'friendship as method' by messaging each other daily through 'what's app messenger' service which is a free instant messaging app available for both Android and iPhone/s. Through this app, we carried out daily check-ins on each other's well-being. As a neophyte artist, I was also keen to take screenshots of my drawings in progress and sent them to Kerry where she provided positive encouragement, reactions, and probed how undertaking this process was impacting me.

Due to our established nine-year friendship, Kerry could identify the state of my mental health in and through the research process. Kerry would check in every Monday morning and ask about the weekend. If I was reclusive at home, she knew my mental health was starting to be affected. Additionally, if my messaged responses to her were short, or I did not respond for a few days, she knew my mental health was affected. While this only occurred once during the process, she carefully suggested (rather than told) me to take some self-care days away from the project and computer. Related to this point, due to our friendship history, she also knew when to provide me with some space (e.g., Friday and Saturday evenings). Being able to identify these unique aspects of my personality and well-being are something that a colleague could either miss or not always be attuned to. As Tillmann (2015) explains, 'friendship as method' demands research to be undertaken with "an ethic of friendship, a stance of hope, reciprocal caring, justice, and even love" (p. 295). As a result of undertaking 'friendship as method', our existing relationship grew and developed into a shared sense of alliance of trust, honesty, safety, generosity, loyalty, understanding, and acceptance towards each other and ourselves (Owton, 2016; Tillmann, 2015).

While employing 'friendship as method' can reconfigure or minimise power imbalances, an important consideration when being trauma-informed

(SAMHSA, 2014, 2023), it does not completely negate it (Garton & Copland, 2010). As the term is used here, 'power' relates to intersecting gender, class, age, socioeconomic class, ethnicity, and (dis)ability, which need to be considered by researchers (Garton & Copland, 2010; Owton & Allen-Collinson, 2014). As Kerry and I are non-disabled, White, cis-gender women, come from similar backgrounds in terms of class/socioeconomic status and were of similar age, power imbalances were somewhat minimised. Kerry is also a trauma survivor and thus able to provide 'authentic peer support' according to the guidelines outlined by SAMHSA (2014, 2023) which recommends 'peers' to be survivors, with lived experience of trauma. This cultural insider status allows for authentic resonance and participation in rich conversations centring on trauma-related topics (McMahon et al., 2022). As NASMHPD (2022) highlights, effective peer support can lead to empowerment which occurs when individuals gain confidence in their own capacity to make decisions leading to enhanced personal strength and efficacy as well as feelings of acceptance. Empowerment is important for trauma survivors (NASMHPD, 2018). There are also emotional demands using 'friendship as method' as it can be distressing to witness struggles and engage in self-reflexive critiques (Tillmann, 2015), and in so doing, it is important to note that we did not use our 'ethic of friendship' to replace a mental health professional, if one of us needed additional care. Below, Kerry provides a vignette in her first-person voice to illustrate a brief example of 'friendship as method' used in this research during Jenny's process.

Chihuahuas, Beaches, and Bonsais … Jenny is grounded when she's with her dogs, having a 'jaunt' at the beach, or tending to her bonsai trees. It might seem strange to notice the non-human as indications of her well-being, but I know if there are no pictures or videos of these for a few days, something's 'up'. When the first drawing comes through, I am stunned … "mate that's amazing … how did you …?" I really take it in – the fleshy folds, the intertwining colour of red. My heart sinks. I can see the pain and anguish on the page. Jenny's text comes, "it's a process. Finn helped me, you know, with his artistic background?" *silence* I look at the image again. It's burned in my brain. I send a video, "it's very powerful. Can you talk me through it, or do you need a break?" No video from Jenny … a short text "the drawing lets me say a lot. More than writing". *silence* for days. Now it's the weekend. I decide to leave it. I keep returning to the drawing. I hope she's ok. Another day lapses, No dogs. No beach. No bonsais. I check in with a picture and text "hope your weekend was good. I was on my run by the pond – ducks are out!" Later a video comes, "working on the auto-ethnography. I'm tired, I was in the house all weekend". I respond, "if you're up for a chat …? Remember this is YOUR story, you can do – or not do – what you want. Maybe a break with the pups?" In a few hours, she texts – "yea. I think I'm good". Short video follows of Ellie – the exalted chihuahua. I know Jenny is processing. No more videos from me. It will be too much. I text, "contact if you need anything".

Choice, Voice, and Empowerment

Historically, trauma survivors and those who experience adverse events are often silenced and provided limited choice to foreground their lived experiences (Delker et al., 2020; NASMHPD, 2022). The Blue Knot Foundation (2020), an organisation that developed guidelines for organisations working with those affected by trauma, outlined that 'choice' means those affected by trauma should be provided with options at all levels of decision making (e.g., therapy, education, research). Although I had considerable choice and options in this research project due to it being self-research and my privilege as a White academic, these points are essential for trauma researchers to consider in the research design. It should be noted that given the subject positions I hold, deciding what to expose in my self-story related to embodied mental health, is not easy. I am always negotiating social, academic, and institutional power. The notion of 'choice' was a key concern in relation to what I wanted to feature in my experiences, and how I wanted my experiences of trauma and abuse to be shared. Arts-based autoethnography enabled me the 'choice' to select from multiple ways and forms of presenting my lived experience such as drawing, poetry, and vignettes. These different representation choices also afforded me control over what I wanted to share and how much detail I provided (McMahon et al., 2022). Providing participants affected by trauma with 'choice' in what they share and how they present their lived experiences means they are actively co-constructing the research (Smith et al., 2022). Boivin and Cohen-Miller (2018) expand on this point noting that enabling participants to construct their lived experience from their point of view and preferred way of telling, instead of confining them to the researchers' perspectives, ensures inclusivity and levelling of power in the research process. As trauma leaves victims feeling powerless, NASMHPD (2022) also supports the need to re-imagine power relationships, saying that there is potential for healing to occur for those affected by trauma when meaningful sharing of power and choice in the decision-making occurs. The levelling of power (SAMHSA, 2023) and enabling choice and voice is therefore an essential TIP to be implemented in and through the research process.

Marginalising survivors' voices does not align with a trauma-informed approach, therefore foregrounding their voice/s is imperative in research (Poole & Greaves, 2012). Empowering my voice was integral to this self-research because as an adolescent athlete subjected to different types of abuse, my voice was suppressed by sporting insiders as I was required to comply with toxic practices or risk being removed from the national team. Trauma researchers have shown that foregrounding silenced voices (i.e., trauma survivors, abuse survivors) has self-awareness and emancipatory potential as the sharing of experience(s) can symbolise a form of resistance, or taking action, against silence (Fivush, 2010; Hernández-Wolfe, 2011). Although a caveat associated with this practice is that the re-telling of stories can result in 'double trauma' (Owton, 2016), therefore it is essential for the research process and subsequent practices be underpinned by evidence-based TIPs. In Delker et al.'s (2020, p. 243) research with women who "shared stories of interpersonal violence to a public audience, giving voice to silence can be seen as part of a developmental progression from trauma victim to survivor and/or advocate", with opportunities to collectively advocate for those in vulnerable positions were shared which, in turn, was healing. Likewise, Pasupathi et al. (2016) found when reflecting on many years of research with survivors of interpersonal violence that the first time that many spoke of the details of their stories, "the telling itself was healing" (p. 53).

One meaningful and authentic way to empower participants in and through the research process is through co-production (Smith et al., 2022). Co-production in qualitative research can vary in terms of what it means and how it is carried out (Williams et al., 2021). In terms of trauma-informed research practice, we envisage co-production to enable trauma participants to have authentic participation in designing research (i.e., co-design), co-production and co-creation of research/data at a minimum. Sharing power in the research process means those with relevant lived experience share the decision-making, and are consulted in data collection, analysis, and representation practices (Smith et al., 2022).

Having some emancipatory benefit (i.e., empowerment) in this self-research was important to me. As a trauma survivor and trauma researcher, one-way transactional research methods (e.g., online questionnaires) and processes (e.g., researcher-led investigations) centring on participants giving their time and 'data' (i.e., lived experiences of trauma through interviews) without consideration for what participants gain from involvement (i.e., benefits), can be perceived as exploitive (Smith et al., 2022). While researchers are not therapists or psychologists, an 'ethics of care' must extend into research practice to ensure that research processes are not one-way transactions (McMahon et al., 2022). In terms of the TIP of empowerment, I implemented arts-based practices due to the successful use of these methods in trauma therapy (Malchiodi, 2023) and their potential to raise my critical consciousness (Leavy, 2018). Such information and studies using the approach, including benefits and caveats, is readily available. After reading these examples, I gained the hope that I could be empowered through my arts-based autoethnographies and other emancipatory benefits could potentially be achieved (i.e., clarity, healing, challenging dominant ideologies). Further, with over 10 years of writing self-stories (i.e., autoethnographies) about my abuse and trauma experiences in sport, and hearing others' stories, I have experienced the impacts of this approach.

Despite my experiences with autoethnography, combining visual/arts and textual methods to construct an arts-based autoethnography was new for me. I was drawn to this approach as researchers have demonstrated its value for healing and empowering participants. Malchiodi (2023) who used *art as therapy* in her trauma-informed care found it to be therapeutic in several ways. For example, victims/participants used several artistic techniques (e.g., integrated movement, sound, art, play, imagery, drama, and other multisensory practices into psychotherapy) to express the details of what occurred in their experience, also allowing them control over how they communicated these harrowing experiences (Malchiodi, 2023). Further, art enabled the participants/victims/survivors the opportunity to express what is often unspeakable, affording them to explore, re-structure, re-frame, and re-story trauma and loss in co-participatory ways (Malchiodi, 2023). Art as a creative action-orientated approach has been shown to provide participants with tools to self-regulate stress and other trauma-related challenges, which is a skill that can be transferred to their everyday lives (Malchiodi, 2023).

The two TIPs outlined above which included *'peer support'* (realised using 'friendship as method') and *'choice, voice and empowerment'* (realised using arts-based autoethnography) were additional considerations to what is generally required to gain ethical approval. Ensuring flexibility and using evidence-based trauma principles in the research process is what Lahman et al. (2011) calls *aspirational ethics* whereby more than the minimum ethical standard is carried out so re-traumatisation is limited.

Conclusions

In closing, we propose three key future directions and ways forward relating to trauma research and TIPs broadly, intertwined with the two methods put forward in this chapter.

1 **Research procedures need to be flexible and adaptable rather than rigid and inflexible**. Ensuring the research process/method is flexible is extremely important because conducting research or working with populations affected by trauma can result in their varied responses (SAMHSA, 2014, 2023). This means that researchers cannot predict participants' reactions beforehand. Therefore, researchers need to be prepared to adapt procedures and processes dynamically and apply evidence-based trauma principles accordingly. The methods put forward in this chapter were beneficial for me as a trauma survivor and included the opportunity to tell my experiences through arts-based methods in multiple ways rather than being restricted to one mode of telling (e.g., narrative only). By enabling the participant to share their experience their way, using different modes of representation means moving away from co-constructed *researcher-led* data to co-constructed *participant-led data* (Boivin & Cohen-Miller, 2018). Towards that end, trauma-informed researchers in sport, exercise, and health settings might consider using

arts-based methods as it foregrounds lived experiences by making trauma symptoms visible. In turn, this broadens the communication and understanding of trauma information (Davies, 2018).

2   Qualitative researchers in sport, exercise, and health contexts carrying out trauma research need to be **mindful of how they communicate information to participants as well as the audience more broadly**. For example, simple but power laden statements such as, "**I [researcher] am going to give you the opportunity …**" or "**this process will allow participants to contribute**" exemplifies inequitable power relations between the researcher and the participant. As NASMHPD (2018) explains, trauma leaves victims feeling powerless, therefore power inequities in the way information is presented and communicated must be considered.

3   **Qualitative researchers need to consider power differentials occurring in all aspects of the research process and should account for, and address them where possible**. The co-production of research affords participants with authentic participation in designing research (i.e., co-design), co-production and co-creation of research data. The sharing or reconfiguring of power from the outset of the trauma research process means those with relevant lived experience share in the decision-making, and are consulted in data collection, analysis, and representation practices (Smith et al., 2022). NASMHPD (2022) warns that if power differentials are not minimised, similar power dynamics to the original trauma/abuse experienced may unintentionally be recreated. This potential impact is something that sits at odds with a trauma-informed approach. In this research, we used 'friendship as method' to reconfigure power relationships in the peer support relationship. Using 'friendship as method' rather than the process of a 'critical friend' approach used broadly in qualitative research in sport, exercise, and health research met my emotional needs as a trauma survivor and addressed power relationships in the research process. 'Friendship as method' is just one way to address power inequities in research relationships, but it is imperative to consider such differentials in all aspects of the research process from the outset.

References

Alexander, K., Stafford, A., & Lewis, R. (2011). *The experiences of children participating in organized sport in the UK*. NSPCC. https://www.research.ed.ac.uk/portal/files/7971883/experiences_children_sport_main_reportwdf85014.pdf.

Barone, T., & Eisner, E. W. (1997). Art-based educational research. In R. M. Jaeger (Ed.), *Complementary methods for research in education* (pp. 73–116). American Educational Research Association Press.

Barone, T., & Eisner, E. W. (2012). *Arts based research*. Sage.

Blue Knot Foundation. (2020). *Organisation guidelines for trauma-informed service delivery*. https://blueknot.org.au/product/organisational-guidelines-for-trauma-informed-service-delivery-digital-download/.

Bochner, A., & Ellis, C. (2016). *Evocative autoethnography: Writing lives and telling stories*. Routledge.

Boivin, N., & Cohen-Miller, A. (2018). Breaking the "Fourth Wall" in qualitative research: Participant-led digital data construction. *The Qualitative Report, 23*(3), 581–592. https://doi.org/10.46743/2160-3715/2018.3136

Coemans, S., & Hannes, K. (2017). Researchers under the spell of the arts: Two decades of using arts-based methods in community-based inquiry with vulnerable populations. *Educational Research Review, 22*, 34–49. https://doi.org/10.1016/j.edurev.2017.08.003

Davies, J. (2018). *Materiality and metaphor: Making trauma visible through an arts-based autoethnography*. Unpublished PhD thesis, Western Sydney University. https://researchdirect.westernsydney.edu.au/islandora/object/uws:49903/

Delker, B., Salton, R., & McLean, K. (2020). Giving voice to silence: Empowerment and disempowerment in the developmental shift from trauma victim to trauma survivor. *Journal of Trauma and Dissociation, 21*(2), 242–263.

Dye, H. (2018). The impact and long-term effects of childhood trauma. *Journal of Human Behaviour in the Social Environment, 28*(3), 381–392. https://doi.org/10.1080/10911359.2018.1435328

Fivush, R. (2010). Speaking silence: The social construction of voice and silence in cultural and autobiographical narratives. *Memory, 18*, 88–98.

Garton, F., & Copland, S. (2010). "I like this interview; I get cakes and cats": The effect of prior relationships on interview talk. *Qualitative Research, 10*(5), 1–10. https://doi.org/10.1177/1468794110375231

Hernández-Wolfe, P. (2011). Decolonization and "mental" health: A Mestiza's journey in the borderlands. *Women & Therapy, 34*(3), 293–306. https://doi.org/10.1080/02703149.2011.580687

Hogue, C. (2006). *The incognito body*. Red Hen Press.

Holman Jones, S., & Adams, T. E. (2023). Autoethnography as becoming-with. In N. K. Denzin, Y. S. Lincoln, G. S. Cannella, & M. D. Giardina (Eds.), *The Sage handbook of qualitative research* (6th ed., pp. 421–435). Sage.

Kavanagh, E., & Brady, A. (2014). A framework for understanding humanization and dehumanization in sport. In D. Rhind, & C. Brackenridge (Eds.), *Researching and enhancing athlete welfare* (pp. 34–43). Brunel University Press.

Kerr, G., Willson, E., & Stirling, A. (2019). *Prevalence of maltreatment among current and former national team athletes*. University of Toronto/AthletesCAN.

Kidder, H. (2019). *How to write a poem: 8 fundamentals for writing poetry*. https://self-publishingschool.com/how-to-write-a-poem

Kirk, D. (1999). Physical culture, physical education, and relational analysis. *Sport, Education and Society, 4*(1), 63–75.

Knowles, G. J., & Cole, A. (2008). *Handbook of the arts in qualitative research: Perspectives, methodologies, examples, and issues*. Sage Publications.

Lahman, M. K., Geist, M. R., Rodriguez, K. L., Graglia, P., & DeRoche, K. K. (2011). Culturally responsive relational reflexive ethics in research: The three Rs. *Quality and Quantity, 45*, 1397–1414. https://doi.org/10.1007/s11135-010-9347-3

Leavy, P. (2018). Introduction to arts-based research. In P. Leavy (Ed.), *Handbook of arts-based research* (pp. 2–22). The Guilford Press.

Malchiodi, C. (2023). Trauma-informed expressive art therapy. In C. Malchiodi (Ed.), *Handbook of expressive arts therapy* (pp. 142–154). The Guilford Press.

McMahon, J. (2010). *Exposure and effect: An investigation into a culture of body pedagogies* (Unpublished Ph.D. thesis). University of Tasmania, Hobart.

McMahon, J., Penney, D., & Dinan-Thompson, M. (2012). Body practices – Exposure and effect of a sporting culture? Stories from three Australian swimmers. *Sport, Education and Society, 17,* 181–206. https://doi.org/10.1080/13573322.2011.607949

McMahon, J., & Barker-Ruchti, N. (2017). Assimilating to a boy's body shape for the sake of performance: Three athletes' body experiences in a sporting culture. *Sport, Education and Society, 22*(2), 157–174. https://doi.org/10.1080/13573322.2015.1013463

McMahon, J., & McGannon, K. R. (2021). I hurt myself because it sometimes helps: Former athletes' embodied emotion responses to abuse using self-injury. *Sport, Education and Society, 26*(2), 161–174. https://doi.org/10.1080/13573322.2019.1702940

McMahon, J., McGannon, K. R., Zehntner, C., Werbicki, L., Stephenson, E., & Martin, K. (2022). Trauma-informed abuse education in sport: Engaging athlete abuse survivors as educators and facilitating a community of care. *Sport, Education and Society.* https://doi.org/10.1080/13573322.2022.2096586

McMahon, J., McGannon, K. R., & Zehntner, C. (Under review). Arts-based methods as a trauma-informed approach to research: Enabling survivors and victims' experiences to be visible and limiting the risk of re-traumatisation. *Methods in Psychology.*

Moon, B. L. (1999). The tears make me paint: The role of responsive artmaking in adolescent art therapy. *Art Therapy, 16*(2), 78–82.

Mountjoy, M., Brackenridge, C., Arrington, M., Blauwet, C., Carska-Sheppard, A., Fasting, K., Kirby, S., Leahy, T., Marks, S., Martin, K., Starr, K., Tiivas, A., & Budgett, R. (2016). International Olympic Committee consensus statement: Harassment and abuse (non-accidental violence) in sport. *British Journal of Sports Medicine, 50,* 1019–1029. https://doi.org/10.1136/bjsports-2016-096121

National Association of State Mental Health Program Directors (NASMHPD). (2018). *Trauma-informed peer support.* https://nasmhpd.org/sites/default/files/TIPS_Training_2018_NASMHPDTemplate_PPT.pdf

National Association of State Mental Health Program Directors (NASMHPD). (2022). *Trauma-informed innovations in crisis services: Empowerment, voice, and choice.* https://www.nasmhpd.org/content/presentation/trauma-informed-innovations-crisis-services-safety-common-ground

Owton, H., & Allen-Collinson, J. (2014). Close but not too close: Friendship as method(ology) in ethnographic research encounters. *Journal of Contemporary Ethnography, 43*(3), 283–305. https://doi.org/10.1177/0891241613495410

Owton, H. (2016). *Sexual abuse in sport: A qualitative case study.* Springer Nature.

Pasupathi, M., Fivush, R., & Hernandez-Martinez, M. (2016). Talking about it: Stories as paths to healing after violence. *Psychology of Violence, 6*(1), 49–56. https://doi.org/10.1037/vio0000017

Phoenix, C. (2010). Seeing the world of physical culture: The potential of visual methods for qualitative research in sport and exercise. *Qualitative Research in Sport, and Exercise, 2*(2), 93–108. https://doi.org/10.1080/19398441.2010.488017

Poole, N., & Greaves, L. (2012). *Becoming trauma informed.* Centre for Addiction and Mental Health.

Rawlins, W. K. (1992). *Friendship matters: Communication, dialectics, and the life course.* Aldine de Gruyter.

Ropers-Huilman, B. (1999). Witnessing: Critical inquiry in a post structural world. *Qualitative Studies in Education, 12*(1), 21–35.

Smith, B., Williams, O., Bone, L., & The Moving Social Work Co-Production Collective (2022). Co-production: A resource to guide co-producing research in the sport, exercise, and health sciences. *Qualitative Research in Sport, Exercise and Health, 15*(2), 159–187. https://doi.org/10.1080/2159676X.2022.2052946

Smith, B., & McGannon, K. R. (2018). Developing rigor in qualitative research: Problems and opportunities within sport and exercise psychology. *International Review of Sport, and Exercise Psychology, 11*(1), 101–121. https://doi.org/10.1080/17509 84X.2017.1317357

Smith, B., & Caddick, N. (2012). Qualitative methods in sport: A concise overview for guiding social scientific sport research. *Asia Pacific Journal of Sport and Social Science, 1*(1), 60–73. https://doi.org/10.1080/21640599.2012.701373

Sparkes, A. C. (1999). Exploring body narratives. *Sport, Education and Society, 4*(1), 17–30. https://doi.org/10.1080/1357332990040102

Sparkes, A. C., & Smith, B. (2014). *Qualitative research methods in sport, exercise, and health: From process to product*. Routledge.

Substance Abuse and Mental Health Services Administration (SAMHSA). (2014). *SAMHSA's concept of trauma and guidance for a trauma-informed approach*. Substance Abuse and Mental Health Services Administration. https://ncsacw.samhsa.gov/userfiles/files/SAMHSA_Trauma.pdf

Substance Abuse and Mental Health Services Administration (SAMHSA). (2023). *Practical guide for implementing a trauma-informed approach*. https://store.samhsa.gov/sites/default/files/pep23-06-05-005.pdf

Tillmann, L. M. (2015). Friendship as method. In L. M. Tillmann (Ed.), *In solidarity: friendship, family, and activism beyond gay and straight* (pp. 287–319). Routledge.

UNICEF. (2010). *Protecting children from violence in sport: A review with focus on industrialized countries*. UNICEF Innocenti Research Centre. http://www.unicef-irc.org/publications/pdf/violence_in_sport.pdf

Williams, O., Tembo, D., Ocloo, J., Kaur, M., Hickey, G., Farr, M., and Beresford. P. (2021). "Co-production Methods and Working Together at a Distance: Introduction to Volume 2." In O. Williams., D. Tembo., J. Ocloo., M. Kaur., G. Hickey., M. Farr, & P. Beresford (Eds.). *COVID-19 and Co-production in Health and Social Care Research, Policy, and Practice (Volume 2): Co-production Methods and Working Together at a Distance* (pp. 1–16). Policy Press.

Chapter 6

Trauma and the Mental Health of Elite Athletes

Andy Smith

Introduction

Trauma is a costly public health problem, common among children, young people, and adults across the world (Emsley et al., 2022). Those who are disproportionately affected by trauma include people experiencing significant socio-economic disadvantage, women, LGBTQ+ groups, minoritized ethnic groups, as well as those who experience poverty, racism, and other forms of discrimination (Emsley et al., 2022). Nearly half of adults have experienced at least one adverse childhood experience (ACE), including childhood physical and emotional abuse, mental illness, and domestic violence (Bellis et al., 2014). Traumatic stress is also associated with increased risk of suicide attempts, suicidal ideation, and self-harm behaviour (including non-suicidal self-harm) in adolescence and young adulthood (Tunno et al., 2021). Trauma experienced during childhood and adolescence can have particularly profound impacts over the life course, including increased risk of depression, addiction, obesity, and heart disease (Bellis et al., 2014; Felitti et al., 1998; SAMHSA, 2014). Consequently, and despite "little evidence of acceptability, effectiveness, and cost effectiveness in the UK context, policies and guidelines at national, regional, and organisational levels recommend implementing TI [trauma-informed] approaches in healthcare organisations and systems" (Emsley et al., 2022, p. 2), though this varies between UK nations.

In addition to the prevalence and impact of societal trauma, sport (especially elite and professional sport) is another important context in which trauma and abuse are common, and researchers have called for trauma-informed approaches in sports organizations, including for mental health benefit (McMahon et al., 2022; Mountjoy et al., 2022). This is especially important given continued concern about the mental health of young elite athletes (e.g., Purcell et al., 2023; Smith, 2023; Walton et al., 2021), adult elite and professional athletes (Reardon et al., 2019; Rice et al., 2016; Smith, 2019), and the consequences of the blurring between athletes' personal and working lives for mental health and other aspects of well-being (e.g., Roderick & Allen Collinson, 2020; Roderick et al., 2017; Smith, 2019). Set in this

DOI: 10.4324/9781003332909-8

context, in this chapter I explore young and adult elite athletes' experiences of trauma and the implications for their mental health. I draw on qualitative interview data from a wider sociological study involving 32 non-disabled UK-based elite athletes (aged 16–33; $n = 31$ self-defined as White) which, it must be noted, was not originally focused on trauma. The emphasis was, instead, placed on the reality of athletes' working lives, and the personal and work-place constraints athletes encountered during their careers. However, upon reflection, athletes' experiences of trauma were indeed hidden in plain sight. It is for this reason, together with the wider lessons which might hopefully be learned from this work that this chapter deliberately draws upon athletes' in-depth qualitative accounts of their sporting and personal lives. I also out-line how trauma-informed practices were implemented into research to best support the athletes involved in this research and to ensure re-traumatization was limited.

The participants whose experiences are reported here were recruited via a non-representative snowball and convenience sampling strategy and were engaged in 17 individual (e.g., athletics track and field, golf, gymnas-tics, and swimming) and team (e.g., football, handball, hockey, and net-ball) sports. The sample included elite athletes who at the time of interview (2009–2013) were members of high-performance development squads, first team players, World Champions, and Olympic medallists. Athletes' com-ments reflected the diversity of trauma which are commonly experienced as a single event, or in multiple instances, over the life course with often profound impacts for their mental health. In some instances, the trauma that athletes experienced in the sporting context occurred because of a diagnosed mental illness, while the mental health problems experienced by others developed during their engagement in elite sports cultures. For example, in the following extract, an athletics field participant (Sarah, fe-male) explained how her diagnosis with bipolar disorder was used publicly by her coach to explain declines in her performance. She said:

> I was diagnosed with bipolar, and I really struggled in certain competi-tions because I just couldn't do it. And I told [coach name], and at first he was fine and when it went wrong [declines in performance] he didn't want it to seem like it was him that had been the problem, so he made sure everybody knew [by disclosing her diagnosis publicly to the rest of the squad] … I suppose it's like a career ending injury, but it's just an injury you can't see, that's the hard bit … If I would have broken my leg no one would question anything.

Other than her partner and mother, Sarah had not previously disclosed her di-agnosis to anyone except her coach and, during an interview, the researcher. The trauma of this coach-led revelation was profound and led Sarah to inter-nalize a deep sense of disappointment, cowardice, and self-stigma about the weakness commonly associated with being diagnosed with a mental illness. This led her to withdraw from an Olympic Games. Sarah explained the impact of her failed attempt to conceal her diagnosis from others:

> I'm a bit disappointed in myself, like I said if it was a physical ... illness you can't really hide it ... At first, I felt a bit of a coward 'cos I thought "I haven't told anybody. I don't want them to think I'm crazy or whatever" ... But [the case of a teammate who attempted suicide following a persistent injury] also made me feel a bit better that I'm not the only one that has given up something because they can't handle it.

Other athletes recalled how their experiences of suicidal ideation resulted from the corrosive workplace relations they had with significant others, including teammates, coaches, and family. When asked about the self-hate and self-questioning which led to his suicidal ideation, Chris (male) pointed to the body shaming he experienced while swimming, which led him to leave the sport to take-up handball:

> I was the younger one. I was like 13 and the rest of them were like 18, 19 ... 'cos I wasn't keeping up with them they bullied me because I wasn't as athletic as them ... just saying oh come on keep up fatty' and stuff like that. 'Cos I was young as well I didn't really feel good ... I just hated myself when I was that age when I was getting bullied in school as well as in swimming. I just hated my whole life. I wasn't happy with it at all. I always complained to my Mum and Dad and said things that I shouldn't have [in relation to suicidal ideation] ... like "I don't like my life at the minute", "Why am I here?", "What am I doing here if I'm just getting bullied?"
>
> (emphases in the original)

Iain, a male gymnast, also described how the challenging longstanding relationship he had with his coach, who was also his father, led him to continually experience self-doubt and depression to such an extent that his friends frequently expressed concern about his safety and welfare:

> It was horrible. It was completely horrible 'cos you didn't want to look at him [Father] because if you looked at him, he might say something ... I'd just put me head down shut my eyes knowing I wasn't asleep just simply because I didn't want to get in a conversation where I know it's gonna relate back to gym and I'm gonna get shouted at ... If you ask all my friends they'll think my Dad is the best person ever. He's funny. If they could, they'd go drinking with him. They think he's great 'cos he goes out of his way for them, makes comments to them ... but it's got to the point where my friend, if someone's jumped off [town name] bridge, he'd text me to

say, "Are you the top of the bridge?" … Sometimes you think it's quite bad that people are texting you "Are you gonna jump off that bridge?", 'cos you think sometimes it just gets too hard.

In addition to athletes' trauma-related suicidal ideation, depression and privatization of distressing emotions were the equally significant, and impactful, challenges encountered in relation to weight management and body consciousness. The following remarks from a female international hockey player (Nicola) captured vividly the "rollercoaster of emotions" which she recalled in relation to the trauma she experienced from coach-related comments about weight maintenance:

> Weight's definitely been an issue for me … It was just a case of [being told by the coach] 'You just need to lose weight, and you need to lose weight, and you need to lose weight'. And it wasn't a case of someone supporting or strategically helping you to do that … it was something I had to address on my own … I don't think I was getting the advice I needed, but then I was watching people that were trying to cut weight in such an extreme way … I would skip meals or I would I would just watch portion sizes or fat content and calories. There were moments that I did get a little bit obsessive about it … Just literally about checking labels and whether it be weighing myself. I would go through phases of weighing myself every day and then panicking about it. I remember getting to a certain point that I had lost quite a bit of weight and feeling quite chuffed and then within a few days my coach [was] saying "You need to lose weight" and … [I thought] "I am never going to win this battle", and then going the other way of over-eating, comfort eating. Just a rollercoaster of emotions.

Another female hockey player, Karen, explained how weight-related trauma and disordered eating was common among her teammates, some of whom lived with anorexia athletica (i.e., engaging a restrictive calorie intake and engaging in excessive exercise), the experience of which was compounded by public daily weighing practices. Karen described these traumatic events by comparing them to practices she encountered early on in her international career:

> We get weighed every morning, but it's all done confidentially [now] … [Previously] we used to stand in a long line in a queue, jump on the scale, [and] the manager would read the weight, shout it out to the physio, and they would write it down. I don't think it was deliberate. I think it was just the quick and easy way to do it. But that certainly upset girls and they felt that they were being compared with other players, and, because we were in a selection situation always for places on the team, they don't like to be compared with other girls in the same position.

Chronic loneliness, which is a significant public health problem, was an additional dimension of the trauma athletes recalled. In the following extract taken from an interview held with Kenny, a male golfer, his experience of loneliness was compounded by the mentally demanding relationship he had with his coach and father:

> Golf is … quite a lonely sport … In terms of the relationship with my dad, I didn't really like it to be honest. I would have valued having a relationship with my dad than a relationship with the coach, 'cos that's essentially what it was. It weren't (sic) really a good relationship with the coach. It was effective, but it weren't (sic) good … Mentally it was quite draining. I suppose it's kind of like living with the same person day in day out; there is only so much one person can stand … When you have a bad day on the course … I just want to forget about it … It weren't really like that; it was like 'Ok, let's go through your holes, what happened.' It's like mentally draining and … it puts more pressure on you.

For other athletes, the experience of perpetual loneliness was associated with the significant degree of routinization and isolation which characterized the reality of elite athletes' lives, and which accompanied occupational hazards including being injured. For example, Liz, a female Olympic field athlete, explained how her life was:

> Lonely, really lonely … pretty much a whole day you spend on your own and I was doing this one week in every three. So you are spending a day there [Holland] travelling pretty much on your own, travelling back pretty much on your own … And then while I'm there, I'm literally just there to train. So I eat, sleep, train, eat, sleep, train and that's all I do, there's nothing else … I remember phoning [partner's name] after the second time I had been there … just crying and being really upset 'cos he [coach] has said 'You won't throw the B standard' … 'Why do I bother?' That was the main thing. Like, 'Why am I doing this sport?'

Greg, a male international Premier League footballer, also described the psychological distress, self-doubt, and emotionality which underpinned his personal trauma as follows:

> I had two bad knee injuries in the same knee with my cartilage … I have been away for a total of six months this year … It's a tough challenge mentally for me, very tough, especially because I live here alone … It's been very hard. The first injury was not the worst, the second was the worst … I found out I was going to be out for four, five months, it was just shit … I had to say 'No' to the national team a few times because of the knee. It was just a very bad time of my life … psychologically. In my head … I was just

thinking many thoughts. Will I be as good? Will I come back? How will I play? Will I be better maybe? How will people think of me? Just loads of thoughts in my head ... Obviously the mental strain, if say you are having a bad time, or you are not playing well, or anything outside of football may not be going right, then [you are just] trying to get through it ... keeping yourself together.

Finally, the profound disappointment, mental anguish, and emotional exhaustion which characterized the hidden traumatic experiences of some elite athletes was summarized by Liz (a female Olympic field athlete):

I don't miss the disappointment and the way it makes you feel. I can't compare that feeling to anything else ... It's disbelief, its emptiness, and you just feel lost, and you almost want to try again but you haven't got any energy ... you can just feel exhausted. But it's not like a feeling of when someone dies or something that makes you really sad. It's more a feeling of disappointment and just inadequacy ... It's like ... if someone got you in a room and just picked apart all your insecurities and told you everything you are rubbish at and called you all the names that really hurt. It's like that. That's the feeling. It's horrible. And the bigger the competition, the worse it is.

Methodology

The research reported above adopted a qualitative approach as part of a cross-sectional study design in which in-depth semi-structured interviews were used to understand the lived realities of elite athletes' working and personal lives. Particular emphasis was placed upon understanding the diverse (but also shared) meanings and interpretations athletes recalled of their lived experiences, their sense-making of these, and how they were understood in the context of their social relations and contexts. Adopting this type of interpretivist approach enabled participants to share their subjective experiences of trauma from the perspective of the "traumatized self," or selves (Miralles et al., 2022), by responding to the researcher's deliberate decision to address potentially traumatic events or experiences directly during the study design planning stage (Jefferson et al., 2021). Although the researcher did not originally set out to explicitly explore athletes' trauma experiences, knowledge of the existing research and insight derived from other sources (e.g., media, autobiographical material) meant that there was a high likelihood that experiences of trauma might be recalled, regardless of the topic being explored (Isobel, 2021). Recognizing that "trauma is widespread, and recovery is possible" (Isobel, 2021, p. 1461), and that it is important to de-stigmatize potentially traumatic experiences, was thus an important feature of assumptions which underpinned the research methodology and design. Also important was the decision to provide participants with an advance summary of the topics to be explored during the research so they could prepare to discuss matters which they were willing and unwilling to reveal (Isobel, 2021; Jefferson et al., 2021; Newman et al., 2006). This practice also had the advantage of allowing the participants to ask questions in advance of being interviewed and make an informed decision about whether to consent to engage in the research given its purpose. Additionally, some participants were high-profile figures whose stories and identities were likely to be of interest to the media and public. Promoting interviewees' agency in this way, being transparent about the potential risks and benefits of engaging in the research and encouraging athletes to disclose (rather than overlook) their lived experience confidentially, helped maximize the ownership interviewees had over the research (Jefferson et al., 2021; Newman et al., 2006).

Upon reflection, adopting co-production approaches to trauma-informed qualitative research would be even more beneficial for participants and researchers (Isobel, 2021; Jefferson et al., 2021). Equitable and experientially informed co-production approaches (see Smith et al., 2023), in particular, can help to embed trauma-informed approaches into all aspects of a study, and enable trauma survivors to share their experiences by disrupting the power and "structural inequities in conventional researcher-participant research partnerships" (Isobel, 2021, p. 1458). Working more equitably with athletes "whose primary contributions are derived from their lived experience" (Smith et al., 2023, p. 160), especially that related to trauma, can also enable participants to shape the design, conduct and evaluation of work which produces more beneficial, equitable, transformative, impactful, and inclusive research outcomes (see Alessi & Kahn, 2023; Isobel, 2021; Jefferson et al., 2021; Smith et al., 2023).

Method

The interviews reported here were undertaken by a White, heterosexual, non-disabled, male researcher whose highest level of previous sporting competition (for team sports) was at regional level. Although I was (am) unable to empathize fully with the culturally specific experiences elite athletes recalled during interviews, as explained below, the research nevertheless reawakened former memories and experiences of trauma which, at least at a general level, were also encountered by interviewees. In hindsight, these former experiences sensitized me to the need to provide interviewees with choice over the physical location or environments in which to be interviewed, so that they felt comfortable disclosing their lived experience (Edelman, 2023; Isobel, 2021). Most athletes preferred to attend audio-recorded semi-structured interviews (lasting 60–90 minutes) held in-person at mutually agreed, physically and culturally safe, locations with the researcher (e.g., university offices, sports clubs, and coffee shops). Two participants requested to be interviewed by telephone because of the location of their training camp which made it difficult to meet with the researcher at a mutually convenient time and space. However, interviews conducted online (i.e., skype) or via telephone have been shown in research (McMahon et al., 2022) to be more predictable for the participants (i.e., particularly those who have experienced abuse or trauma) so they experienced less anxiety because their environment was more stable.

Providing participants with choice over the types of research environments is crucial for trauma survivors since it can help to minimize the replication of contexts in which trauma can occur and enable them to engage in the research on their terms (Isobel, 2021). Potentially trauma-sensitive settings can include work or social spaces where participants can be judged/influenced by others (including powerful authority figures), enclosed spaces where physical distancing is difficult to manage, locations which trigger unwanted psychological and emotional thoughts or which are geographically isolated, or spaces where significant others (e.g., family, friends, teammates) can overhear conversations involving experiences of which they might not be aware (Edelman, 2023; Jefferson et al., 2021). Being flexible to accommodate the needs, experiences, and preferences of trauma survivors, and ensuring they feel culturally and physically safe, is thus crucial for qualitative trauma research. This is especially true for interview-based qualitative studies, including the one reported here, intended to enable athletes to discuss the reality of their lived experience, which in the context of trauma can also enable them to share their stories of trauma by performing their 'traumatized self' or selves (Miralles et al., 2022).

In this study, in-depth semi-structured interviews enabled athletes to discuss trauma and resilience as simultaneous experiences of vulnerability and strength (Isobel, 2021; Jefferson et al., 2021; Miralles et al., 2022). Interviewees were encouraged to challenge the many common sense, often taken-for-granted and mis-guided, assumptions others have of them as often high-profile, public figures (Roderick & Allen Collinson, 2020; Roderick et al., 2017), by comparing them to "how their lives really are." This was deliberately intended to reassure athletes that the researcher did not uncritically accept the dominant (usually unambiguously positive) discourses which typically characterize discussions of elite athletes' lives, and that the focus should instead be on their insider experiences or perspectives. This practice not only increases interviewees' sense of ownership and control over the research but can also help ensure that the trauma recalled is understood in the appropriate cultural context (in this case, elite sport) and is disclosed in culturally safe ways (Edelman, 2023). Where appropriate, the researcher used examples of relevant athlete media interviews and stories, or autobiographical extracts (McMahon et al., 2022; Smith, 2019), as prompts to aid these discussions. In some cases, the examples used were media reports on the athlete themselves so that they were able to "give their side of the story." This approach appeared empowering for interviewees and enabled them to articulate their actual, rather than perceived or reported, experiences of trauma. In other instances, examples of other athletes' experiences were used to encourage interviewees to begin discussing general "public issues" (e.g., concern about athlete mental health) before exploring these more sensitively in relation to their own "personal troubles" (e.g., experiences of trauma and mental health) (Mills, 2000).

These techniques helped to build trust and rapport with interviewees which was important given the sensitive and often upsetting accounts athletes gave relating to their trauma. Indeed, several interviewees broke down in tears when discussing their experiences, especially of depression, bullying, and suicidal ideation. In such cases, athletes' emotional displays were bound-up with their concerns about "being believed" and about communicating the genuine impact their experiences had on them physically, psychologically, and socially. I thus spent (often quite considerable) time listening to the athlete, reassuring them that they were being believed, and that it must have been difficult to share their experiences. I also assured participants that being able to manage their experiences was a source of strength or resilience, rather than weakness, which is often a concern of trauma survivors (Edelman, 2023). Recognizing the impact trauma had on athletes' lives, repeatedly offering opportunities to pause interviews, and re-visiting informed consent and the use of, and right to withdraw, data were also important principles used to ensure that interviewees felt safe (Edelman, 2023; Isobel, 2021; Newman et al., 2006).

Forgetting Oneself: Vicarious Trauma and Researcher Mental Health

As a result of undertaking this investigation, I was inadvertently impacted in various ways by listening to athletes recount their trauma histories. It was certainly difficult not to appear visibly impacted by the accounts athletes gave during the interview, but it was often after the interviews ended and following the completion of the study when the emotional costs of the research manifested (Brackenridge, 1999). Listening to athletes recall experiences of anxiety, depression, and suicidal ideation and behaviour evoked sleeping memories, embodied in one's habitus, which had been encountered directly, and indirectly through relations with others, since childhood. Much of these trauma histories were compounded by what was effectively the vicarious trauma (i.e., a shift in one's worldview after prolonged exposure to others' trauma experiences) encountered, first, during this study, and in subsequent work. These impacts were often managed (or not) privately, in unexpected and unplanned ways, and in retrospect could have been anticipated but they were not. Instead, I experienced occasional, at times prolonged, periods of mental health challenges and distress attributable partly to previous trauma histories, but also to "what one [was] thinking and feeling [was] related to listening to participants' trauma narratives"

(Alessi & Kahn, 2023, p. 148). I certainly under-estimated the unexpected longer-term impacts of listening and being exposed to athletes' traumatic accounts. In retrospect, additional protections beyond the expected ethical requirement of consulting a mental health professional were needed to manage the impacts interviews had on my trauma history and to help avoid secondary traumatization (e.g., after hearing an interviewee's trauma stories once), compassion fatigue (the physical, emotional, and psychological impacts of helping others experiencing trauma), and vicarious trauma (Alessi & Kahn, 2023; Berger, 2021; Edelman, 2023).

The failure to anticipate the longer-term emotional impacts of the research is partly understandable despite the "critical need for qualitative researchers to be trauma-informed in their work" (Alessi & Kahn, 2023, p. 122). Until recently few detailed discussions exist about how to conduct qualitative research using a trauma-informed approach (Alessi & Kahn, 2023; Edelman, 2023; Isobel, 2021; Jefferson et al., 2021). Nevertheless, the next section reflects upon how two trauma-informed practices – *safety* and *cultural, historical, and gender issues* – were addressed in the research.

Trauma-Informed Practices Applied to Research

Safety

Safety is a critical feature of all trauma-informed qualitative research, especially interview-based work (Alessi & Kahn, 2023; Isobel, 2021), which can risk re-traumatizing participants. The evidence indicates, however, that when well-managed, this risk can be minimized, and most trauma survivors do not experience these effects (Edelman, 2023; Isobel, 2021; Jefferson et al., 2021). This appeared to be the case in the present study, where participants were encouraged to discuss the emotional highs and lows of their lived experience as an athlete, and if they were willing, any traumatic events identified. As noted earlier, some participants became emotional and cried during the interviews, but this did not appear to equate to harm (Isobel, 2021). Instead, it appeared a consequence of the techniques implemented at the outset to maximize participant safety and trust, and a willingness among athletes to disclose highly sensitive information to the researcher.

Before interviews took place, as noted earlier, these techniques included paying particular attention to the safety and confidentiality of the settings or environments in which interviews were held (Alessi & Kahn, 2023; Edelman, 2023; Isobel, 2021). Being clear about the focus of the research (e.g., outlining the topics to be discussed in advance), being predictable in one's actions in relation to constant consent-checking and choice (e.g., about what or what not to say), and verbally emphasizing the importance of interviewees' voices and stories (Edelman, 2023; Isobel, 2021; Newman et al., 2006), were also important in reassuring athletes about what would happen, why, and how. Designing questions which were semi-structured in nature to ensure coverage of particular themes while providing sufficient flexibility for interviewees to address the nuances of their lived experience does, of course, risk re-traumatization of participants. However, it was *how* and *when* they were asked which appeared to matter. Being "adequately prepared to make circumstantial decisions about whether to ask certain questions" (Isobel, 2021, p. 1462) after revelations of often widespread, but individually felt, traumatic experiences, and focusing on how athletes negotiated these, were important in facilitating safety.

During interviews, it was essential to address the power relations which are typically skewed in favour of the researcher, rather than participant, and can replicate features of traumatic experiences. To help mitigate this, and maximize relational safety, the researcher continually reminded athletes that the intention was to understand the nature and complexity of their experiences rather than to judge them (Alessi & Kahn, 2023; Reeves, 2015; Sweeney et al., 2018; Tunno et al., 2021). Formally recognizing the sensitive and distressing nature of athletes' experiences, inviting interviewees to return to the line of questioning at a later stage, and encouraging pauses using simple grounding techniques (e.g., having a drink) were also used to promote athlete safety and agency (Edelman, 2023; Isobel, 2021). Observing and responding to non-verbal cues during interviews also appeared helpful in minimizing distress and the potential for secondary traumatization through unintentionally reinforcing feelings of shame, embarrassment, and stigma. These cues included changed body language (e.g., fidgeting, nail biting, freezing), facial expression (including signs of crying or anxiety), and signs of disassociation (e.g., sudden changes in mood) (Alessi & Kahn, 2023; Isobel, 2021; Reeves, 2015; Tunno et al., 2021). Ending interviews with questions relating to positive, rather distressing, experiences was also deliberately intended to focus athletes' attention on how they successfully navigated any instances of trauma (Alessi & Kahn, 2023; Edelman, 2023; Isobel, 2021). Indeed, Alessi and Kahn (2023, p. 146) argue "it is the responsibility of the qualitative researcher to leave participants feeling empowered, not broken or overly exposed by the time the interview … winds down."

Once interviews were completed, athletes were encouraged to share any further unstructured thoughts, reminded of the availability of relevant developmentally sensitive services to support their immediate and continued safety (Tunno et al., 2021), and reassured about how, where, and why their information will be used (Edelman, 2023; Isobel, 2021). Invitations to check-in with them after a few days were also provided, as were the researcher's contact details, should they wish to follow anything up. While these are common research practices, "through a TI [trauma-informed] lens they allow for a return to the present, validation of feelings of uncertainty and transparency of processes that reinforces the protection of their words and experiences" (Isobel, 2021, p. 1464).

Self-Safety

Earlier I recalled how completing this research evoked sleeping memories of former trauma histories related to mental health, and that much of this was experienced once the research had been completed, but occasionally after particularly challenging interviews. It also impacted my post-research mental health. On reflection, having a more effective framework in place for self-care throughout the research process was, and is, important to help prevent traumatization, compassion fatigue, and vicarious trauma (Alessi & Kahn, 2023; Newman et al., 2006). A self-care framework can also support researchers' vicarious post-traumatic growth (Berger, 2021). In this regard, Brackenridge's (1999) self-management framework, developed in response to the many demands her ground-breaking work on sexual abuse in sport had on her well-being, is a useful starting point. She identifies three overlapping matters relevant to trauma-informed qualitative research. First, *managing* myself recognizes the many impacts sensitive research can have on researchers. Further, how these can and need to be managed depends on the self-identification of strategies which researchers feel will best support them in their particular research context, in my case, mental health and sport. Second, managing *(by) myself* refers to the often highly individualized nature of one's research, which for Brackenridge was compounded by the lack of collaborators working in the field. This was true to an extent when I was conducting my research, but the fact that the memories reawakened were then known primarily to myself exacerbate feelings of isolation and re-traumatization. Working in teams, sharing concerns, joint supervision, and identified opportunities for regular review, reflection, and discussion with support networks are among the strategies that may assist trauma researchers when conducting similar research (Berger, 2021; Isobel, 2021; Jefferson et al., 2021). The third strategy identified by Brackenridge is managing my*self/selves*, which refers to ways of balancing one's personal, political, and scientific self. Brackenridge (1999) benefitted from the involvement of a trained counsellor/friend who routinely reminded her of the central goal of the research; namely, its scientific one of advancing understanding in the field. Other personal and political motivations are important, including when the researcher – as I did – felt the need to respond to questions about one's own research expertise and credibility, and requests to reveal details of findings and study participants (Brackenridge, 1999). Difficult as that can be, remaining focused on the advancement of scientific understanding which provides a more secure basis on which more effective policy and organizational change can be made, should remain uppermost in one's mind (Brackenridge, 1999).

Cultural, Historical, and Gender Issues

According to Sweeney et al. (2018, p. 323), researchers need to adopt a broad-based understanding of trauma which accounts for "community, social, cultural and historical traumas such as racism, poverty, colonialism, disability, homophobia and sexism and their intersectionality." Trauma-informed qualitative research involving in-depth semi-structured interviews should thus be interviewee-centred and individualized, but also culturally and situationally specific, if survivors' engagement in it is to be maximized and as beneficial as possible (Isobel, 2021; Jefferson et al., 2021; Reeves, 2015; Sweeney et al., 2018). In this study, the researcher sought to fully account for the intersectional characteristics of interviewees' lives and how the multiple traumas athletes recalled interrelated with other social determinants of health, especially mental health. This consideration involved encouraging interviewees to explore the cultural language, values, norms, ideologies, and behaviours which existed in their respective sports, and how these shaped their lived experience and related trauma. However, recognizing the differential experiences interviewees had of their life worlds, including traumatic life events and symptoms in their working and personal lives, was challenging. What was traumatic to one person was not necessarily traumatic to another (SAMHSA, 2014). It was therefore necessary to explore different perspectives, voices, and experiences which characterized athletes' power relations during the interviews, as well as how athletes were positioned – and positioned themselves – in multiple categories (e.g., as an athlete, as ill, as a woman, as a partner) simultaneously (Isobel, 2021). This exploration was important, and being intersectional in one's approach is "inherently TI" because it considers "the relations of power that affect people across their lives and influence their experiences" (Isobel, 2021, p. 1465). In this study, these power relations were explored through agreed lines of interview questioning, and relevant case studies of participants' experiences using autobiographical accounts or media interviews (McMahon et al., 2022; Smith, 2019), to stimulate non-stigmatizing conversations and reflections about the lived realities of athletes' diverse sporting and cultural contexts. This approach emerged out of a concern with finding out as much as possible about athletes' lives before the interviews, but it can also be beneficial for establishing whether participants have "encountered interpersonal, historical, or stigma-related traumas" (Alessi & Kahn, 2023, p. 137).

Given the significance of intersectionality for trauma research, it is important that this and cultural competence (i.e., being aware of, and respecting, others' cultural values, beliefs, and practices) is embedded throughout all stages of the research process, from sample recruitment through to project design, data analysis, and dissemination (Edelman, 2023; Jefferson et al., 2021). Although it was difficult to recruit a diverse sample of interviewees (particularly for gender, ethnicity, and race) in this study, wherever possible qualitative researchers should endeavour to be as culturally competent as possible by recruiting participants and interviewers with diverse experiences and identity characteristics, particularly where social justice and inequality are central concerns (Edelman, 2023). Ensuring "research contexts are culturally appropriate in supporting participation, minimising re-traumatisation, and promoting resilience" (Edelman, 2023, p. 73) is also important for enhancing cultural safety (i.e., safeguarding the well-being of others who may have different cultural values, beliefs, and practices) and ensuring cultural variation in trauma research (Jefferson et al., 2021). Recognizing that safety is socially and structurally produced, and that "oppression and cultural, historical, racial, and systemic trauma may affect participants' ability to safely and comfortably engage" (Jefferson et al., 2021, p. 7) in trauma research, also requires diverse culturally acceptable forms of local support to be identified for participants even if they do not engage in the research (Jefferson et al., 2021). This recognition is important not only for developing more inclusive and participatory approaches to co-produced research. It is also practically important because it can help researchers avoid "intervention-generated inequality" (Edelman, 2023, p. 67) where "health inequalities are worsened when interventions are inadvertently developed to be most inclusive of those facing least adversity" (Edelman, 2023, p. 67) from trauma and other social problems. Using interviewers of the same gender and cultural background (e.g., sport, country) who can draw upon relevant culturally specific language during interviews might thus be one effective strategy worth considering (McMahon et al., 2022).

Conclusions

The trauma-informed principles for qualitative research enabled trauma survivors to recount their experiences in safe and supportive ways. In closing, I have three key future research directions which readers might wish to consider:

1 Qualitative research with diverse groups of trauma survivors might include interview-based investigations (including in-depth semi-structured, narrative, or unstructured interviews) which incorporate case studies of media interviews and publicly circulated stories, or other cultural artefacts including autobiographical extracts (McMahon et al., 2022; Smith, 2019), to enable participants to share (in-person or online) their lived experiences and stories of trauma. Qualitative research which prioritizes the voices and trauma histories of sports workers (e.g., athletes, coaches, support staff, volunteers) is also needed across all levels of sport (from community/recreational to elite and professional sport), particularly as part of equitable experientially informed approaches to co-production of trauma research.
2 Ongoing evaluations of trauma-informed policies and practices (e.g., education programmes) implemented in sport are also needed to ensure they are effective, not doing harm, and remain appropriate to participant need (McMahon et al., 2022). This focus includes research on "provider perceptions of trauma-informed care and the efficacy of trauma-informed interventions [which] can establish the most feasible and effective ways

to implement changes to practice" (Reeves, 2015, pp. 707–708). Indeed, while there is "no one-size-fits-all" policy and set of approaches, there will likely be many challenges in the universal implementation of trauma-informed practices in sports organizations. Such an approach is necessary to "ensure that the unique needs of trauma survivors as patients are met, and mitigate barriers to care and health disparities experienced by this vulnerable population" (Reeves, 2015, p. 708). However, also important are the development of critiques of existing policies and place-based practices, including through discourse or narrative analysis, and the implications of those critiques for developing more effective trauma-informed practices.

3 Finally, more attention needs to be paid to researcher well-being in trauma-informed qualitative research (Alessi & Kahn, 2023; Berger, 2021; Jefferson et al., 2021). Consideration needs to be given to the different types of self-management strategies (e.g., Brackenridge, 1999) which work best to support different groups of researchers, engaging different groups of trauma survivors (directly and indirectly), with different kinds of experiences, in their work. This should go beyond the minimum standards of ethical practice which typically requires mental health professional support to be available for researchers to access. In particular, given the often complex nature of trauma experiences which can be evoked at any time (often unexpectedly), more specialized support needs to be made available to researchers on an on-going basis for them to access in their preferred ways.

References

Alessi, E. J., & Kahn, S. (2023). Toward a trauma-informed qualitative research approach: Guidelines for ensuring the safety and promoting the resilience of research participants. *Qualitative Research in Psychology, 20*(1), 121–154.

Bellis, M. A., Hughes, K., Leckenby, N., & Lowey, H. (2014). National household survey of adverse childhood experiences and their relationship with resilience to health-harming behaviors in England. *BMC Medicine, 12*, 72.

Berger, R. (2021). Studying trauma: Indirect effects on researchers and self – And strategies for addressing them. *European Journal of Trauma and Disassociation, 5*, 100149.

Brackenridge, C. (1999). Managing myself: Investigator survival in sensitive research. *International Review for the Sociology of Sport, 34*(4), 399–410.

Edelman, N. (2023). Trauma and resilience informed research principles and practice: A framework to improve the inclusion and experience of disadvantaged populations in health and social care research. *Journal of Health Services Research & Policy, 28*(1), 66–75.

Emsley, E., Smith, J., Martin, D., & Lewis, N. (2022). Trauma-informed care in the UK: Where are we? A qualitative study of health policies and professional perspectives. *BMC Health Services Research, 22*, 1164.

Felitti, V. J., Anda, R. F., Nordenberg, D., Williamson, D. F., Spitz, A. M., Edwards, V., Koss, M. P., & Marks, J. S. (1998). Relationship of childhood abuse and household dysfunction to many of the leading causes of death in adults. *The Adverse Childhood Experiences (ACE) Study. The American Journal of Preventive Medicine, 14*(4), 245–258.

Isobel, S. (2021). Trauma-informed qualitative research: Some methodological and practical considerations. *International Journal of Mental Health Nursing, 30*(S1), 1456–1469.

Jefferson, K., Stanhope, K. K., Jones-Harrell, C., Vester, A., Tyano, E., & Hall, C. D. X. (2021). A scoping review of recommendations in the English language on conducting research with trauma-exposed populations since publication of the Belmont report; Thematic review of existing recommendations on research with trauma-exposed populations. *PLoS ONE, 16*(7), e0254003. https://doi.org/10.1371/journal.pone.0254003

McMahon, J., McGannon, K. R., Zehntner, C., Werbicki, L., Stephenson, E., & Martin, K. (2022). Trauma-informed abuse education in sport: Engaging athlete abuse survivors as educators and facilitating a community of care. *Sport, Education and Society*. https://doi.org/10.1080/13573322.2022.2096586

Mills, C. W. (2000). *The sociological imagination*. Oxford University Press.

Miralles, M., Lee, B., & Dörfler, V. (2022). Guest editorial: Investigating trauma: Methodological, emotional and ethical challenges for the qualitative researcher. *Qualitative Research in Organizations and Management: An International Journal, 17*(4), 397–405.

Mountjoy, M., Vertommen, T., Denhollander, R., Kennedy, S., & Majoor, R. (2022). Effective engagement of survivors of harassment and abuse in sport in athlete safeguarding initiatives: A review and a conceptual framework. *British Journal of Sports Medicine, 56*(4), 232–238.

Newman, E., Risch, E., & Kassam-Adams, N. (2006). Ethical issues in trauma-related research: A review. *Journal of Empirical Research on Human Research Ethics, 1*(3), 29–46.

Purcell, R., Henderson, J., Tamminen, K. A., Frost, J., Gwyther, K., Kerr, G., Kim, J., Pilkington, V., Rice, S. M., & Walton, C. (2023). Starting young to protect elite athletes' mental health. *British Journal of Sports Medicine, 57*(8), 439–440.

Reardon, C., Hainline, B., Aron, C. M., Baron, D., Baum, A. L., Bindra, A., Budgett, R., Campriani, N., Castaldelli-Maia, J. M., Currie, A., Derevensky, J. L., Glick, I. D., Gorczynski, P., Gouttebarge, V., Grandner, M. A., Han, D. H., McDuff, D., Mountjoy, M., Polat, A., … Engebretsen, L. (2019). Mental health in elite athletes: International Olympic Committee consensus statement (2019). *British Journal of Sports Medicine, 53*(11), 667–699.

Reeves, E. (2015). A synthesis of the literature on trauma-informed care. *Issues in Mental Health Nursing, 36*(9), 698–709.

Rice, S., Purcell, R., DeSilva, S., Mawren, D., McGorry, P., & McGrath, A. (2016). The mental health of elite athletes: A narrative systematic review. *Sports Medicine, 46*(9), 1333–1353.

Roderick, M., & Allen Collinson, J. (2020). 'I just want to be left alone': Novel sociological insights into dramaturgical demands on professional athletes. *Sociology of Sport Journal, 37*(2), 108–116.

Roderick, M., Smith, A., & Potrac, P. (2017). The sociology of sports work, emotions and mental health: Scoping the field and future directions. *Sociology of Sport Journal, 34*(2), 99–107.

Smith, A. (2019). Depression and suicide in professional sport. In M. Atkinson (Ed.), *Sport, mental illness, and sociology* (pp. 79–96). Emerald.

Smith, A. (2023). Sport, youth, and elite development. In L. Wenner (Ed.), *The Oxford handbook of sport and society* (pp. 637–653). Oxford University Press.

Smith, B., Williams, O., Bone, L., & the Moving Social Work Coproduction Collective (2023). Co-production: A resource to guide co-producing research in the sport, exercise, and health sciences. *Qualitative Research in Sport, Exercise and Health, 15*(2), 159–187.

Substance Abuse and Mental Health Services Administration (SAMHSA). (2014). *SAMHSA's concept of trauma and guidance for a trauma-informed approach.* SAMHSA.

Sweeney, A., Filson, B., Kennedy, A., Collinson, L., & Gillard, S. (2018). A paradigm shift: Relationships in trauma-informed mental health services. *BJPsych Advances, 24*, 319–333.

Tunno, A. M., Inscoe, A. B., Goldston, D. B., & Asarnow, J. R. (2021). A trauma-informed approach to youth suicide prevention and intervention. *Evidence-Based Practice in Child and Adolescent Mental Health, 6*(3), 316–327.

Walton, C., Rice, S., Hutter, V., Currie, A., Readon, C., & Prucell, R. (2021). Mental health in youth athletes: A clinical review. *Advances in Psychiatry and Behavioral Health, 1*(1), 119–133.

Chapter 7

Embracing Trauma-Informed Practices in Athlete Disordered Eating Research

Anthony Papathomas, Maria Luisa Pereira Vargas, and Erin Prior

Introduction

Athlete disordered eating, which spans unhealthy eating attitudes and behaviours to clinical eating disorders, is prevalent across a range of sports (de Bruin, 2017). Based on the premise that weight is indirectly proportional to performance, athletes engage in stringent, and sometimes extreme dieting behaviours in the name of athletic success. Some sport cultures condone and promote dangerous eating practices to the point that obsessive dietary control is *expected* of athletes (Papathomas, 2018). The literature is replete with stories of coaches fanatically monitoring athlete weight and body fat (e.g., McGannon & McMahon, 2019; McMahon et al., 2012), and shaming them into further weight loss through derogatory comments about appearance (e.g., Papathomas & Lavallee, 2010). Against this backdrop, disordered eating represents a practice that most athletes *must* do to succeed. This chapter challenges this normalisation of athlete disordered eating and draws on our own published qualitative data to argue that in extreme cases it can be a form of psychological trauma. Reflecting on our own research practices, we critically inspect how our preferred methodologies and methods negotiated traumatic eating disorder experiences and the impact on researcher and participant. Finally, we explore the ways trauma-informed research practices can better serve athletes with disordered eating experiences and those who support them to ensure re-traumatisation is limited.

Is Disordered Eating a Form of Trauma?

Eating disorders, at the extreme end of the disordered eating continuum, are severe, persistent, debilitating mental illnesses that ravage the minds and bodies of those who live with them. Anorexia nervosa, for example, involves an intense fear of weight gain and extreme self-starvation, both of which occur in the face of dangerously low body weight (American Psychiatric Association [APA], 2022). Without intervention, the body's organs will shut down and anorexia nervosa remains one of the deadliest mental illnesses despite the

DOI: 10.4324/9781003332909-9

young age of most patients (Mehler et al., 2022). Bulimia nervosa is broadly characterised by regular repeat binge-purge cycles, whereby vast and contextually inappropriate quantities of food are hurriedly consumed before being expelled from the body, often through self-induced vomiting (APA, 2022). Although bulimia is less life-threatening than anorexia nervosa, bingeing can lead to intolerable feelings of guilt, shame, and self-loathing (Davis et al., 2022). Across both these eating disorder types, comorbidities include depression, anxiety, and substance abuse (Keski-Rahkonen & Mustelin, 2016). There is also an increased prevalence of self-harm, suicide ideation, and suicide attempts (Sohn et al., 2023). These brutal outcomes point to an experience that is overtly traumatic rather than normative.

Trauma is often a precursor to eating pathology and these potentially causal events cannot be divorced from the wider eating disorder experience. For example, many individuals living with an eating disorder are also survivors of childhood sexual abuse, physical abuse, and emotional abuse (Caslini et al., 2016). Up to a quarter of eating disorder patients also experience posttraumatic stress disorder, a comorbidity that intensifies the severity of eating disorder symptoms (Rijkers et al., 2019). The link is hypothesised to occur because eating disorder behaviours, such as self-starvation, bingeing, and purging, have a strong capacity to help individuals escape trauma-related thoughts and emotions (Trottier & MacDonald, 2017). Whether as a cause or a consequence, trauma is, seemingly, inextricably linked to the eating disorder experience. It is a link that led Brewerton (2019) to call for more *trauma-informed care and practice* in the treatment of eating disorders as a root to better treatment adherence and outcomes. This call should extend to research contexts, particularly researchers who work with people experiencing eating disorders where trauma often prevails.

Athlete Eating Disorders as Trauma

Although most athlete disordered eating experiences are subclinical, cases of clinically severe athlete eating disorders may include trauma. In this section, I (the first author) draw on my own qualitative research to illustrate that trauma can, and does, envelop the lives of athletes living with eating disorders. Specifically, I refer to three single-participant studies informed by life history and narrative approaches to research (i.e., Papathomas & Lavallee, 2006; Papathomas & Lavallee, 2012b; Papathomas & Lavallee, 2014). Each study involved repeated face-to-face interviews with an athlete, taking place over several weeks, and amassing between 6 and 11 hours of data. The extensive time spent on one person's experience enabled interviews to move at a slower pace, digressions to be encouraged and followed up on, and the fullness of life to be explored and made sense of. This type of research can deliver contextually rich data that supports revisiting through a fresh trauma-informed lens (Riessman, 2008).

My first foray into athlete eating disorder research was my Master's thesis, a life history study of Mike, a male soccer player living with bulimia nervosa (Papathomas & Lavallee, 2006). Prior to submitting the manuscript to the Journal of Loss and Trauma, I pondered whether it was a suitable outlet; was this about trauma? I had interviewed a close friend in this study, a friend I felt I already knew well, and his was not a life I deemed traumatised, at least not in the clinical sense. The term features in the paper, but often erroneously as a synonym for a difficult event: "in what was a hugely traumatic experience, he visited his doctor and was put on a nine-month waiting list (for cognitive behavioural therapy)" (p. 164). The visit to the doctor was deeply stigmatising for Mike but "hugely traumatic" does a disservice to genuine trauma and it is not a term I would choose again. On the other hand, some of the data within the article suggests elements of trauma defined his experience:

> Life became a real uphill struggle to the point when it crossed my mind that I've got this forever and it's going to get the better of me and this might be, ultimately, what is the end of me.
>
> (Papathomas & Lavallee, 2006, p. 147)

Although no overt reference to trauma is made in the above example, Mike's suggestion that his eating disorder might be what is "the end of me" perhaps hints at the high mortality rates in eating disorders or even the prevalence of suicide ideation in this population. I did not seek to clarify this at the time, however. The *friendship as method* approach presents many benefits, but it may also have limitations; for some researchers, it may be difficult to probe trauma in people they are close to. In this example, could I have probed for clarification on what Mike meant by "the end of me"? Had a more trauma-informed approach been used at the time, I may have been more prepared to see, manage, and explore declarations that hint at sensitive topics like suicide.

The second single-participant study explored the experiences of Beth, a competitive tennis player with experiences of anorexia nervosa (Papathomas & Lavallee, 2012b). Around our third interview, Beth disclosed she had been groomed and sexually abused by her tennis coach for several years. Although she offered numerous competing explanations for her eating disorder, Beth connected it to her abuse in the following extract:

> It was because I hadn't told my parents about what had happened, you know, with the abuse issue and I thought they'd disown me so I thought that if I made myself really ill and then they found out (about the abuse) then maybe they wouldn't hate me so much or they'd see how much I was suffering.
>
> (Papathomas & Lavallee, 2012b, p. 310)

Beth's story was a story about shame, stigma, self-blame, confusion, and anger. It was a difficult story to hear, and this particular interview with her was much shorter than those before and those after.

As a researcher interested in athlete eating disorders, my focus centred on weight loss for performance gains, and I was not ready for a story about sexual abuse, despite the established links between abuse and eating disorders. I can vividly remember Beth asking me: "have I disgusted you?" My reaction to her experience potentially contributed to her feelings of shame. Thankfully, as we were early in the research process, with several more hours of conversation to come, I was able to reassure Beth that although I *was* disgusted by the actions of a sexual abuser, I was not disgusted with her. The extra time also allowed me to prepare for discussing such sensitive content and to support Beth to continue to tell her story.

In the final example of athlete eating disorders and trauma, I interviewed Holly who played elite basketball and continued to self-starve at the time of interviews. Holly described a childhood where she felt bullied by a schoolteacher and alienated by her parents. For Holly, nothing was enough to meet the perceived expectations of the adults around her. She alluded to barely communicating with her family for long periods of time and to experiencing depression as well as disordered eating. Neglect is a recognised form of abuse, but it was not clear whether this is what had occurred for her. At the time, it was not something I sought to explore further as part of my research process into disordered eating in sport. So, although Holly's experiences may well have been traumatic, my conversations with her, and later, my analysis and writing, were not alert to this. This speaks to the need to approach research into disordered eating in sport, and mental health more generally, through a trauma-informed lens. Specifically, evidence-based trauma-informed research practices ensure that participant trauma is more likely to be heard, witnessed, supported, and documented. This is not to say that narrative approaches cannot be effective in researching trauma, but rather that they are not inherently designed for such a purpose. The hallmarks of quality narrative inquiry align with many trauma-informed research principles, and the two approaches are perfectly compatible. The following section identifies how the narrative tradition and associated methods can support the delivery of trauma-informed research.

Narrative and Trauma: Methodological and Ethical Considerations

Within this section we define narrative inquiry and its fundamental tenets, before considering its potential benefits when researching with athletes experiencing trauma. We also suggest ways narrative research can support others to learn more about the trauma associated with athlete disordered eating. We also reflect on ethical concerns that arise when seeking to research trauma from a narrative perspective.

What Is Narrative Inquiry?

Narrative inquiry involves collecting and analysing stories, which are considered the primary way in which life is made meaningful (Polkinghorne, 1988). Personal stories about life events offer rich context, deep subjectivity, and explanations imbued with meaning (Papathomas, 2016). People engage in a creative process of *emplotment* – organising life events into an order that makes sense to them (Ricoeur, 1984). These stories are personal but always collaboratively formed through interactions with others (e.g., family, friends, researchers), thereby providing insight into a teller's social and cultural worlds (Smith, 2010). Stories are also performative and identity constituting; we tell stories that communicate particular facets of who we are and/ or would like to be; as well as silencing stories that misalign with a sense of self (McAdams, 2018). To this end, although abstract and subject to constant revision, we live by the stories we tell, they guide our thoughts, feelings, and motives (Holstein & Gubrium, 2000). Overall, narrative approaches to research foreground experiential meaning, how that meaning is constructed, and its implications for identity and action. Narrative research sensitises to the needs of participants, delivering narrative opportunities (Papathomas & Lavallee, 2012a, 2012b), and *witnessing* their testimonies (Frank, 1995). Narrative research often prioritises marginalised communities and can serve as activism for social justice, including for those living with mental illness. For these reasons, narrative inquiry and the methods used within it, hold great potential to impact research into trauma and to serve those who live with it.

Narrative Research in Action

Doing good narrative inquiry requires an underpinning commitment to the importance of narratives to human life (Papathomas, 2016). Narratives provide templates with which to organise life events into a coherent story; thereby giving meaning to the events we live through. When events are traumatic, our capacity to make sense through story can be life-changing, or even lifesaving (Papathomas & Lavallee, 2012b). A narrative scholar researching trauma must design their study according to the collection of participant stories. Reviewed literature, research questions, recruitment strategy, chosen methods, and analysis must be informed by the foundational assumption that stories of trauma impact the thoughts, feelings, and actions of the traumatised. From a literature standpoint, it is important to explore literature beyond dominant medical perspectives on trauma to embracing text that deliver compassionate, person-focused, experiential accounts. This exploration will ensure the research focus is not tokenistic, a mere nod to personal stories within the strict framework of the medical model. Appropriately engaging with wider trauma literature will also ensure that research questions are appropriately grounded in the needs of participants who live with trauma. Questions might address the types of stories participants tell about trauma, how these stories are co-constructed within social and cultural interactions, and the ways stories work for or against the teller. Storytelling methods might embrace dominant forms such as semi-structured or unstructured interviews, but also alternative approaches such as life writing, creative writing, and visual storytelling. Choice with regard to how trauma is told by the participant is indeed one of the six trauma-informed principles outlined by SAMHSA (2014a). From an analysis standpoint, the story structure and performance, that is the mechanics of how it is put together and the way it is delivered for others, can provide insights into how trauma is constructed and reproduced, and may even prompt ideas as to how it may be overcome. These considerations, across all phases of the research process, ensure a methodologically and philosophically coherent study that honours stories of trauma and the participants who tell them.

Narrative Inquiry: Trauma-Informed Benefits

Those with experiences of trauma have had their voices silenced and diminished (SAMHSA, 2014a). Narrative methodologies can provide participants with the agency and autonomy to tell their stories. For example, narrative or life story interviewing places a great emphasis on the autonomy of participants to "tell it in their own words" (Riessman, 2008). A narrative opportunity is an opportunity to provide a means for identity reconstruction and renewed understandings of the self (i.e., the trauma-informed principle of empowerment). For example, returning to Holly (Papathomas & Lavallee, 2014), the research experience, re-reading transcripts, allowed her to reflect on the focus of her life: "I start seeing trends when I'm speaking, like I talk about obviously achieving and failing a lot and I think that definitely linked with how I felt about myself" (p. 691). Similarly, Beth's story (Papathomas & Lavallee, 2012b) offers an example of how narrating trauma may lead to new insights for the participant with therapeutic implications. Discussing the impact of telling others of her sexual abuse by a tennis coach, Beth stated:

> I've been more open with some people about it and I've managed to tell a couple of people, and you as well, and in doing that I've kind of realized people's reactions and the fact, OK well it was weird of him and it was wrong and I wasn't to blame. That's helped me so much.
> (Papathomas & Lavallee, 2014, p. 305)

For Beth, seeing a negative response to her story about her abuser's actions helped reinforce that he was the perpetrator of a crime against a child and that she did nothing wrong; an important step towards adjusting to the trauma of abuse (Feiring & Cleland, 2007).

Using Narrative to Promote Learning

Narrative analysis has great potential for assisting others to learn more about trauma by placing meaning and context at the centre of insights in contrast to dominant approaches which present an exclusive symptom focus. For example, returning to Beth's story (Papathomas & Lavallee, 2012b), the uncertainty associated with many of her narrative explanations show us that abuse and anorexia are difficult experiences to integrate into a life story and therefore difficult to make sense of. These insights were only made possible through acknowledging the storied experiences of these athletes and embracing how people make sense of their experiences within their social world. Narrative is a useful tool for others to learn more about how, and if, people make sense of trauma (Winning, 2020). These others can include mental health practitioners, sporting organisations, and other athletes with similar experiences with trauma who perhaps do not see their experiences reflected elsewhere.

Narrative research also holds great potential as an educational tool about trauma through varied storied forms, such as visual narratives through art and illustrated stories (e.g., Busanich et al., 2016) or creative non-fictions in the form of composite vignettes (e.g., Cavallerio, 2021; McGannon & McMahon, 2022). Visual narratives can allow explorations into visuals that tell stories, whilst creative non-fiction practices such as composite vignettes contain a range of different experiences from various people fused together into one single story (Spalding & Phillips, 2007). These accessible representations of experience can help overcome the taboo of trauma in sport, a subculture where vulnerability is downplayed, and tales of toughness dominate (Papathomas, 2018). Narrative's immersive qualities make it capable of bringing forth these silenced stories, so that others can be educated of the experiences portrayed within them. For example, McMahon (2013) presented coaches with athlete stories of abuse, with the aim of challenging coach practices in the short and long term. Douglas and Carless (2008) used written stories and poems to communicate to coaches about various athlete experiences of elite golf. On hearing these stories, coaches were prompted to engage in reflective practice about their own coaching activities. These works highlight the value of narrative as a potential educative tool resulting in social change by engaging audiences, eliciting emotional responses, and ultimately educating people about trauma in sport.

Towards Trauma-Informed Athlete Eating Disorder Research

We now discuss examples of where trauma-informed principles feature in our narrative research on disordered eating in sport. We make specific reference to the principles of Safety, Empowerment, Voice and Choice, and Trustworthiness and Transparency (SAMHSA, 2014a). We also argue for the development of a body of work into athlete eating disorders that explicitly adheres to these principles and embraces trauma-informed practices as a guide to all elements of the research process.

Establishing Safety in Research Processes

Those who participate in research who have experienced trauma or mental illness are considered a "vulnerable" population (Seedat et al., 2004). Although, vulnerable is a contested term – those considered vulnerable may not view themselves as vulnerable (Wilson & Neville, 2009). Therefore, researcher practice must be trauma-informed and sensitive to participant vulnerability and work to ensure safety. Institutional ethical guidelines, which focus on whether vulnerable groups are at risk of being harmed by the processes in a study, may not go far enough in this regard. Rigid, pre-prescribed processes that seek to standardise safety cannot always account for unexpected harms that can arise during participation in a research study (Palmer, 2016). Ensuring researcher practice centres on evidence-based trauma-informed principles can ensure the risk of re-traumatisation is limited for the participants. In turn, aspirational ethics can be achieved (e.g., higher than the minimum ethical requirements) (Lahman et al., 2011). Commitment to aspirational ethics requires balancing the interests in the aims of the research, with the obligations towards the care and safety of participants. In our efforts to achieve aspirational ethics, we have noticed many instances of unexpected potential harm required management in the moment. For example, deciding whether to listen to a story about sexual abuse, and later whether to include it in our analysis, despite sexual abuse not featuring in the institutional ethics application (Papathomas & Lavallee, 2012b). In this case, cutting off a participant who had chosen to open up about a personal trauma was considered more harmful than allowing them to relay the story and potentially revisit painful memories (Palmer, 2016). Even with hindsight, it is difficult to be certain the correct decision was made, but the participant did express the benefits of having told her story in later interviews. What is more certain, a deep knowledge and appreciation of the core trauma-informed principles could have facilitated making a good (ethical) decision at the time (Bath, 2008; SAMHSA, 2014a, 2014b). Balancing ideas of empowerment (the participant controlling how the story is told) versus notions of participant safety (what is the psychosocial impact of telling trauma?) is trauma-informed ethical work.

We have primarily used interviews as the main data collection tool to explore athlete disordered eating and found the pre-planning of interviews to be an important step in commitment to athlete safety. Ensuring the questions asked are open and able to provide narrative opportunities is a necessary component of this (see Empowerment, voice, and choice section below). We also must consider *how* questions are asked and how we respond. In line with recommendations by Isobel (2021a), it is important that the research team is knowledgeable concerning eating disorders in sport and that this knowledge is used to respond appropriately during interviews. In terms of our research specifically, this would involve having a good prior understanding to athlete eating disorders, which presents nuanced experiential differences to eating disorder experiences in the general population (Papathomas & Lavallee, 2010). Regardless of the precautions taken and the knowledge possessed, athletes still may become severely distressed during the interview and later. It is important that researchers are prepared to assist participants in these situations (Palmer, 2016). For instance, in our experiences, we have had to be constantly prepared to make circumstantial decisions about whether to ask certain questions, allow a participant to continue discussing a sensitive topic, or encourage participants to expand on a topic, as well as whether to discontinue an interview (Isobel, 2021b; Jones, 1998).

Without knowledge or experience of how trauma may impact people and their social interactions, there is a risk of re-traumatising participants (SAMHSA, 2014a). Further, researchers may avoid asking certain questions due to worries about causing participants further distress, which can result in superficial data (Alessi & Kahn, 2023). Therefore, we recognise that those with less experience in conducting research with vulnerable populations need to be adequately supported by an experienced member of the research team who has trauma knowledge. For example, in our dynamic of working as part of a research team, the first author (an experienced senior academic researcher) provided constant feedback and support to the second and third authors (early career researchers) in their PhDs exploring athlete mental illness by looking over transcripts to ensure open-ended appropriate questions, encouraging further reading into the topic area to develop knowledge, looking over transcripts and opportunities to de-brief post-interviews. These processes not only ensured safety of participants by ensuring researchers are capable to ask appropriate questions and respond adequately to avoid harm to participants, but also that researchers are adequately prepared and supported to explore potentially upsetting topics. By considering how to keep athletes we interview safe, we served as active listeners, able to evoke stories of experience with thoughtful questioning and by providing a comfortable environment for participants (Bath, 2008).

Enhancing Participants' Empowerment, Voice, and Choice

Speaking to others is known to help people make sense of their experiences (Sandick, 2012) and gather new meanings from past experiences (Hirsch, 2020), with narrative interviews considered a particularly useful tool in this regard (Papathomas & Lavallee, 2012b). Although the resurfacing of difficult emotions is not entirely avoidable when discussing sensitive topics (see Kavanagh et al., 2017), participants can be appreciative of the opportunity to share their experiences and find value in sharing their stories (Stirling &

Kerr, 2009). Therefore, by working in a trauma-informed way as researchers, to establish safe, comfortable environments and offer opportunities for connection (see Bath, 2008), participants can feel empowered when sharing their stories. As such, researchers should ask open questions that encourage storytelling. This approach to research not only aims to avoid further harm but strives to provide a beneficial experience for participants.

Conducting trauma-informed research requires the recognition that participants may have experienced trauma and carefully considering the tensions that exist between protecting and empowering participants (Giorgio, 2013). As mentioned in the section above, ethical considerations centre around whether individuals are at risk of being harmed by participating in a study (Isobel, 2021b). Although these protections are important, there is a risk of disempowering individuals by assuming vulnerability and neglecting to recognise a person's agency in choosing whether to participate in research. A trauma-informed qualitative researcher should recognise the autonomy of participants and the need for choice and empowerment (Harris & Fallot, 2001). Therefore, it is not necessary to completely avoid any topic that may be distressing to participants, as a trauma-informed approach assumes individuals have control over what they choose to share and what they do not (Isobel, 2021b). The role of the researcher is to enact in a trauma-informed way, such that participants can feel able to share or not share aspects of their stories.

Traumatic experiences that have a lasting impact may result in feelings of powerlessness (Yatchmenoff et al., 2017). Therefore, an important aspect of trauma-informed research is avoiding re-inducing this experience and instead implementing practices and procedures that restore power. Although it comes with challenges and barriers, co-production offers the potential for many benefits, one of which being the empowerment of individuals who choose to share their stories through research (Smith et al., 2023). Co-production disrupts the structural inequities between researcher and participant – an important goal when working with individuals disempowered by trauma (Isobel, 2021a). Through co-production, participants can draw upon their experiences to meaningfully inform, influence, or lead the direction of research projects (Smith et al., 2023). This approach may present different ways of exploring eating disorders in sport as participants with lived experience can identify research priorities and questions that are relevant, timely and meaningful to them. Therefore, a trauma-informed approach to research perhaps contrasts with the typical research process where researchers – who may be somewhat detached from certain issues – determine the direction of research projects (Smith et al., 2023).

Although there can be benefits to sharing experiences surrounding mental health, there can often also be consequences to not disclosing mental health concerns. For example, athletes not disclosing eating disorders may feel the burden of secrecy (Pettersen et al., 2008), avoid seeking appropriate professional help (Hepworth & Paxton, 2007), and experience a lack of social support (Papathomas & Lavallee, 2010). By not sharing their experiences, athletes may also be deprived of an opportunity to make sense of their lives and identities. Therefore, researchers are implored to engage with trauma-informed approaches to facilitate therapeutic and cathartic opportunities for participants (Pichon et al., 2022).

Striving for Transparency to Build and Maintain Participant Trust

When conducting trauma-informed research, researchers should strive for transparency with the goal of building and maintaining trust with participants (see SAMHSA, 2014a). This practice is fundamental not only to improving participants' experiences of engaging with research but also to produce high-quality qualitative research (Smith et al., 2023). One example of how we have ensured transparency within our research is by sharing the topics that may be discussed with participants prior to data collection. This can involve broadly sharing the topic areas in a participant information form and/or sharing potential interview questions prior to the commencement of interviews so there are no surprises and participants are prepared for the line of questioning that is to come. We have noticed taking these steps can help participants feel more comfortable when engaging in interviews and build a rapport and trust between researcher and participant. This is particularly relevant for those who have experienced an eating disorder, as asking certain questions without warning might shock participants and may risk re-traumatisation.

In further consideration of trust, we have taken advantage of our networks and friendships where pre-existing rapport and trust has already been built, as mentioned in the opening of this chapter (e.g., Papathomas & Lavallee, 2006). Conversations, compassion, and vulnerability unique to friendships can help gain insight into more sensitive and vulnerable topics (Tillmann-Healy, 2003). Our friendships with participants put us in a position where feelings of comfort and trust were heightened, which allowed them to share their stories comfortably. This tool may also ease concerns of power imbalances between a participant and a researcher. A power imbalance is particularly pertinent for those who have experienced trauma, as power imbalances may have previously existed and been exploited leading to the experience of trauma (Alessi & Kahn, 2023). Therefore, utilising friendship as a method may dissipate such inherent imbalances and thus reduce the risk of potential harm and re-traumatisation.

We understand that not all researchers have pre-established connections to participants when exploring trauma. As an alternative, we also encourage the use of narrative research methods and life story/history interviewing which can encourage a rapport, comfort, and trust to be built over time. For instance, in our research, athletes were interviewed over a period of months which aided in rapport and trust to be built with the lead researcher in a way that is more difficult to achieve with a one-off structured interview which launches into topic areas without much lead-in time (e.g., Papath-omas & Lavallee, 2006, 2012a, 2012b, 2014). However, we understand that time-constraints may limit researchers' ability to build rapport in this way. A possible solution is engaging in a short informal interview prior to the main interview, where participants can become accustomed to the interview experience (Papathomas & Lavallee, 2010). This approach further enhances the transparency of the research process and can increase rapport and trust between the participant and the researcher.

Considering the trauma-informed principles of (a) safety, (b) empowerment, voice, and choice, and (c) transparency and trustworthiness, conducting re-search in a trauma-informed way not only benefits participants and minimises the risk of them experiencing re-traumatisation (Isobel, 2021b), but it also provides opportunities to further develop knowledge and insight into eating disorders in sport. Papathomas and Lavallee (2012a, p. 391) make the case that:

> the more athlete accounts available in the literature, the more colour added to our understanding of the many facets of life with an eating dis-order [with] much to learn from the deeply personal, idiosyncratic stories people tell.

Without considering evidence-based trauma-informed principles (SAMHSA, 2014a) and their application to research prior to data collection, researchers may leave themselves feeling unprepared when sensitive topics are discussed. This may result in interviews concluding prematurely; a missed opportunity to hear more about an athlete's eating disorder experience and for them to share their story.

What Is the Relevance of Trauma-Informed Practice to the Applied World?

Much like researchers need to consider their practices when working with those who have experienced trauma, this is also the case for applied prac-titioners. If sporting organisations do not have the knowledge or trauma-informed expertise to engage survivors safely and effectively, they may unintentionally re-traumatise and cause further harm to athletes (Mountjoy & Verhagen, 2022; SAMHSA, 2014a). This compounding of athlete trauma would be at odds with the International Olympic Committee (IOC) con-sensus statement that centralises the notion that all people have a right to engage in sport free from harm (Mountjoy et al., 2016). Therefore, trauma-informed practice must be prioritised, and this needs to be supported by trauma-informed research.

When conducting trauma-informed research with a focus on disordered eating, it is fundamental to consider how to ensure our research can inform applied practice (e.g., the support of athletes with eating disorders). Participant stories have the power to guide professionals towards improved trauma-informed care (Brewerton, 2019). Therefore, by conducting research in a trauma-informed way to encourage the sharing of participant stories, researchers play an important role in informing those who work in applied settings. This may also align with participants' reasons for taking part in the research. In some cases, participants may want to publicly tell their story to researchers to make their experiences available to those who have the ability to affect policy and practice (Owton & Sparkes, 2017). Thus, when presenting findings and proposing recommendations, researchers should consider not only how their trauma-informed work contributes to theoretical knowledge but how it can bridge the research-practice gap and guide those working in applied settings, ensuring athlete experiences can be accessed by those responsible for organisational change.

There is a pressing need to work more cohesively across research, policy, and practice (Prior et al., 2022). Applied practitioners often look to research to provide an evidence-based framework for their own work (Gardner & Moore, 2006). Therefore, researchers adopting a trauma-informed approach to studying athlete eating disorders should communicate trauma-informed best practice to applied practitioners and organisations. For example, reflections may include how a trauma-informed approach provided an environment of "felt safety" by promoting trust and building a connection with an athlete participant (Bath, 2008). Researchers could also share how they understand and attend to the specific needs of individuals who have experienced trauma (i.e., having a safe space without judgement; power in decision-making; a space where they can be heard rather than silenced; a space where fears and emotions can be shared) (see McMahon et al., 2022). By sharing experiences of implementing trauma-informed care guidelines (e.g., Bath, 2008; SAMHSA, 2014a, 2014b) researchers can increase awareness of the impact of trauma and encourage practitioners to consider how they can work in a trauma-informed way.

Finally, Isobel, (2021a) recommend ensuring findings are accessible to the community of people who participate in your research. If athletes with eating disorders can access the stories of others, this may inform their personal narrative, helping them produce new meaning and understand their lives (Papathomas & Lavallee, 2012b). This in turn may help athletes to articulate their own stories and share them with those supporting their mental health. With practitioners gaining insight from trauma-informed research, this goes some way to align them with SAMHSA's four assumptions: that those working with people affected by trauma need to "realise" how widespread trauma is, "recognise" the signs and symptoms of trauma, "respond" by putting theory into practice, and "resist" doing further harm (SAMHSA, 2014a). In sum, researchers should consider how conducting their research in a trauma-informed way can be of benefit to those working within sport and thus, athletes living with eating disorders.

Summary and Conclusions

Trauma is recognised as both a cause and a consequence of eating disorders, yet athlete-focused research is rarely considered through a trauma-informed lens. Although qualitative approaches such as narrative share commonalities with trauma-informed work, an overt grounding in trauma-related concepts is absent. Research into athlete disordered eating therefore stands much to gain from embracing trauma-informed practices. Future research might first consider exploring the experiences of disordered eating athletes who identify as traumatised or living with trauma, thereby improving knowledge of what athletes go through and also fighting against the idea it is a normal part of elite sport. There is value to exploring how such trauma-informed research resonates with applied practitioners and better equips them to manage athlete disordered eating. Finally, reflexive pieces that articulate researcher and participant experiences may illuminate the benefits and challenges of studying athlete disordered eating in a trauma-informed way.

References

Alessi, E. J., & Kahn, S. (2023). Toward a trauma-informed qualitative research approach: Guidelines for ensuring the safety and promoting the resilience of research participants. *Qualitative Research in Psychology, 20*(1), 121–154.

American Psychiatric Association (APA). (2022). *Diagnostic and statistical manual of mental disorders* (5th ed., text rev.). https://doi.org/10.1176/appi.books.9780890 425787

Bath, H. (2008). The three pillars of trauma-informed care. *Reclaiming Children and Youth, 17*(3), 17–21.

Brewerton, T. D. (2019). An overview of trauma-informed care and practice for eating disorders. *Journal of Aggression, Maltreatment & Trauma, 28*(4), 445–462https://doi.org/10.1080/10926771.2018.1532940

Busanich, R., McGannon, K. R., & Schinke, R. J. (2016). Exploring disordered eating and embodiment in male distance runners through visual narrative methods. *Qualitative Research in Sport, Exercise and Health, 8*(1), 95–112.

Caslini, M., Bartoli, F., Crocamo, C., Dakanalis, A., Clerici, M., & Carrà, G. (2016). Disentangling the association between child abuse and eating disorders: A systematic review and meta-analysis. *Psychosomatic Medicine, 78*(1), 79–90.

Cavallerio, F. (Ed.). (2021). *Creative nonfiction in sport and exercise research*. Routledge.

Davis, H. A., Keel, P. K., Tangney, J. P., & Smith, G. T. (2022). Increases in shame following binge eating among women: Laboratory and longitudinal findings. *Appetite, 178*, 106276.

de Bruin, A. K. (2017). Athletes with eating disorder symptomatology, a specific population with specific needs. *Current Opinion in Psychology, 16*, 148–153.

Douglas, K., & Carless, D. (2008). Using stories in coach education. *International Journal of Sports Science & Coaching, 3*(1), 33–49.

Feiring, C., & Cleland, C. (2007). Childhood sexual abuse and abuse-specific attributions of blame over 6 years following discovery. *Child Abuse & Neglect, 31*(11–12), 1169–1186.

Frank, A. (1995). The wounded storyteller: Body, illness. *Ethics*. Chicago: University of Chicago Press.

Gardner, F., & Moore, Z. (2006). *Clinical sport psychology*. Human Kinetics.

Giorgio, G. (2013). Trust. Listening. Reflection. Voice: Healing traumas through qualitative research. *Counterpoints, 354*, 459–474.

Harris, M. E., & Fallot, R. D. (2001). *Using trauma theory to design service systems*. Jossey-Bass/Wiley.

Hepworth, N., & Paxton, S. J. (2007). Pathways to help-seeking in bulimia nervosa and binge eating problems: A concept mapping approach. *International Journal of Eating Disorders, 40*(6), 493–504.

Hirsch, T. (2020). Practicing without a license: Design research as psychotherapy. In *Proceedings of the 2020 CHI Conference on Human Factors in Computing Systems* (pp. 1–11).

Holstein, J. A., & Gubrium, J. F. (2000). The self we live by: Narrative identity in a postmodern world. New York: Oxford University Press.

Isobel, S. (2021a). Is trauma informed care possible in the current public mental health system? *Australasian Psychiatry, 29*(6), 607–610.

Isobel, S. (2021b). Trauma-informed qualitative research: Some methodological and practical considerations. *International Journal of Mental Health Nursing, 30*, 1456–1469.

Jones, D. W. (1998). Distressing histories and unhappy interviewing. *Oral History, 26*(2), 49–56.

Kavanagh, E., Brown, L., & Jones, I. (2017). Elite athletes' experience of coping with emotional abuse in the coach–athlete relationship. *Journal of Applied Sport Psychology, 29*(4), 402–417.

Keski-Rahkonen, A., & Mustelin, L. (2016). Epidemiology of eating disorders in Europe: Prevalence, incidence, comorbidity, course, consequences, and risk factors. *Current Opinion in Psychiatry, 29*(6), 340–345.

Lahman, M. K., Geist, M. R., Rodriguez, K. L., Graglia, P., & DeRoche, K. K. (2011). Culturally responsive relational reflexive ethics in research: The three Rs. *Quality & Quantity, 45*, 1397–1414.

McAdams, D. P. (2018). Narrative identity: What is it? What does it do? How do you measure it? *Imagination, Cognition and Personality, 37*(3), 359–372.

McGannon, K. R., & McMahon, J. (2019). Understanding female athlete disordered eating and recovery through narrative turning points in autobiographies. *Psychology of Sport and Exercise, 40*, 42–50.

McGannon, K. R., & McMahon, J. (2022). (Re) Storying embodied running and motherhood: A creative non-fiction approach. *Sport, Education and Society, 27*(8), 960–972.

McMahon, J. (2013). The use of narrative in coach education: The effect on short-and long-term practice. *Sports Coaching Review, 2*(1), 33–48.

McMahon, J., McGannon, K. R., Zehntner, C., Werbicki, L., Stephenson, E., & Martin, K. (2022). Trauma-informed abuse education in sport: Engaging athlete abuse survivors as educators and facilitating a community of care. *Sport, Education and Society, 28*(8), 958–971.

McMahon, J., Penney, D., & Dinan-Thompson, M. (2012). 'Body practices—Exposure and effect of a sporting culture?' Stories from three Australian swimmers. *Sport, Education and Society, 17*(2), 181–206.

Mehler, P. S., Watters, A., Joiner, T., & Krantz, M. J. (2022). What accounts for the high mortality of anorexia nervosa? *International Journal of Eating Disorders, 55*(5), 633–636.

Mountjoy, M., Brackenridge, C., Arrington, M., Blauwet, C., Carska-Sheppard, A., Fasting, K., Kirby, S., Leahy, T., Marks, S., Martin, K., Starr, K., Tiivas, A., & Budgett, R. (2016). International Olympic Committee consensus statement: Harassment and abuse (non-accidental violence) in sport. *British Journal of Sports Medicine, 50*(17), 1019–1029.

Mountjoy, M. L., & Verhagen, E. (2022). '# BeTheChange': The responsibility of sports medicine in protecting athletes from harassment and abuse in sport. *BMJ Open Sport & Exercise Medicine, 8*(1), e001303.

Owton, H., & Sparkes, A. C. (2017). Sexual abuse and the grooming process in sport: Learning from Bella's story. *Sport, Education and Society, 22*(6), 732–743.

Palmer, C. (2016). Ethics in sport and exercise research: From research ethics committees to ethics in the field. In *Routledge handbook of qualitative research in sport and exercise* (pp. 338–351). Routledge.

Papathomas, A. (2016). Narrative inquiry: From cardinal to marginal … and back? In *Routledge handbook of qualitative research in sport and exercise* (pp. 59–70). Routledge.

Papathomas, A. (2018). Disordered eating in sport: Legitimized and stigmatized. In *Sport, mental illness, and sociology* (Vol. 11, pp. 97–109). Emerald Publishing Limited.

Papathomas, A., & Lavallee, D. (2006). A life history analysis of a male athlete with an eating disorder. *Journal of Loss and Trauma, 11*(2), 143–179.

Papathomas, A., & Lavallee, D. (2010). Athlete experiences of disordered eating in sport. *Qualitative Research in Sport and Exercise, 2*(3), 354–370.

Papathomas, A., & Lavallee, D. (2012a). Eating disorders in sport: A call for methodological diversity. *Revista de Psicología del deporte, 21*(2), 387–392.

Papathomas, A., & Lavallee, D. (2012b). Narrative constructions of anorexia and abuse: An athlete's search for meaning in trauma. *Journal of Loss and Trauma, 17*(4), 293–318.

Papathomas, A., & Lavallee, D. (2014). Self-starvation and the performance narrative in competitive sport. *Psychology of Sport and Exercise, 15*(6), 688–695.

Pettersen, G., Rosenvinge, J. H., & Ytterhus, B. (2008). The "double life" of bulimia: Patients' experiences in daily life interactions. *Eating Disorders, 16*(3), 204–211.

Pichon, L. C., Teti, M., & Brown, L. L. (2022). Triggers or prompts? When methods resurface unsafe memories and the value of trauma-informed photovoice research practices. *International Journal of Qualitative Methods, 21*, 16094069221113979.

Polkinghorne, D. E. (1988). *Narrative knowing and the human sciences*. Suny Press.

Prior, E., Papathomas, A., & Rhind, D. (2022). A systematic scoping review of athlete mental health within competitive sport: Interventions, recommendations, and policy. *International Review of Sport and Exercise Psychology*, 1–23.

Ricoeur, P. (1984). *Time and narrative* (Vol. 1). University of Chicago Press.

Riessman, C. K. (2008). *Narrative methods for the human sciences*. Sage.

Rijkers, C., Schoorl, M., van Hoeken, D., & Hoek, H. W. (2019). Eating disorders and posttraumatic stress disorder. *Current Opinion in Psychiatry, 32*(6), 510–517.

SAMHSA. (2014a). *SAMHSA's concept of trauma and guidance for a trauma-informed approach* (pp. 12–17). U.S. Department of Health and Human Services.

SAMHSA. (2014b). *A treatment improvement protocol (TIP 57): Trauma-informed care in behavioral health services.* U.S. Department of Health and Human Services.

Sandick, P. A. (2012). Speechlessness and trauma: Why the International Criminal Court needs a public interviewing guide. *Northwestern Journal of International Human Rights, 11,* 105.

Seedat, S., Pienaar, W. P., Williams, D., & Stein, D. J. (2004). Ethics of research on survivors of trauma. *Current Psychiatry Reports, 6*(4), 262–267.

Smith, B. (2010). Narrative inquiry: Ongoing conversations and questions for sport and exercise psychology research. *International Review of Sport and Exercise Psychology, 3*(1), 87–107.

Smith, B., Williams, O., Bone, L., & Collective, T. M. S. W. C. P. (2023). Co-production: A resource to guide co-producing research in the sport, exercise, and health sciences. *Qualitative Research in Sport, Exercise and Health, 15*(2), 159–187.

Sohn, M. N., Dimitropoulos, G., Ramirez, A., McPherson, C., Anderson, A., Munir, A., Patten, S. B., McGirr, A., & Devoe, D. J. (2023). Non-suicidal self-injury, suicidal thoughts and behaviors in individuals with an eating disorder relative to healthy and psychiatric controls: A systematic review and meta-analysis. *International Journal of Eating Disorders, 56*(3), 501–515.

Spalding, N. J., & Phillips, T. (2007). Exploring the use of vignettes: From validity to trustworthiness. *Qualitative Health Research, 17*(7), 954–962.

Stirling, A. E., & Kerr, G. A. (2009). Abused athletes' perceptions of the coach-athlete relationship. *Sport in Society, 12*(2), 227–239.

Tillmann-Healy, L. M. (2003). Friendship as method. *Qualitative Inquiry, 9*(5), 729–749.

Trottier, K., & MacDonald, D. E. (2017). Update on psychological trauma, other severe adverse experiences and eating disorders: State of the research and future research directions. *Current Psychiatry Reports, 19,* 1–9.

Wilson, D., & Neville, S. (2009). Culturally safe research with vulnerable populations. *Contemporary Nurse, 33*(1), 69–79.

Winning, J. (2020). Trauma, illness and narrative in the medical humanities. In C. Davis, & H. Meretoja (Eds.), *The Routledge companion to literature and trauma* (pp. 266–274). Routledge.

Yatchmenoff, D. K., Sundborg, S. A., & Davis, M. A. (2017). Implementing trauma-informed care: Recommendations on the process. *Advances in Social Work, 18*(1), 167–185.

Chapter 8

Researching Abuse in Women's Artistic Gymnastics

A Trauma-Informed Approach

Natalie Barker-Ruchti

Introduction

Since the release of the Netflix documentary *Athlete A* (Cohen, 2020), women's artistic gymnastics (WAG) has gained mainstream media attention as a sport where gymnasts are physically, psychologically, and sexually abused. In its wake, the documentary's calling out of WAG's culture has empowered hundreds of current and former gymnasts to voice their experiences of abuse and its damaging consequences. Today, the hashtag gymnastalliance has grown into an unprecedented online sports #MeToo movement on the social media platforms Instagram and Twitter.

Since the 1980s, researchers have shown that WAG harms gymnasts through serious injuries and life-long physical debilitation, stunted growth, delayed puberty/menarche, disordered body/self-image, self-harm, eating disorder, and even death (Barker-Ruchti & Schubring, 2016; Cavallerio et al., 2016; Neves et al., 2017; Tan et al., 2014). Researchers have also demonstrated that an authoritarian coaching model prevents gymnasts from developing competencies such as independence and self-determination (Barker-Ruchti, 2008; Barker-Ruchti & Tinning, 2010). Moreover, researchers have identified that harm occurs because of gender ideology, the idealisation of a pre-pubescent gymnast body, the cultivation of an authoritarian coach-gymnast relationship, and the normalisation of violent coaching methods (Barker-Ruchti et al., 2020; Kerr et al., 2019; Way, 2021). Alarmingly, it is presently documented that WAG's culture and its devastating consequences are tolerated and normalised by federations, clubs, coaches, and other stakeholders (Novkov, 2019; Ryan, 2013; Way, 2021). In the case of the USA Gymnastics sex abuse scandal, which first broke in 2016, this tolerance provided the medical doctor Larry Nassar with carte blanche to sexually abuse girl gymnasts for decades.

Despite this existing body of literature, WAG scholarship is only beginning to consider the sport's harmful practices and consequences from the perspective of trauma. This delay may be surprising, given that the evidence on the harm gymnasts experience reflects the definition of trauma, such as the one developed by Huang et al. (2014) for the US Department of Health

DOI: 10.4324/9781003332909-10

and Human Services agency, Substance Abuse and Mental Health Services Administration (SAMHSA):

> Individual trauma results from an event, series of events, or set of circumstances that is *experienced* by an individual as physically or emotionally harmful or life threatening and that has lasting adverse *effects* on the individual's functioning and mental, physical, social, emotional, or spiritual well-being.
>
> (p. 7, emphasis in original)

Moreover, and equally important to address, is the limited available guidance on *how* to conduct trauma-informed research with women's gymnasts. As increasingly more researchers are interested in the topic of abuse in WAG, it is vital that researchers understand what trauma-informed research practices involve and how such an approach should be implemented. If not, researchers may risk that their findings do not fully capture the nuances of trauma events, experiences, and effects, that they inadvertently (re)traumatise research participants, and that they are, themselves, negatively affected by the research process and findings (Alessi & Kahn, 2023).

To address the paucity of literature on how to conduct trauma-informed research in WAG, the purpose of this chapter is to present how I adopted trauma-informed practices in and through the qualitative research project *#gymnastalliance: An international study on women's gymnasts speaking out about abuse*. I will begin by presenting the #gymnastalliance study, its participants, and their ongoing trauma effects. In the second part, I outline the trauma-informed practices that I applied in the research. To do this, I draw on Alessi and Kahn's (2023) five trauma-informed research guidelines for qualitative research.

The #Gymnastalliance Study

The #gymnastalliance study is grounded in the conceptualisation that digital technologies and social media movements (e.g., the #MeToo movement) afford women opportunities to speak out about abuse and facilitate the act of disclosing experiences because those speaking out can gain public recognition, empathy, and solidarity (Clark, 2016; Clark-Parsons, 2021; Suk et al., 2021). When current and former gymnasts began to take to Instagram and Twitter to speak out about their experiences of abuse upon the release of the *Athlete A* documentary, social media appeared to have this positive influence and effect (Seanor et al., 2023; Willson et al., 2023). The gymnasts' speaking out gained momentum across countries and the reactions to the disclosures included acknowledgement, empathy, and solidarity.

The #gymnastalliance study started in January 2021, upon receiving funding from the Swedish Research Council for Sport Science and gaining ethical approval from the Swedish Ethical Review Authority. The purpose of the study was to understand the experiences of gymnasts' speaking out through five overarching questions: (1) What methods do gymnasts use to speak out about abuse (e.g., social media, mainstream media, and other outlets)? (2) What abusive behaviours and practices do they disclose when speaking out? (3) What influenced the gymnasts to speak out now? (4) How do gymnasts experience their speaking out? and (5) What demands do they request for the future?

To recruit research participants, I adopted a purposeful sampling strategy, with the criteria being current or former gymnasts who anonymously or by using their name had spoken out about abuse through social and/or traditional media since June 2020, or other forums (e.g., lawyer/law firm, ombudsman, reporting agency, public investigation into abuse, and police). Recruitment occurred through posting a call on my Twitter account (@barkerruchti), which the Swedish Ethical Review Authority had approved (see Figure 8.1) as well as forwarding the Tweet call to relevant individuals and organisations. Twenty-one former gymnasts contacted me, of which 19 consented to participate in the study.

The qualitative research method that I used to understand the experiences of the gymnasts' speaking out was individual semi-structured online interviews using the computer-mediated communication program Zoom (Smith & Sparkes, 2016). An interview schedule consisting of six topics structured the interview: (1) entrance into and career in WAG; (2) life after retirement; (3) realisation that WAG experiences are abusive; (4) decision to speak out about the abuse (publicly or otherwise); (5) meanings made from speaking out; and (6) demands for change and hopes for the future. At the time of writing this chapter (November 2022–June 2023), the project is in the data analysis and writing-up phase.

Research Participants

The research participants of the #gymnastalliance study included 19 participants in total, 18 of which were former women's artistic gymnasts and 1 was a former rhythmic gymnast. They were citizens of 12 countries on four continents and spoke five different languages. Throughout 2021, participants were between 20 and 50 years old and had retired from gymnastics between two to 30 years ago. All had trained at an elite-level. Five of the women had competed in major international competitions (e.g., World Championships and Olympic Games), 14 had either remained in an elite-level training group without reaching the international competition level or had left elite-level gymnastics before reaching the age of 15 years.

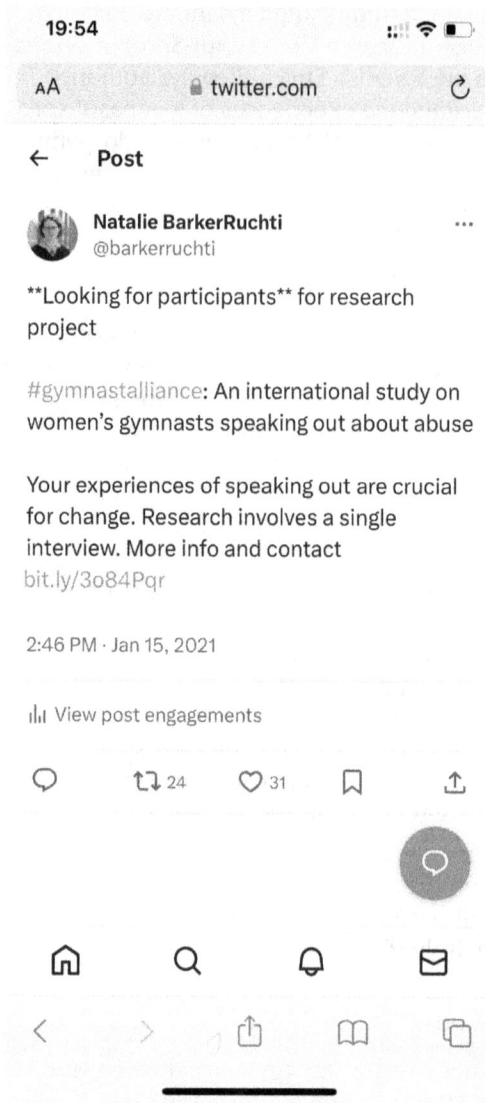

Figure 8.1 #gymnastalliance recruitment call on Twitter.

At the time of participating in the study, 13 of the participants had publicly spoken out about their experiences of abuse. Some had also used other avenues, including an ombudsman, a legal expert, an investigation, and the police. Two of the 19 had only spoken out through an ombudsman or an investigation, and four used the #gymnastalliance study to speak out for the first time.

Each of the 19 former gymnasts' stories reflects what research findings have evidenced for years as they entail all forms of physical and psychological abuse defined by sports science scholars (e.g., Fortier et al., 2020; Mountjoy et al., 2016). Both male and female coaches were identified as the abusers. Three of the former gymnasts also recounted sexual abuse by their respective male coaches, two of which have since been convicted and sentenced to imprisonment. The former gymnasts' stories are also characterised by ongoing medical, psychological, and psychiatric treatment since leaving gymnastics. Finally, it was only after the USA Gymnastics sex abuse media coverage, including the *Athlete a* documentary, that most of the research participants' realised that their experiences were abusive and reflected a global phenomenon. For *all* 19 interviewees, regardless of age, location, level of gymnastics, and time since retirement, the trauma effects of their gymnastics participation remain ongoing.

The Ongoing Trauma Effects

The women's ongoing trauma effects disclosed in interviews are of physical, cognitive, emotional, mental health, behavioural, relational, educational, professional, and economic nature. Most of the ongoing effects are direct causes of WAG participation, such as hyperextended knees, slipped vertebra bones, reconstructive surgeries, eating disorders, depression, and no positive gymnastics memories. Other effects have occurred because of re-traumatisation experiences later in life, including not being listened to or believed when reporting abuse. Finally, some of the ongoing trauma effects relate to re-victimisation, such as through a violent partner or being publicly discredited when reporting abuse to gymnastics organisations. To exemplify the gymnasts' ongoing trauma effects, I offer in the following quotations from participants.

In terms of physical effects, Becky, who entered in gymnastics in 1977, said the following:

> My knees are hurting. My hips are hurting. My ankle's done. It doesn't hold anymore. I can fall anytime and I'm afraid to hurt myself further. I've got arthrosis everywhere. I can't even stand up for a big amount of time so, I'm aching 24-hours-a-day.

Similarly, Zoë, who started competitive gymnastics in 1994, described physical trauma effects:

> It's my ankles that hurt when I'm having a mentally stressful time … It's gym injuries that hurt, which I don't know what that means. I don't know if it's psychological or if those are the most broken parts of my body.

As with physical effects, cognitive, emotional, and mental health effects are extensive and experienced by all 19 women. Drew, seven years retired, described the cognitive effect of memory loss:

> I had four years of high school, where I remembered nothing [from her time in WAG] ... And then at 18, I started to remember everything and that was when my mental health really went downhill ... And so that led to me being in therapy. From 18 to 22 was when I've really had to work on my mental health. I developed post-traumatic stress disorder. I have an eating disorder, anxiety, depression, and I have a service dog.

Another cognitive effect that several interviewees described is dissociation (Thomson et al., 2011). Maria, who left gymnastics in the early 1990s, provided the following insight:

> I disappeared, I vanished into thin air. I didn't want to talk or know anything about anyone. A year after undergoing surgery, I began to hang out with some of my closest [gymnastics] friends, but I wasn't so sure, because inside of me, the wound was still open .... So, [20] years went by, I moved into something else ... but that wasn't me. It was like the sport and gymnast part was something else, that was another [Maria] ... the attention was put elsewhere, it's like [gymnastics] never existed for me.

Like Maria, recently retired Ruth described the ongoing mental health effects she experiences:

> I really hit a low point at the beginning of this year, and I went back to therapy, and I was ... diagnosed with generalized anxiety disorder, so I take anti-anxieties and antidepressants, just to function in my life and be able to go to work and relate with people ... My therapist came to the conclusion that this abuse that was inflicted over and over again is the main source of my condition because I'm scared of everything. Like I literally, I can't drive, I have panic attacks when I drive, for example. I'm working on it, but all this, it's overwhelming.

The women also recounted extensive behavioural and relational effects from gymnastics. Most of the interviewees described that they wanted to withdraw from their gymnastics communities (e.g., Maria's quote above). A further issue many mentioned was distrust and/or suspicion, a common ongoing relational trauma effect (Collins & Long, 2003). Relational effects were also experienced for several of the interviewees when registering complaints about abuse. Nic, who described that her coaches had forced her out of elite gymnastics in 2016, explained her reaction to her gymnastics federation downplaying her experiences:

> I was outraged and disappointed. Because there are so many of us in [her country] who have spoken out. There are so many of us who went to the [gymnastics] federation and who spoke to the coaches. And they're now acting as if none of it is true and as if they didn't know anything about.
>
> (the abuse they had reported)

In addition to disbelief, Drew (quoted earlier above) described how she and her family were threatened for speaking out publicly:

> They [people at my gymnastics club] found my home address. They contacted former teammates to get my mobile number. They had my email address. They were sending me messages via Instagram. They sent my [parent] a threatening letter at [their] work … it just got really bad really quickly.

Finally, the interviewees recounted educational, professional, and economic effects because of ongoing health and well-being problems. These effects have included struggles at school and university, temporary and/or a long-term inability to work, and medical and therapy costs. Several of the former gymnasts also spoke of how they had entered gymnastics coaching, judging, and gymnastics governance, but left these roles because the WAG culture had weighed too heavy on them. Ruth (also quoted above) remembered:

> I continued coaching [recreational gymnastics] while I was at university … there was competitive gymnastics going on, so I saw a lot of stuff again that reminded me of my experience. And although I never said anything, you know, it was there, me just feeling uncomfortable seeing it happen. Children crying because they're too scared to do stuff and not being treated particularly nicely, pressure being put on for no reason.

While restricted space only allows for some excerpts of the data, the interview data drawn on in this section offers significant longitudinal insight into how the WAG participation continues to affect the women and their lives. In order to generate a research encounter that motivates trauma survivors to participate and allows them to openly and safely recount their experiences, without re-traumatising effects, a trauma-informed approach is vital.

The #Gymnastalliance Trauma-Informed Research Practice

While the #gymnastalliance movement on social media included hundreds of current and former gymnasts speaking out about their experiences of abuse and its damaging consequences, I knew from earlier research that gymnasts are reluctant to verbalise their experiences (Barker-Ruchti, 2008; Barker-Ruchti & Schubring, 2017). Thus, it was clear to me that I needed to adopt a qualitative research approach that would involve a *trustworthy* research process and create a *safe* research environment. I found relevant literature in Kahn and Alessi (2020) and Alessi and Kahn's (2023) trauma-informed research guidelines, which they had developed based on research with multiple marginalised queer and transgender migrants in South Africa. While others have developed guidelines (e.g., Huang et al., 2014), I found Alessi and Kahn's (2023) discussion of trauma specific to historically and structurally marginalised individuals particularly relevant to the women's gymnastics context of women's gymnasts (Barker-Ruchti, 2008; Barker-Ruchti et al., 2020; Way, 2021). In the following, I introduce Alessi and Kahn's (2023) five trauma-informed research guidelines for qualitative research – (1) preparing for community entry; (2) preparing for the interview; (3) extending safety and trust to the interview; (4) knowing when to change course to avoid re-traumatisation; and (5) committing to self-reflection and self-care – and outline how I attempted to follow these guidelines in the #gymnastalliance study.

Preparing for Community Entry

Alessi and Kahn's (2023) first guideline urges qualitative researchers to learn about the impacts of traumatic events and historical trauma on research participants and their communities. To achieve this impact, the two authors propose a collaboration with community partners (e.g., activist groups and victim/survivor support organisations) or the engagement of an advisory board comprised of representatives from the affected population to understand more deeply how trauma impacts survivors in different ways. Where this collaboration is not possible, researchers are advised to consult available information on survivors, such as through literature, social media, and other media forms (e.g., biographies and film). What Alessi and Kahn (2023, p. 136) want to highlight is the importance of researchers understanding "how trauma manifests in the community and how [a research interview or an interviewer] may reactivate trauma based on historical events and current social conditions."

When formulating the project application for the Swedish Research Council for Sport Science in 2020, I was in the fortunate position to already have had gained in-depth knowledge of WAG (e.g., Barker-Ruchti, 2008; Barker-Ruchti & Schubring, 2016; Barker-Ruchti & Tinning, 2010). I was further fortunate to be able to draw on experience from engaging in the gymnast activist organisation Gymnasts4Change and the athlete support organisation Safesport Sweden. Finally, by the time the project could start in January 2021, I had read many Instagram and Twitter posts by current and former gymnasts, had scanned the reactions to these posts, and collected media reports that were emerging in response to gymnasts' disclosures. In sum, and in relation to Alessi and Kahn's (2023) guideline for how to prepare for community entrance, I felt that I had come to understand the mechanisms that enable the abuse of gymnasts, the practices of physical and psychological abuse coaches employ, the culture of threat and silence and the bystander effect, and gymnasts' experiences of abuse and its life-long consequences. Through my research, I had also come to recognise that WAG's mechanisms, culture, and lack of adult interference to protect gymnasts prevents gymnasts from wanting to engage in a research interview (Barker-Ruchti & Schubring, 2017). The following four guidelines that Alessi and Kahn (2023) outline are thus crucial to fully capture the nuances of trauma events, experiences, and effects, to not re-traumatise and re-victimise the research participants, and to avoid being negatively affected by the research process and findings.

Preparing for the Interview

Alessi and Kahn's (2023) second guideline focuses on the safety and trust required in the research environment. The guideline relates specifically to external safety during the research encounter, relational safety, which extends to researcher-research participant relationship, and internal safety, which relates to research participants' capacities to decide, control, and set boundaries. As survivors of abuse may "be reluctant to ask questions, feel unable to stand up for their rights, might not even know what their rights are, and may even agree to continue with research activities despite feeling uncomfortable" (Alessi & Kahn, 2023, p. 140), external, relational, and internal safety is paramount.

To prepare for the #gymnastalliance interviews, I adopted three strategies: A pilot interview (external safety), a communication protocol (relational safety), and radical transparency (internal safety). The pilot interview involved an interview with an athlete, who had spoken out about her experiences of abuse in another aesthetic sport. While researchers traditionally conduct pilot interviews to refine data generation tools, such preparatory work also offers a means to foreshadow possible challenges and risks, and how best to prepare for these to protect both the interviewee and interviewer (Malmqvist et al., 2019). In the context of trauma research, I felt that it was not only important for me to test the semi-structured interview guide, but also to gain feedback from an abuse victim on what the online interviews would be like for both the interviewee and myself. I noticed, for example, that the interviewee at times avoided eye contact with me, faltered when speaking, and that her skin colour around her throat and chest became red when she described abusive experiences. When reflecting on the pilot interview, the interviewee commented that she was glad to sit in her home environment and of the degree of anonymity that the Zoom encounter created, something that other trauma scholars have recognised as essential to conducting research with trauma survivors (e.g., McMahon et al., 2022). The pilot interviewee also offered information on what had helped her and could help her to deal with the reactions, such as having time to recover, being asked if she is ok or would like to take a break, and the researcher acknowledging the challenge of speaking about experiences relating to abuse.

The communication protocol that I had developed served as a schedule for when and what to relate to the research participants. While clear and transparent communication is a standard research practice, the protocol I had developed detailed each communication step and the contents that needed to be communicated to participants. I had learned from Alessi and Kahn (2023), for instance, that it is important that research participants receive information about the interview structure and questions in advance of the interview so that they are able to gauge what could be upsetting during the interview (Alessi & Kahn, 2023). Such predictability is "salient for trauma survivors, for whom uncertainty and unpredictability may trigger memories, thoughts, emotions, and bodily sensations associated with past victimisation or feelings of helplessness" (Alessi & Kahn, 2023, p. 139).

The third strategy, to be radically transparent, entails not overselling the impact research can have in the current moment or the future. At the end of each interview, I mentioned to the research participants that it would likely take considerable time (i.e., years) for publications from the #gymnastalliance research to emerge. I further let the participants know that the research can contribute to, but may not achieve, structural and cultural change.

Extending Safety and Trust to the Interview

The third of Alessi and Kahn's (2023) trauma-informed qualitative research guidelines entails measures that sustain and strengthen research participants' safety *during* the data production moment. The elements of this guideline concern the nuances of the interview structure, the purpose of the interview, the mitigation of re-traumatisation, and the follow-up with victims after the data production moment.

In terms of the interview structure, Alessi and Kahn (2023) recommend a gradual approach of stressful questions. To ease interviewees into the interview, I used a "welcome address" to greet and thank the interviewees, which recapped the project information that I had communicated to the research participants via email. I also repeated that the interview could be stopped at any time and could be continued at another time when they felt they were able. I also asked the women if they had questions to ensure any concerns they had were foregrounded, a contrast to what they would have experienced in the coach-athlete relationship. Finally, I alerted participants when I would start the Zoom recording. The interview then began with me inviting the research participants to recount their early years in gymnastics. I assumed that since most gymnasts enter the sport at a local club that offers recreation or toddler type gymnastics classes, remembering back to those experiences would be an easy, low stress, start to the interview. This proved indeed to be the case. The gymnasts remembered their early times in WAG as a fun time during which they had fallen in love with the sport.

In terms of the purpose of the interview, Alessi and Kahn (2023) highlight that the purpose of a data generation moment in trauma-informed research is to gather information on interviewees' experiences and the meanings attached to them. Therapeutic benefits, although possible, are *not* its goal (see also Rossetto, 2014). To remain on the data gathering purpose, it is important for the researcher to be "fully present when asking questions and express empathy, curiosity, and cultural humility," and to refrain from reassuring interviewees, and evaluating and "normalizing" their experiences and feelings (Alessi & Kahn, 2023, p. 143).

I did not find it difficult to stay present in the interviews. The interviewees were incredibly open, and their stories were captivating. The interviews were also very emotional and I found it natural to cry with the interviewees, apologise for their trauma, and thank them for their courage to speak with me and share their experiences, reactions that Campbell and colleagues (2009) argue may positively affect the interviewees. When reading through the interview transcripts, I did notice, however, that I had at times reassured the women that there was nothing wrong with their anguish and that what they recounted was consistent with what I had heard from others. According to Alessi and Kahn (2023), such comments should be avoided as they normalise abuse survivors' experiences and feelings. Instead, Alessi and Kahn (2023, p. 143) recommend responses such as: "How do you manage to live with nightmares [or other ongoing trauma effects]; what have you tried?" and "How do you understand what is happening to you?" An additional reaction can be to offer resources on trauma recovery and support services, but Alessi and Kahn (2023) recommend that such resources be provided at the end of the research encounter.

Mitigating re-traumatisation is most crucial in relation to an interviewee reliving instead of recounting past experiences. As used here, recounting refers to storying past experiences, while reliving refers to losing touch with the present and being pulled back to the time of abuse (Alessi & Kahn, 2023). Such reliving, and thus re-traumatisation, may occur if the researcher reminds the interviewee of authority figures that exploited, betrayed, oppressed, or neglected them and/or if interviewees are pulled back to any actual event(s) of abuse. The active empowerment of the interviewee to set their boundaries around disclosure, and changing the course of the interview, are presented by Alessi and Kahn (2023, p. 144) as crucial means to "circumvent a trauma re-enactment in the researcher-participant relationship."

In the interviews that I conducted throughout my research investigation, I felt that the interviewees freely recounted their gymnastics and speaking out about their abuse experiences. Where I did notice reservations was in the interviews with the women who had suffered sexual abuse. The three interviewees were guarded in describing the types of abuse they had suffered and in disclosing perpetrator names, and I did not press the interviewees to provide further details. Instead, I sought to enable the interviewees to have control over what they were willing to share or not (McMahon et al., 2022). This is not to say that I did not ask follow-up questions, and in several instances, when the interviewees were emotional, I momentarily waited (also to manage my emotions) before asking the interviewee if she wished to take a break or continue the interview at a later time. In two instances, the research participants took up my offer to continue the interview on a later day of their choosing.

The last element to extend safety into the research encounter included extending an ethics of care after the interview. This practice involved me following-up with research participants to check on their well-being and if needed, offer access to relevant resources (e.g., lists of support organisations and education resources). I began this process by emailing the 19 women the day after their interviews to show my appreciation for their participation while also checking on their well-being. If the interviewees had discussed any matters where I felt they could be best supported through relevant supporting organisations, I provided them with contact details and carried out a soft introduction for them. Alessi and Kahn (2023) explain how this practice is particularly helpful for "participants who are isolated, as this can contribute to trauma reactivity after the interview" (p. 145). Indeed, several of the research participants had not yet connected with other WAG survivors and in those instances, I provided them with contact details to WAG activist groups, reporting services (e.g., national investigations), and other relevant WAG abuse survivor information.

Knowing When to Change Course to Avoid Re-Traumatisation

Alessi and Kahn's (2023) fourth research guideline focuses on the researcher ensuring that the interview is an *empowering experience,* which the two authors define to mean feeling empowered and not broken or overly exposed by the end of the interview. This practice demands that the researcher changes course when participants become stuck in traumatic experiences (see reliving of trauma experiences above) or express little hope for the future. It is the researcher's responsibility to bolster "participants' natural coping strengths with questions that support their capacity to recognise and mobilise their own resilience (through questions such as "You have clearly been through so much. So, tell us how you managed to stay strong?" and "Thank you for sharing such difficult experiences. You have made it so far, how did you do it?" (Alessi & Kahn, 2023, p. 146). Concluding the interview in this way is particularly important.

During the 19 interviews, although the former gymnasts did express frustration and sadness over what they had experienced, I did not perceive their responses in the interviews as overly pessimistic or expressing feelings of hopelessness. In contrast, I found that the women were extraordinarily resilient and a key motivation for them to participate in the interview was to contribute to transforming WAG. To reinforce this resilience, I ended the interview with questions on the women's demands for change and hopes for the future. I found that this directed the interviewees' thoughts away from their experience of abuse to considering how they could turn their experiences into useful future endeavours (e.g., social action). The following quotation from Becky exemplifies how the interviewees reacted to the closing question:

> Oh, I want every child safe in the sport, and loving it [laughter]. You know, the way I loved it before I was affected. It's such a great sport. And that's my big dream, and if there's anything I can do to enable that dream to go forward, then I will. And I get very excited when I find other people with a similar approach to things, and who love the sport as much as I do.

In general, the research participants' correspondence with me after the interview indicated that the women felt empowered by the research encounter. Ruth, for instance, wrote:

> I wanted to thank you for giving your time and care to me today, and allowing me to share my story, and hopes, and hurts, in an understanding and safe environment … it was such an insightful and meaningful experience meeting you and talking.

Several interviewees also acknowledged that they felt the interview had given them an opportunity to be part of something bigger, as Maria wrote:

> What a pleasure it was to speak with you yesterday. Thank you very much for the time you took to hear my story and your ability to listen, I know that isn't easy. Although I was drained after our call, I also felt strangely good … lighter perhaps, very heard and that I was contributing to solving this decades old problem.

Committing to Regular and Radical Self-Reflection and Self-Care

This fifth and last of Alessi and Kahn's (2023) guidelines for conducting trauma-informed research focuses on researcher self-reflection and self-care. The guideline includes, on the one hand, standard parameters of reflexivity, such as to attend to the influence gender identity and age, personal experiences, and emotional resonance with a study topic have on research activities and outcomes. On the other, Alessi and Kahn (2023) expand the guideline to a trauma-informed reflexivity, which demands that researcher(s) assess their own trauma histories, question their motivations for engaging in trauma research, and attend to emerging emotions before, during, and after conducting the research. Relating to this, Alessi and Kahn (2023) outline that researchers should consider what self-care strategies they can employ to manage vicarious trauma.

As mentioned above, the WAG research I had conducted prior to the #gymnastalliance study had offered in-depth knowledge of the sport. As my PhD research also entailed an auto-ethnographic study, it had also offered me opportunities to explore my gymnastics past (Barker-Ruchti, 2011). While my experiences did not result in trauma as described by the 19 interviewees, it had created affinity for others' experiences of abuse. My embodied gymnastics-self had also afforded insider knowledge of what it might "feel" like to be an elite gymnast. I am, however, cognisant that gymnasts' circumstances that I had seen when participating in the sport, and have examined in my research, are the key driver behind my motivation to conduct research with this population.

Attending to my emerging emotions before, during, and after conducting the research has taken me on a roller-coaster. When gymnasts began to speak out about abuse in June/July 2020, I was elated. A dam wall seemed to have broken and I was hopeful that the increasing media attention would finally result in change for the better (e.g., gymnastics being safer as a sport). I felt an intense urge to contribute to this potential, and this was the context from which I developed the #gymnastalliance research proposal. During the data collection phase in 2021, the interviews with the 19 women were distressing and discussions with colleagues and reflections became important self-care activities. What I also found useful during this phase was spreading the interviews over the space of a year, and opportunities to present early analysis of #gymnastalliance data (e.g., conferences and workshops). Since completing data generation, the emotions that I continuously need to manage are my ongoing perceived responsibility to publish, and the restrictions that ethical and publishing protocols create when it comes to presenting the 19 women's stories of trauma.

Conclusions

The #gymnastalliance movement has shown that the abuse women's gymnasts experience has ongoing and lasting trauma effects. While WAG research is today extensive, scholarship is only beginning to recognise this abuse and the harmful effects from the perspective of trauma. Trauma-informed WAG research is entirely new, and I thus conclude this chapter by providing three recommendations for conducting trauma-informed qualitative research in WAG and sport, exercise, and health contexts. First, I recommend that researchers use any means available to them to *prepare* for research with trauma populations. This does not need to go as far as conducting ethnographic research to understand a cultural context that causes trauma. However, knowing the lived realities of gymnasts, as well as the history and culture of WAG, were central preparations for me to develop and conduct a trauma-informed qualitative study. I further believe that these preparations and the insider knowledge I had gained enabled me to build trust and credibility with the research participants. This trust resulted in gaining rich data on the nuances of trauma events, experiences, and effects, prevent inadvertent (re)traumatisation, and make the interview a positive experience for the research participants. Indeed, I would argue that it was the preparations that were most valuable for the research I have conducted.

Second, I recommend that researchers allocate additional *time* (and thus also resources) to conduct trauma-informed research. Additional time is necessary because trauma research demands extensive preparation and reflections, reflexivity, and self-care. For me, the spread of the interviews over 12 months ended up being a valuable and needed self-care strategy. Indeed, a shorter timeframe might have resulted in me experiencing vicarious trauma, which would negatively have impacted my ability to manage the continued research.

Third, I recommend that researchers intending to study trauma do so adopting a *longitudinal* perspective. Although trauma can be caused by single events or circumstances specific to a life phase, trauma effects are most likely ongoing. They shape lives. With regard to WAG, as most gymnasts enter this sport as children, and thus experience abuse during childhood and adolescence, as was the case for the 19 former gymnasts in the #gymnastalliance study, the longitudinal perspective is particularly important. As suggested here, a longitudinal perspective would entail the research method (i.e., interview) to cover the entire athletic life, from entrance into to retirement from sport, and the research participants' lives afterwards.

References

Alessi, E. J., & Kahn, S. (2023). Toward a trauma-informed qualitative research approach: Guidelines for ensuring the safety and promoting the resilience of research participants. *Qualitative Research in Psychology, 20*(1), 121–154. https://doi.org/10.1080/14780887.2022.2107967

Barker-Ruchti, N. (2008). "They must be working hard": An (auto-)ethnographic account of women's artistic gymnastics. *Cultural Studies-Critical Methodologies, 8*(3), 372–380. https://doi.org/10.1177/1532708607310799

Barker-Ruchti, N. (2011). *Women's artistic gymnastics: An (auto-)ethnographic journey.* gesowip.

Barker-Ruchti, N., & Schubring, A. (2016). Moving into and out of high-performance sport: The cultural learning of an artistic gymnast. *Physical Education and Sport Pedagogy, 21*(1), 69–80. https://doi.org/10.1080/17408989.2014.990371

Barker-Ruchti, N., & Schubring, A. (2017). People in contexts. In M. L. Silk, D. L. Andrews, & H. Thorpe (Eds.) *Routledge handbook of physical cultural studies* (495–504). Routledge.

Barker-Ruchti, N., Schubring, A., & Stewart, C. (2020). Gendered violence in women's artistic gymnastics: A sociological analysis. In M. Lang (Ed.), *Routledge handbook of athlete welfare* (57–68). Routledge.

Barker-Ruchti, N., & Tinning, R. (2010). Foucault in leotards: Corporeal discipline in women's artistic gymnastics. *Sociology of Sport Journal, 27*(3), 229–250. https://doi.org/10.1123/ssj.27.3.229

Campbell, R., Adams, A. E., Wasco, S. M., Ahrens, C. E., & Sefl, T. (2009). Training interviewers for research on sexual violence: A qualitative study of rape survivors' recommendations for interview practice. *Violence Against Women, 15*(5), 595–617. https://doi.org/10.1177/1077801208331248

Cavallerio, F., Wadey, R., & Wagstaff, C. R. (2016). Understanding overuse injuries in rhythmic gymnastics: A 12-month ethnographic study. *Psychology of Sport and Exercise, 25*, 100–109. https://doi.org/10.1016/j.psychsport.2016.05.002

Clark, R. (2016). "Hope in a hashtag": The discursive activism of #WhyIStayed. *Feminist Media Studies, 16*(5), 788–804. https://doi.org/10.1080/14680777.2016.1138235

Clark-Parsons, R. (2021). "I see you, I believe you, I stand with you": #MeToo and the performance of networked feminist visibility. *Feminist Media Studies, 21*(3), 362–380. https://doi.org/10.1080/14680777.2019.1628797

Cohen, B. (2020). *Athlete a (film)*. Actual Films. Distributed by Netflix.

Collins, S., & Long, A. (2003). Working with the psychological effects of trauma: Consequences for mental health-care workers – A literature review. *Journal of Psychiatric and Mental Health Nursing, 10*(4), 417–424. https://doi.org/10.1046/j.1365-2850.2003.00620.x

Fortier, K., Parent, S., & Lessard, G. (2020). Child maltreatment in sport: Sashing the wall of silence: A narrative review of physical, sexual, psychological abuses and neglect. *British Journal of Sports Medicine, 54*(1), 4–7. https://doi.org/10.1136/bjsports-2018-100224

Huang, L. N., Flatow, R., Biggs, T., Afayee, S., Smith, K., Clark, T., & Blake, M. (2014). *SAMHSA's concept of trauma and guidance for a trauma-informed approach*. Substance Abuse and Mental Health Services Administration.

Kahn, S., & Alessi, E. J. (2020). Whose story is it, anyway? Supporting sexual and gender minority asylum seekers in the preparation of their trauma narratives. In M. Jaffe, M. Conti, J. Longhofer, & J. Floersch (Eds.) *The social work and LGBTQ sexual trauma casebook: Phenomenological perspectives* (pp. 45–64). Routledge.

Kerr, R., Barker-Ruchti, N., Schubring, A., Cervin, G., & Nunomura, M. (2019). Coming of age: Coaches transforming the pixie-style model of coaching in women's artistic gymnastics. *Sports Coaching Review, 8*(1), 7–24. https://doi.org/10.1080/21640629.2017.1391488

Malmqvist, J., Hellberg, K., Möllås, G., Rose, R., & Shevlin, M. (2019). Conducting the pilot study: A neglected part of the research process? Methodological findings supporting the importance of piloting in qualitative research studies. *International Journal of Qualitative Methods, 18*, 1–11. https://doi.org/10.1177/1609406919878341

McMahon, J., McGannon, K. R., Zehntner, C., Werbicki, L., Stephenson, E., & Martin, K. (2022). Trauma-informed abuse education in sport: Engaging athlete abuse survivors as educators and facilitating a community of care. *Sport, Education and Society*, 1–14. https://doi.org/10.1080/13573322.2022.2096586

Mountjoy, M., Brackenridge, C., Arrington, M., Blauwet, C., Carska-Sheppard, A., Fasting, K., Kirby, S., Leahy, T., Marks, S., Starr, K., Tiivas, A., & Budgett, R. (2016). International Olympic Committee consensus statement: Harassment and abuse (non-accidental violence) in sport. *British Journal of Sports Medicine, 50*(17), 1019–1029. https://doi.org/10.1136/bjsports-2016-096121

Neves, C. M., Filgueiras Meireles, J. F., Berbert de Carvalho, P. H., Schubring, A., Barker-Ruchti, N., & Caputo Ferreira, M. E. (2017). Body dissatisfaction in women's artistic gymnastics: A longitudinal study of psychosocial indicators. *Journal of Sports Sciences, 35*(17), 1745–1751. https://doi.org/10.1080/02640414.2016.1235794

Novkov, J. (2019). Law, policy, and sexual abuse in the# MeToo movement: USA Gymnastics and the agency of minor athletes. Journal of Women, *Politics & Policy, 40*(1), 42–74. https://doi.org/10.1080/1554477X.2019.1563412

Rossetto, K. R. (2014). Qualitative research interviews: Assessing the therapeutic value and challenges. *Journal of Social and Personal Relationship, 31*(4), 482–489. https://doi.org/10.1177/0265407514522892

Ryan, J. (2013). *Little girls in pretty boxes: The making and breaking of America's elite gymnasts and figure skaters*. Doubleday.

Seanor, M. E., Giffin, C. E., Schinke, R. J., Coholic, D. A., & Larivière, M. (2023). Pixies in a windstorm: Tracing Australian gymnasts' stories of athlete maltreatment through media data. *Sport in Society, 26*(3), 553–572.

Smith, B., & Sparkes, A. C. (2016). Interviews: Qualitative interviewing in the sport and exercise sciences. In B. Smith, & A. C. Sparkes (Eds.) *Routledge handbook of qualitative research in sport and exercise* (pp. 125–145). Routledge.

Suk, J., Abhishek, A., Zhang, Y., Ahn, S. Y., Correa, T., Garlough, C., & Shah, D. V. (2021). #MeToo, networked acknowledgment, and connective action: How "empowerment through empathy" launched a social movement. *Social Science Computer Review, 39*(2), 276–294. https://doi.org/10.1177/0894439319864882

Tan, J., Bloodworth, A., McNamee, M., & Hewitt, J. (2014). Investigating eating disorders in elite gymnasts: Conceptual, ethical and methodological issues. *European Journal of Sport Science, 14*(1), 60–68. https://doi.org/10.1080/17461391.2012.728632

Thomson, P., Kibarska, L. A., & Jaque, S. V. (2011). Comparison of dissociative experiences between rhythmic gymnasts and female dancers. *International Journal of Sport and Exercise Psychology, 9*(3), 238–250. https://doi.org/10.1080/1612197X.2011.614850

Way, A. K. (2021). Cruel optimism as organizing strategy in USA Gymnastics: The threat of high-stakes organizations in precarious times. *Human Relations, 76*(2). https://doi.org/10.1177/00187267211054689

Willson, E., Taylor, A., Kerr, G., & Stirling, A. (2023). Discussing safe sport in the digital space: the #gymnastalliance movement. *International Journal of Sport and Exercise Psychology*, 1–20. https://doi.org/10.1080/1612197X.2023.2231949

Part III

Trauma and Disability, Injury, Chronic, and Life-Threatening Diagnosis

Chapter 9

Trauma-Informed Narrative Interviewing after Limb Amputation

Learning to Put on the Brakes

Melissa Day and Ross Wadey

Introduction

This chapter focuses on our experiences of doing research with individuals who have experienced lower limb amputation along with those who support them (i.e., family, National Health Service, various charities). We began this research almost a decade ago, and our programme of research has allowed us to engage in individual interviews, focus groups, visual and written methods, along with immersing ourselves in a variety of environments, from the hospital to sporting arenas. We have observed the hard reality of life in a rehabilitation centre and experienced (somewhat inevitable) defeat on the wheelchair basketball court. Working in this way, with a range of participants, has enriched our understanding of both ethical and compassionate ways of researching lower limb loss. Put simply, we have moved from understanding *what* should be done (i.e., understanding guidelines for trauma-informed practice) to *how* this might be accomplished in practice. In this chapter, we aim to unpack the process of our practice and how it was trauma-informed, outlining the benefits of our methods but also incorporating a confessional element that reflects how our practice can continue to improve.

Despite the traumatic nature of amputation, there is relatively little literature that has explored amputation through a trauma lens. Instead, the focus of research has been on understanding psychological responses to amputation (e.g., depression, anxiety), some of which may be recognisable as symptoms of Post-Traumatic Stress Disorder (PTSD) (e.g., Horgan & MacLachlan, 2004). Yet for us, as researchers who ask about experiences of amputation, it has been important to consider not only the amputation itself as a traumatic event, but the cumulative trauma that may be present in a life story before, during, and after amputation.

In the United Kingdom (UK) where our work is located, there are five primary causes of lower limb amputation: sepsis, complications arising from peripheral arterial disease, serious trauma, neoplasm (e.g., cancer), or a deformation of the limb (NHS, 2016). Given these causes, for some individuals, amputation occurs as a planned necessity in the context of a chronic medical

DOI: 10.4324/9781003332909-12

illness, whereas for others amputation is necessitated by the sudden onset of infection or acute injury. Yet, despite suggestions that PTSD is relatively rare (<5%) in those whose surgery follows a chronic illness (Cavanagh et al., 2006), our research has outlined the complex emotional process associated with storying amputation as a 'cure' to chronic pain. While amputation may provide a release from chronic pain and lead to improvements in subjective well-being during rehabilitation, the day-to-day struggles of life after limb loss often only becomes apparent after returning home (Sanders et al., 2020). Thus, where amputation is not the 'cure' that had been hoped for, individuals may be left questioning their choice of elective surgery and unable to move forward in life. For example, as one participant in our research on rehabilitation described:

> I wish I'd looked into it more beforehand, but I'd believed what my head told me [amputation would solve pain] … I was a very angry lady, I was very bitter.

> *Where was that anger coming from?*

> Because I couldn't walk and I could see people that could walk and mine was a planned amputation, it wasn't a traumatic amputation … I just couldn't walk, I couldn't do it and I didn't understand it. I had all this anger, I was moody, I wanted to thump people, I mean I didn't obviously, but it was just red, it overtook me. People were saying you need to move on, and I couldn't, I just couldn't.

In comparison, individuals experiencing emergency amputation have less time to envisage the future post-amputation and less autonomy in the decision-making process. Research has consistently shown that these individuals report significantly higher depressive symptoms (e.g., Darnall et al., 2005) and demonstrate higher prevalence of PTSD and greater use of avoidant coping strategies (e.g., Cavanagh et al., 2006). Stories we have heard from participants following emergency amputation often revolve around one single moment of realisation, for example:

> Some of the people I know, they've gone home, they felt a bit ill, they've passed out at home, and then they've woken up in hospital with their legs amputated. You wake up to 'we're sorry, but we've had to take your legs off otherwise you would have died'. How's that for a bombshell.

> *It's hard to contemplate how much your world would change at that moment …*

> And a lot of people fall apart at that moment, don't want to go out, don't want to see anyone, just feel so down and depressed.

The two participants' quotes above illustrate that experiences of amputation and the type of trauma described can be remarkably different. While both are stories about embodied trauma, planned amputation is often told *through* an already wounded body. Emergency amputation is often told *about* an event that happened to the body. Both types of story depict trauma and both depict a loss of hope, but vary by *where* in the story these are located and *how* the story is told.

In addition to considering the traumatic nature of amputation, it is also important to consider iatrogenic trauma, which is bodily and psychic trauma created in the course of practicing health and wellness care (Burstow, 2003). As Eales and Goodwin (2022) describe, those concerned with helping can (and do) cause harm, despite good intentions. Further, trauma can be magnified when injury is denied, minimised, or not accommodated by others (Burstow, 2003). Thus, the responses of others post-amputation are crucial, yet many primary care providers report discomfort discussing trauma and its health effects, and feel unprepared to do so (Green et al., 2011). Perhaps one of the most shocking elements of our work with this population has been the stories we have listened to from participants being unheard and consequently un-helped in medical contexts. For example:

> One particular [limb] centre had discharged me and said that there was nothing that they could do for me, find somebody else to help you, we can't help you. I was distraught. I was driving down the motorway crying my eyes out to my husband on the phone saying 'I don't know what to do' … It's horrible because you fight and you fight and you fight and they blame you, a lot of the people blamed me that I didn't try hard enough, I didn't wear it [prosthetic leg] for long enough, I didn't behave myself, I drank too much.

The example above provides an illustration of insidious trauma and how such an approach may play out in practice by 'being expected to answer "what is wrong with you" questions daily' (Eales & Goodwin, 2022, p. 143).

Finally, in understanding the stories of those who have undergone amputation, it is also important to recognise that the trauma experience is embodied. As the term is used here, 'embodiment' refers to an awareness and responsiveness to bodily sensations. While other types of trauma may be time-limited (e.g., experiencing a robbery), the loss of a limb can provide a permanent physical reminder that positions the individual as never entirely 'post-traumatic' (Cordova, 2008). Thus, as Hefferon and Kampman (2020) outlined, physical trauma can lead to a heightened corporeal awareness, situating the body first and foremost in consciousness. Further, as Frank (1995) suggested 'people telling illness stories do not simply describe their sick bodies; their bodies give their stories their particular shape and direction' (p. 27). Consequently, as researchers we need to not only ask stories about the body but make the body a familiar topic of conversation during interviews. Such 'body storytelling' can be achieved by listening to how the body is described, while considering how this description may change over time, and over the course of trauma experiences. Yet as Frank warns, while the body is 'simultaneously cause, topic, and instrument of whatever new stories are told' (p. 2), 'actually hearing traces of the body in the story is not easy' (p. 2) for anyone who listens. We learned from our own early experiences of interviewing, that neglecting the physical body in discussions of trauma can leave stories feeling incomplete for our participant. One very memorable interview taught us that ignoring the physical body may lead to fragmented or incomplete stories:

> Mel: Is there anything you feel has been missing from what we have talked about today?
>
> Participant: I know we are going to talk again, but before we do, I'm surprised you didn't ask me more about this … [picks up prosthetic leg and puts it on the café table]. I think we've skirted around it and you've never really asked me directly how it feels to wear this or how it feels when I look at my leg. I want to tell you about it. I want you to know what it's like to have this.

Lessons such as the one above provided us with enhanced awareness of asking about the physical body, and the value of incorporating the body into conversations about trauma. Further, this interview made us reflect on elements of body conversations that we, as researchers, have found uncomfortable, either because they are unfamiliar to us (e.g., asking how it feels to live in a body after limb loss) or because they may prompt graphic conversations (e.g., talking about blisters incurred while wearing the prosthesis). Working as a research team has helped us to debrief and reflect on embodied conversations and conversations about trauma experiences that we have with our participants. In doing this, our aim was to normalise talking about the impact of trauma on the researcher (Berger, 2021) while continually improving our practice.

Methodology/Method

While we have used a variety of methods to collect data (e.g., interviews, visual and written methods), much of our work with individuals who have experienced amputation and subsequent trauma is underpinned by narrative inquiry. Narrative inquiry rests on the premise that human life is storied and that narrative is, therefore, both a method of knowing and an ontological condition of social life (Smith & Sparkes, 2006). While individuals may tell specific stories about their experiences to make sense of their lives, narratives refer to the general overarching plot lines which people rely on to tell these stories. Thus, as Smith and Sparkes (2009) outline, narratives are a constructed form or template, which contain a point, characters, and a plot of events that evolves sequentially over time. These narrative templates function as resources which people may use to construct big and small stories. While narrative inquiry has most often focused on big stories that contain a central plot, McGannon et al. (2022) advocated for the value of small stories, that is shorter tales or snippets of information. Typically underpinned by ontological relativism and epistemological social constructionism, narrative inquiry has been well used to explore experiences of sport, exercise, and health (Papathomas, 2017). Despite the potential value of narrative inquiry, we were initially cautious about the application of this methodology in trauma research. Drawing on seminal theories concerning the development of PTSD such as Van der Kolk's (1994) psychobiological theory and Brewin's (2014) dual representation model of PTSD, trauma memories are uniquely encoded in autobiographical memory and therefore separated from the overall memory network. Trauma memories are held at the level of the amygdala and therefore reside 'beneath' the level at which conscious narrative processing takes place (Currier & Neimeyer, 2006). Consequently, memories of trauma can be difficult to recall and often lack any sequence and coherence, resulting in a fragmented narrative.

Before defining this 'fragmented' narrative, it is important to first outline the practice of narrative scholars, allowing us to show why fragmentation may be problematic. In general, narrative scholars seek out personal experience stories, gleaned through methods that allow the narrator to offer their own world view such as life story interviews (Papathomas, 2017). The practice of narrative interviewing aims to encourage and stimulate the participant to tell a story about some significant event in their life and social context (Jovchelovitch & Bauer, 2000). In telling these stories, people rely on cultural templates or frameworks, that guide the shape of the story told. Thus, narratives are organised and can be identified through common features. As Smith and Sparkes (2009) suggested 'a narrative is taken to mean a complex genre that routinely contains a *point* and *characters* along with a *plot* connecting *events* that unfold *sequentially* over *time* and in *space* to provide an overarching *explanation* or *consequence*' (p. 2).

The process of integrating events from the past into a comprehensible account is termed emplotment (Neimeyer & Levitt, 2001). In narrative terms, emplotment enables the individual to make sense of past events, providing the capacity to organise life events into a meaningful story. Yet trauma can elude the ability to attain emplotment, leaving the individual with no way to make sense of their life. An example of eluded emplotment is perhaps best represented by Arthur Frank's chaos narrative. As Frank (1995, p. 97) describes:

> Chaos is the opposite of restitution: its plot imagines life never getting better. Stories are chaotic in their absence of narrative order. Events are told as the storyteller experiences life: without sequence or discernible causality. The lack of any coherent sequence is why chaos stories are hard to hear; the teller is not understood as telling a "proper" story.

Given the potential lack of plot and resulting fragmentation, why then use a methodology that focuses on storytelling to understand experiences of trauma? To answer this question, it is first important to consider the nuanced meaning of the term 'fragmented' and reflect on whether fragmentation prohibits narrative research. Crespo and Fernández-Lansac (2016) proposed that there are two fundamental dimensions of fragmentation: disorganisation (the order of specific structural elements) and incoherence (the degree to which the report is weakly articulated or incomprehensible). While some studies have aimed to code or rate incoherence and/or disorganisation (e.g., Bennett & Wells, 2010), in our experience these dimensions are not consistent throughout an interview or series of interviews (i.e., some parts of the interview discussion may be disorganised while others may be organised) and the use of categorical thinking and coding is therefore problematic. Further, in our experience, while some participants may struggle to make sense of their amputation and tell a coherent life story, when asked about smaller, everyday experiences (e.g., taking children to school), the coherence of the story may be improved, making the story both easier to tell and to understand. Put another way, when participants struggle to tell 'big' stories that have a central plot, they may be more able to tell 'small' stories (e.g., shorter text segments, focus on everyday and/or mundane experiences) that can feed into big story narratives (McGannon et al., 2022). In most of our work we use multiple interviews, and thus the use of small stories can become particularly pertinent, allowing us to start to make connections between small stories and life narratives with our participants over time.

It is also important to acknowledge that while fragmented stories may be difficult to hear and difficult to follow, such stories mirror the participant's life experiences and sense making process. If the investigator's purpose is to understand trauma, then it is important to recognise that trauma is incomprehensible and disorganised and not always easily understood by the participant and researcher. Fragmented stories tell of trauma as it is experienced: chaotic, distressing, and unimaginable. If we are to research experiences of trauma, then as researchers we need to be okay with fragmentation. Our aim should not be to organise what is fragmented but to sit *with* disorganisation. As Frank (1995) writes, while those telling stories of chaos certainly need help, the first step of those who care is to be 'willing to become witnesses to the story' (p. 110).

In line with our suggestions above, it is important for researchers to acknowledge the potential for fragmentation in people's stories, and therefore plan for this when conducting trauma interviews. In doing this acknowledgement, Gemignani's (2014) origami metaphor of narrative interviews is helpful:

We can think about the narrative interview as an origami. Initially, the origami is in the paper as potential: that is, the paper can or cannot become an origami .... The "final" memory that we researchers "collect" emerges in the process of folding, unfolding, and refolding of emotions, expectations, related memories, intuitions, poetic readings, contexts, and fields of power that constitute "memory-ing."

(p. 132)

Our narrative interviews on trauma start from the position that the participant has control over whether the paper becomes an origami or not. Further, unlike more structured interviewing that may guide participants to produce a particular shape or form of origami that is recognisable to the researcher, we follow the participant's direction of folds and unfolds.

To do this, there is one main 'feature' of our interviews that is particularly pertinent. Near the start of our interview, we aim to locate and understand the participant's 'safe place' or memory of a 'safe' experience. This technique draws on the work of trauma therapists such as Babette Rothschild (2003) who advocate the use of methods to 'apply the brakes before they [participant] use the accelerator' (p. 18) and the need to identify internal (e.g., imagery ability) and external (e.g., cue given by interviewer) resources that may assist in doing this. In describing her therapeutic trauma work, Rothschild notes that it is advisable to apply the brakes (expanded on further below) periodically in every session. This practice allows for adjusting the level of arousal experienced by participants and works to reduce the 'pressure' that can be experienced when describing trauma. We draw on Rothschild's (2003) work when interviewing to ensure that as interviewers we know how to apply the brakes, as and when needed. To do this, near the start of the interview we focus discussions around safe or supportive encounters. In finding out what some might deem 'background information' we look for descriptions of times when participants have felt supported or have felt safe and focus specifically on understanding these experiences in more depth, creating a vivid picture that we can return to at points during the interview. In particular, we ask questions about the finer details of the safe or supportive experience (e.g., descriptions of the location, emotions experienced, and words to describe the relationship). These descriptions can then be used to put on the brakes at points where needed in the interview. Alessi and Kahn (2022) present a similar suggestion, of asking 'resilience' questions to change course when needed (e.g., what has helped you to survive until now?). Yet, gathering these descriptions before this moment provides a safety net allowing us to guide discussions back to safety, even when the participant feels 'stuck'. In doing this practice, we are cautious that many of the people we interview have difficult family relationships or have struggled to maintain friendships following the amputation (Day, 2013). Consequently, in developing this initial description of a safe place or experience, our questions need to be sensitive and follow the participant's lead.

On paper, acquiring information about safe places or experiences might sound like an achievable and uncomplicated step for a qualitative researcher, yet we also offer a warning. We have found that some of our participants want to accelerate the interview quickly before we, as inter-viewers, have sufficient understanding of applying the brakes. In doing this, they 'drop in' or 'sandwich' information about their trauma experi-ences while we ask opening questions about supportive experiences. For example:

> There's one gentleman, Simon (pseudonym), he's down there [points into sports hall]. I couldn't afford to come to this event [sport weekend] but he has paid for me and he won't take any money back. Without him, I wouldn't have done anything. I'd still be sitting indoors, putting on weight and feeling sorry for myself. Feeling suicidal all the time. I mean since my accident, I've tried suicide three times, because I don't want to live like this. I've got no help, I've got no-one. But he pushed me to try and do things and I do actually enjoy myself, it does really help me.

In such instances we often witness participants expressing relief (e.g., taking a deep breath, relaxing their body posture) that they have 'offloaded' trauma information that they would like to bring into the interview. Yet without know-ing how to 'apply the brakes', proceeding with discussions of trauma may be dangerous for the participant and researcher. Our strategy here is first to ac-knowledge what has been said (i.e., noticing rather than ignoring the trauma experience) and asking permission to return to this later in the interview. For example, in this case:

> You've opened up a lot for us to talk about there and it sounds as though you have been through some very difficult and lonely times. If it is ok with you, we can talk about these low times today, but as a start point I'd like to know a little more about Simon. [waits for response] … Can you tell me about a sport or activity that he's pushed you to try …'.

Our conversation then proceeds to gain a vivid picture of these supportive and enjoyable experiences which can be used later in the interview to 'apply the brakes' if needed. We also make sure that we come back to his experiences of suicide and provide an opening to talk about this later in the interview. At times, the flow of conversation may not naturally lead us back to this point, but we note that it is important to return to what we have said we would ask about. In line with Alessi and Kahn's (2022) recommendations, qualitative researchers discussing trauma must be predictable (doing what they say they will) and consistent (over time). Thus, when the flow of conversation pauses, we direct back to this experience, for example:

> I'm cautious that we've been discussing X today but at the start of the inter-view you opened up about some really difficult times. Is it ok to go back to these or would you prefer to continue as we are?

By asking such questions, we aim to empower participants to choose the direction of conversation but remain reliable and predicable as interviewers.

Applying Trauma-Informed Practices to Our Research

In this next section of the chapter, we outline how we implemented evidence-based trauma-informed practices to our research with participants who have experienced limb amputation. While trauma-informed approaches do not necessarily directly address trauma, they provide a 'universal precautions' approach in which one expects the presence of trauma in the lives of individuals. Our research drew from expert recommendations on trauma-informed practices (e.g., SAMHSA, 2014) and published work that has applied such practices (e.g., Alessi & Kahn, 2022; Goodwin & Tiderington, 2022; McMahon et al., 2023; Roche et al., 2020). One of the strengths of using a trauma-informed approach to guide the research process is that guidelines such as SAMHSA provide key principles (i.e., safety, trustworthiness and transparency, peer support, collaboration and mutuality, empowerment, and cultural, historical, and gender issues) rather than a prescribed set of practices. These guidelines can therefore be applied by researchers to a range of settings, including narrative interviews. In the section below, we unpack how these guidelines underpinned our research process, specifically when working with individuals post-amputation using narrative interviews.

Preparation for the Research

As part of our preparation for engaging in research we started by spending time in physical spaces (e.g., hospital waiting rooms, rehabilitation gyms, organised sports events for individuals post-amputation) where we learned about the physical environment related to amputation (Sanders et al., 2020; Wadey & Day, 2018) prior to conducting our research. In line with SAMHSA's (2014) guidelines, those experiencing trauma often perceive the world as 'unsafe' and may be in a constant state of arousal, yet at the point of embarking on this research, we had limited understanding of this specific world and consequently what/who held the potential to make it unsafe. To ensure that our research participants felt physically, socially, and psychologically safe, we needed to understand the spaces these participants typically inhabited, how these looked, felt, and smelled, and what sounds and conversations took place. To supplement our observations, we also read newspaper articles, magazines, autobiographies, and online blogs or community discussions which provided us with an understanding of contemporary difficulties that may be experienced and influential figures who had experienced similar trauma. We also engaged in conversations with medical practitioners (e.g., physiotherapists, occupational therapists) and charity founders to understand multiple perspectives. We further sought additional training outside of sport (e.g., Tavistock and Portman Clinic, UK; Wealden Institute, UK) to understand a range of trauma therapies and approaches to working with trauma.

Preparing for the research through observations, readings, and conversations helped us to create safety for participants in two ways. First, these practices impacted the planning and development of the research by allowing us to thoroughly consider procedural aspects of the research process that might be re-traumatising for participants (see below for changes implemented in practice). Second, these practices provided cultural understanding for us who, as researchers, may have been deemed 'outsiders' by our participants. Similar to the practice of McMahon et al. (2022) who recognised the importance of understanding specific beliefs, norms, values, spoken or unspoken rules in a specific context when exploring trauma, it was important for us to recognise specific language and terminology related to the context (e.g., ampuversary: the anniversary of an amputation). This recognition allowed us to converse in ways that were familiar to our participants as well as ensuring that our interview questions were contextually relevant.

Planning and Conducting Narrative Interviews

In planning for interviews, we considered the physical, social, and psychological safety of participants (SAMHSA, 2014) through adherence to four trauma-informed guidelines relating to relational safety: be predictable (i.e., do what you say you are going to do), be consistent (i.e., do what you say you will do over time), be accepting (i.e., do not shame, judge, or stigmatise others), and be accountable for your actions (acknowledge when mistakes are made and attempt to remedy them) (Alessi & Kahn, 2022). There were a number of procedural steps we took in planning and conducting our interviews that allowed us to adhere to these trauma-informed guidelines:

1 We provided details on the location of the interview, including features that might assist in avoiding re-traumatisation (e.g., the room is well-lit, the room has a window looking out over the park, the room includes tea and coffee making facilities). Where possible, participants were also provided with a photo of the interview space in the information letter. The aim of providing this additional information about the physical location was to enhance transparency (i.e., telling and even showing what the environment would look like) and consequently ensure participants could make an informed choice regarding their own sense of safety prior to consenting to take part in the research.
2 To further enhance trustworthiness and transparency (SAMHSA, 2014) we provided guidance on how long the interview would last and kept roughly to this length. This allowed for predictability of interviews and the amount of trauma information discussed in one interview. In line with McMahon et al. (2022), being trustworthy meant stating precisely what we intended

to do and following through with what we had stated. There were times that this was challenging. For example, on occasions participants would 'drop in' trauma-related information in the final ten minutes, knowing that the interview was nearly finished. When this occurred, we ensured the participant felt heard (e.g., acknowledging what had been said without rushing to close the interview) and invited them to revisit this in the next interview. For this reason, we found multiple interviews to be beneficial in our trauma research, rather than changing time boundaries and potentially reducing trust and predictability. It was also important to be consistent and predictable with the support we could offer (e.g., informing participants when and how we would follow-up and keep to this practice) after and in-between multiple interviews to maintain trustworthiness and professional boundaries.

3 To facilitate participant choice during interviews, we started questions with 'is it ok if we discuss …' and 'would you like to talk more about …'. This type of question was used to continually remind participants of their choice and power to remain involved in the research. As McMahon et al. (2022) highlighted in their trauma-informed work, trauma survivors have historically been diminished in voice and choice and thereby providing choice during interviews may empower the participant. In line with this approach, while we also re-iterated that participants could stop or pause the interview at any time, it was important to recognise that asking to stop may be difficult for those who have had limited previous opportunities to speak up in such a way. Thus, when appropriate, we took the lead in slowing the pace of the interview or pausing for some time out.

In addition to using these aforementioned procedural steps, we also considered how to structure our narrative interview content to avoid re-traumatisation. There is limited research concerning how to conduct or structure narrative interviews on traumatic experiences and consequently the approach outlined below is based on reflections of our own practice and understandings gained over time when conducting trauma research.

When we look back on our earlier practice, we tended to invite participants to tell chronological stories, choosing an appropriate start point and asking questions that would allow the participant to tell their story. This type of chronological story was familiar to us, it was how we told everyday (non-traumatic) stories, and it was how we ourselves, as research students, learned about the practice of narrative interviewing. Yet as outlined in Day and Martinelli (2016), using a chronological approach to hearing the participant's story can mean that 'during the early stages of an interview when rapport may be at its weakest, participants could be asked to discuss aspects of the story that they may find most difficult' (p. 16). In line with SAMHSA (2014) guidelines, using this chronological approach runs the risk of asking participants to share stories of trauma before establishing safety or demonstrating trustworthiness and transparency. Consequently, we no longer use a chronological approach and instead structure our narrative interviews based on 'chapters' rather than the whole story. We have found this approach fits particularly well when stories are fragmented as it allows the individual to consider a collection of small stories rather than starting out by telling a big story. Thus, now we often begin narrative interviews using the following invitation:

> I'd like you to imagine that rather than talking through your whole life story from start to end, you could divide up your story into a number of different chapters. There might, for example, be a chapter around amputation or a chapter around learning to ride a bike again [waits for participant response]. In our time today, if it's ok with you, I'd like to explore one of these chapters. It can be any chapter that you like, perhaps something that you'd like to talk about today or something that feels right as a start point.

Where we have used multiple interviews, participants are invited to consider which chapter they would like to talk about in their subsequent interview. In our experience, some participants will choose to start at the beginning, preferring to tell a chronological story, others will start at the end, describing how their life is now, while some will 'jump' around, choosing stories across time points. What is important here is that the order becomes the participant's choice rather than the interviewer's preference for traditional types of story-telling. As SAMHSA (2014) guidelines outline, it is important to recognise and build upon participant strengths and experiences, thereby fostering empowerment. As the term is used here, 'empowerment' refers to the degree to which participants feel a sense of agency and control over the interview process. Structuring narrative interviews in chapters has allowed us to maintain the research focus, while simultaneously allowing the research participant to control the topic, pace, and order of conversations across multiple interviews.

Our final consideration after interviewing was the well-being of participants and ourselves as researchers. We found that engaging in thorough preparation work (i.e., observing, reading, having conversations with physiotherapists and other hospital staff) prior to commencing the research facilitated better support provision to participants post-interview. Spending time gathering contextual knowledge and understanding prior to the project not only enhanced our research design but provided us with knowledge of resources and support available to this particular community. Rather than recommending support that we were unfamiliar with, we were able to provide more personal suggestions for support or resources, that were context specific, trauma-informed and which we ourselves found useful.

It is also important to acknowledge that studying trauma and engaging in trauma-focused interviews can and does impact us as researchers. Berger (2021) suggests that trauma work can have both positive impacts (e.g., experiencing vicarious growth) and negative impacts (e.g., vicarious trauma, behavioural and cognitive reactions). As researchers we have made new friends and witnessed or heard about many positive events (e.g., sporting achievements, the birth of a grandchild), yet there are negative impacts to our work. We both recall very vividly the story of one participant who became involved in a road accident while out for a run. This story impacted us both in a similar way, often thinking about this participant and his story when crossing the road and changing our own road safety behaviours as a consequence. Reflecting on how this story impacted us, we became aware that trauma stories focusing on every day or familiar events were very relatable and challenged some of our own assumptions of safety. We also became aware that the nature of our research can result in the need to complete interviews with multiple participants discussing trauma across a short period of time (e.g., while attending sporting/activity weekends). Recognising the cumulative effects of hearing trauma stories is important and where trauma-heavy content is expected, personal measures for self-care need to be put in place (e.g., taking breaks as needed, using each other for support and debriefing, planning time out such as exercise or hobbies the following day) (Berger, 2021). What has become clear to us when conducting trauma research, is that working as a research team allows us to support each other. Further, as our work has progressed, we have developed a clear philosophy of practice (e.g., prioritising well-being) that guides the way we work and communicate with each other.

Conclusions

To conclude this chapter, we present three ways in which research practice might move forward in becoming trauma-informed:

1   Trauma-informed practice is valuable for all who engage in research, not just those working with specific trauma populations. There is a critical need for researchers to be aware of what it means to be trauma-informed, and to utilise evidence-based trauma-informed practices (e.g., SAMHSA, 2014) to guide research practices with *all* research participants, regardless of what has been disclosed in the research process. In this chapter, we outline the numerous additional considerations that informed our research process with a trauma population, yet many of those participating in research have experienced undisclosed trauma or have not been asked about their trauma experiences because it is not within the scope of the study. Trauma-informed guidance from SAMHSA (2014) highlights that trauma is widespread and harmful. Thus, we need better consideration of the research environment and role of the researcher across all sport, exercise, and health research disciplines and how participating in research might inadvertently re-traumatise. Trauma-informed practice should therefore become part of standard training requirements across sport, exercise, and health disciplines.

2 At present there is limited research into how to conduct trauma-informed qualitative interviews. Therefore, it may be beneficial to expand our consideration of *how* to conduct interviews that ask about trauma (e.g., how to avoid creating power differences, how to maximise choice; SAMHSA, 2014). Second, we might make better use of therapeutic literature on trauma, for example the existing body of literature on narrative therapy. Authors such as Polkinghorne (2004) describe how narrative therapists look to extract the dominant story, hold it out for examination, and then assist the client in deconstructing the story using a variety of techniques. In this chapter, we have demonstrated how Rothschild's (2003) 'putting on the brakes' technique may be applied in a research context. While practicing therapy with individuals who have experienced traumatic events is very different to conducting research with them, there is much we could learn from those who work therapeutically with trauma stories, particularly regarding how to protect participants from re-traumatisation while helping them to share stories.
3 While we focused on the interview process in this chapter, it is imperative to consider what happens beyond the research interview. Qualitative procedures such as member reflections whereby participants are asked to comment on and reflect on results may pose additional challenges, often presenting results pertaining to trauma experiences virtually (i.e., by email or online discussion) to participants and asking for reflections. Thus, we need to consider the research process in its entirety, from preparing the study through to gaining member reflections on results and how participants' experiences are represented.

References

Alessi, E. J., & Kahn, S. (2022). Toward a trauma-informed qualitative research approach: Guidelines for ensuring the safety and promoting the resilience of research participants. *Qualitative Research in Psychology*. https://doi.org/10.1080/1478088 7.2022.2107967

Bennett, H., & Wells, A. (2010). Metacognition, memory disorganization and rumination in posttraumatic stress symptoms. *Journal of Anxiety Disorders, 24*, 318–325. http://dx.doi.org/10.1016/j.janxdis.2010.01.004

Berger, R. (2021). Studying trauma: Indirect effects on researchers and self- and strategies for addressing them. *European Journal of Trauma and Dissociation*. https://doi.org/10.1016/j.ejtd.2020.100149

Brewin, C. R. (2014). Episodic memory, perceptual memory, and their interaction: Foundations for a theory of posttraumatic stress disorder. *Psychological Bulletin, 140*(1), 69–97. https://doi.org/10.1037/a0033722

Burstow, B. (2003). Towards a radical understanding of trauma and trauma work. *Violence Against Women, 9*, 1293–1317. http://doi.org/10.1177/1077801203255555

Cavanagh, S. R., Shin, L. M.,Karamouz, N. Rauch, S. L (2006) Psychiatric and emotional sequelae of surgical amputation. *Psychosomatics, 47*, 459–464. https://doi.org/10.1176/APPI.PSY.47.6.459

Cordova, M. (2008). Facilitating posttraumatic growth following cancer. In S. Joseph & A. Linley (Eds.), *Trauma, recovery, and growth: Positive psychological perspectives on posttraumatic stress* (pp. 185–206). John Wiley.

Crespo, M., & Fernández-Lansac, V. (2016). Memory and narrative of traumatic events: A literature review. *Psychological Trauma: Theory, Research, Practice, and Policy, 8*(2), 149–156. https://doi.org/10.1037/tra0000041

Currier, J., & Neimeyer, R. A. (2006). Fragmented stories: The narrative integration of violent loss. In E. K. Rynearson (Ed.), *Violent death* (pp. 85–100). Routledge.

Day, M. (2013). The role of initial physical activity experiences in promoting post-traumatic growth in Paralympic athletes with an acquired disability. *Disability and Rehabilitation*, 1–9. https://doi.org/10.3109/09638288.2013.805822

Day, M., & Martinelli, L. (2016). The complexities of narrating athletic injuries. *Qualitative Methods in Psychology Bulletin, 22*, 14–21.

Darnall, B. D., Ephraim, P., Wegener, S. T., Dillingham, T., Pezzin, L., Rossbach, P., & MacKenzie, E. J. (2005). Depressive symptoms and mental health service utilization among persons with limb loss: Results of a national survey. *Archives of Physical Medicine and Rehabilitation, 86*, 650–658. https://doi.org/10.1016/j.apmr.2004.10.028

Eales, L., & Goodwin, D. L. (2022). Addressing trauma in adaptive physical activity: A call to reflection and action. *Adapted Physical Activity Quarterly, 39*, 141–159. https://doi.org/10.1123/apaq.2020-0129

Frank, A. (1995). *The wounded storyteller*. University of Chicago Press.

Gemignani, M. (2014). Memory, remembering, and oblivion in active narrative interviewing. *Qualitative Inquiry, 20*(2), 127–135. https://doi.org/10.1177/1077800413510271

Goodwin, J., & Tiderington, E. (2022). Building trauma informed research competencies in social work education. *Social Work Education, 41*, 143–156. https://doi.org/10.1080/02615479.2020.1820977

Green, B. L., Kaltman, S.,Frank, L., Glennie, M., Subramanian, A., Fritts-Wilson, M., Neptune, D., & Chung, J. (2011). Primary care providers' experiences with trauma patients: A qualitative study. *Psychological Trauma: Theory, Research, Practice, and Policy, 3*, 37. https://doi.org/10.1007/s11606-018-4810-2

Hefferon, K., & Kampman, H. (2020). Taking an embodied approach to post-traumatic growth research and sport. In R. Wadey, M. Day, and K. Howells (Eds.), *Growth following adversity in sport: A mechanism to positive change* (pp.131–143). Routledge.

Horgan, O., & MacLachlan, M. (2004) Psychosocial adjustment to lower-limb amputation: A review. *Disability and Rehabilitation*, 837–850. https://doi.org/10.1080/09638280410001708869

Jovchelovitch, S., & Bauer, M. W. (2000). Narrative interviewing. In M. W. Bauer & G. Gaskell (Eds.), *Qualitative researching with text, image, and sound: A practical handbook*. (pp. 57–74). SAGE Publications.

McGannon, K. R., Graper, S., & McMahon, J. (2022). Skating through pregnancy and motherhood: A narrative analysis of digital stories of elite figure skating expectant mothers. *Psychology of Sport and Exercise, 59*. https://doi.org/10.1016/j.psychsport.2021.102126

McMahon, J., McGannon, K. R., Zehntner, C., Werbicki, L., Stephenson, E., & Martin, K. (2023). *Trauma-informed abuse education in sport: engaging athlete abuse survivors as educators and facilitating a community of care*, 28, 958–971. https://doi.org/10.1080/13573322.2022.2096586

Neimeyer, R. A., & Levitt, H. (2001). Coping and coherence: A narrative perspective on resilience. In S. Snyder (Ed.), *Coping with stress* (pp. 47–67). Oxford University Press.

NHS. (2016). *Amputation.* https://www.nhs.uk/conditions/amputation/

Papathomas, A. (2017). Narrative inquiry: From cardinal to marginal … and back? In B. Smith & A. Sparkes (Eds.), *Routledge handbook of qualitative research in sport and exercise.* Routledge.

Polkinghorne, D. E. (2004). Narrative therapy and postmodernism. In L. E. Angus & J. McLeod (Eds.), *The handbook of narrative and psychotherapy: Practice, theory and research* (pp. 53–68). Sage.

Roche, P., Shimmin, C., Hickes, S., Khan, M., Sherzoi, O., Wicklund, E., Lavoie, J. G., Hardie, S., Wittmeier, K., & Sibley, K. (2020). Valuing all voices: Refining a trauma-informed, intersectional, and critical reflexive framework for patient engagement in health research using a qualitative descriptive approach. *Research Involvement and Engagement, 19,* 42. https://doi.org/10.1186/s40900-020-00217-2

Rothschild, B. (2003). *The body remembers: Unifying methods and models in the treatment of trauma and PTSD.* W. W. Norton and Company.

Substance Abuse and Mental Health Services Administration. (2014). SAMHSA's concept of trauma and guidance for a trauma informed approach. HHS publication no. (SMA) 14–4884. Rockville: Substance Abuse and Mental Health Services Administration. https://store.samhsa.gov/product/samhsas-concept-trauma-and-guidance-trauma-informed-approach/sma14-4884

Sanders, P., Wadey, R., Day, M., & Winter, S. (2020). Narratives of recovery over the first year after major lower limb loss. *Qualitative Health Research, 30,* 2049–2063. https://doi.org/10.1177/1049732320925794

Smith, B., & Sparkes, A. C. (2006). Narrative inquiry in psychology: Exploring the tensions within. *Qualitative Research in Psychology, 3,* 169–192. https://doi.org/10.1191/1478088706qrp068oa

Smith, B., & Sparkes, A. (2009). Narrative inquiry in sport and exercise psychology: What can it mean, and why might we do it? *Psychology of Sport and Exercise, 10,* 1–11. https://doi.org/10.1016/j.psychsport.2008.01.004

Van der Kolk, B. A. (1994). The body keeps the score: Memory and the evolving psychobiology of posttraumatic stress, *Harvard Review Psychiatry, 1,* 253–265. https://doi.org/10.3109/10673229409017088

Wadey, R., & Day, M. (2018). A longitudinal examination of leisure time physical activity following amputation in England. *Psychology of Sport and Exercise, 37,* 251–261. https://doi.org/10.1016/j.psychsport.2017.11.005

Chapter 10

Trauma and Spinal Cord Injury

Reflections from Research into Physical Activity and Sport

Toni Louise Williams and James Brighton

Introduction

Spinal cord injury (SCI) is the term given to the neural damage to the spinal cord and is typically experienced as a *traumatic* event impacting the physical, psychological, social, and emotional worlds that people inhabit. According to the World Health Organization (2020), the majority of traumatic SCIs are due to preventable causes including road traffic accidents, falls, violence, and work and sports-related injuries. Given these causes, people are most at risk of SCI during adolescence (15–19 years), young adulthood (20–29 years), and older age (60+ years) with the ratio of men to women with SCI at least 2:1. Damage to the spinal cord affects the conduction of neurological signals across the site(s) of lesion resulting in temporary or permanent changes in sensory, motor or autonomic function below the level of injury (Singh et al., 2014). The degree of resulting impairment depends upon injury location and whether the spinal cord is partially ruptured or completely severed. Damage to the thoracic vertebrae can result in immediate impairment in the legs, trunk, and pelvic organs (known as paraplegia), whereas injury to the cervical vertebrae also impacts arm and hand function, swallowing and speech (known as quadriplegia or tetraplegia) (Ahuja et al., 2017).

Following SCI, people are also at risk of developing debilitating and life-threatening secondary health conditions. These health conditions include urinary tract infections, pressure ulcers, obesity, chronic pain, respiratory dysfunction, and cardiovascular disorders and put people at risk for poor mental health, increased disability, and a decreased life expectancy (Canning & Hicks, 2014; Krause & Saunders, 2011). Not only is the act of acquiring SCI traumatic, but losses related to the consequences of injury (e.g., physical functioning, bladder and bowel control, employment, social role, identity, previously valued activities) and associated conditions (e.g., surgery) that are experienced during rehabilitation present further enduring traumatising experiences (e.g., Day, 2013; Pollard & Kennedy, 2007; Smith, 2013). Considering the above, in this chapter we draw on extracts from our own empirical research with people who have acquired SCI and their experiences in

DOI: 10.4324/9781003332909-13

physical activity (PA) (Toni) and sport (James) to explore responses to such a traumatic life event over time. In doing so, we reflect on conceptual, methodological, and method-based considerations in undertaking research in SCI, trauma, PA, and sport to limit the possibility of causing further trauma to those people involved in our research. As each approach is outlined, we shift to the first-person voice to share each researcher's experiences. We conclude with suggestions for trauma-informed approaches to future research with people with SCI.

Toni's Research: A Critical Approach to Physical Activity for People with SCI

My research focuses on taking a critical approach to PA promotion for people with acquired SCI. There is a growing body of research focusing on PA for people with SCI based on the established benefits of exercise to health and well-being. Being physically active, whether that be generally wheeling, exercising in the gym, or playing sport, has been shown to alleviate or prevent many of the health and well-being complications associated with SCI (van Der Scheer et al., 2017). Further, psychological benefits to well-being include perceived enjoyment, reduced depression, enhanced life satisfaction, and the promotion of positive experiences following SCI known as post-traumatic growth (Brighton, 2020; Day, 2013; Williams et al., 2014). The impact of traumatic SCI and the perceived benefits to both physical and mental health from regular PA participation can be illustrated by a participant called 'Robert' who acquired SCI at the age of 45 following a car accident:

> Well I've had with my diet a two stone weight loss and psychologically its [adapted exercise programme] helped me a lot. It's something in my life, whereas I have a lot of lonely boring days. Yeah, takes my mind of things, because when I have loads of time on my hands and not doing anything, I'm inactive. I think of the accident and my life in general and it's kind of depressing. So this has helped me psychologically because I was on anti-depressants and I've come off them now ... but when I did come here, initially I had pain medication, bladder and bowel [issues] and some other important things. But a lot of those issues have been addressed now since I've been doing this [adapted exercise programme], I feel a lot better.
>
> (Williams, 2018, p. 230)

Although Robert highlights perceived benefits of PA to managing ongoing traumatic experiences associated with his injury, the promise of PA as a panacea for health and well-being issues following SCI aligns with the dominant *exercise is medicine* narrative (Papathomas et al., 2015; Williams et al., 2018a). The *exercise is medicine* movement reproduces the late modern neoliberal ideal, by calling on healthcare providers to prescribe PA as a means to control clinical health issues and urges individuals to take responsibility for their physical and psychological health and exercise for their own good (see Cairney et al., 2018). Yet, despite the promise of health and well-being gains through PA, people with SCI face multiple personal, social, environmental, cultural, and political barriers to leading an active lifestyle (Williams et al., 2014). Facing such barriers can be traumatising when people with SCI are unable to access PA opportunities they wish to pursue, or face discrimination and exclusion in sport and exercise spaces (e.g., Richardson et al., 2017). The exercise is medicine initiative thereby ignores the numerous interacting inequalities impacting sport, exercise, and PA participation for people with SCI (Williams et al., 2018a). Exercise is medicine also reproduces ableist ideologies of 'fixing' and 'controlling' the disabled and traumatised body entrenched in the medical model of conceptualising disability (Brighton et al., 2021). I will further draw on these critical insights from my research of the role of PA in the lives of people with SCI and trauma-informed methodological considerations in this chapter.

James' Research: SCI, Sport, and Identity

While Toni's research focused on PA, my research centred on using ethnographic methodologies in exploring the traumatic embodied experiences of people who have acquired SCI and their subsequent involvement in disability sport (e.g., Wheelchair Rugby, Wheelchair Basketball, and Athletics). This work has highlighted how participation in disability sport can provide resistance to common medically informed, and normative stereotypes of disability, assist in the development of valued body-self relationships and identities, and improve fitness and social opportunity (e.g., Brighton, 2014, 2020; Sparkes et al., 2018, 2021). These points are demonstrated from the following quote from 'Jack' on his experiences of attending a gym five years post-SCI:

> It wasn't until I went to my local gym that I could come to terms with myself. That's what did it for me, I'm not saying that works for everybody I'm not saying it can't …. Whatever it might be that helps you turn that corner but for me it was sport and going down my local gym. And it was like a snowball, that domino effect from going down the gym to someone saying why don't you join the [athletics] club now, you'd be great you know, being a great role model and then you know … from there my jigsaw puzzle, I started putting together a few pieces … I got down [the gym] and I started training and I was like "wow". I found myself. I am back. I had found my comfort zone. This is where I wanted to be, this is what I was born to do, to train. That's all I wanted to do, to train. I was gladiator. I couldn't do anything else; I wasn't born to do anything else.
>
> (Brighton, 2020, p. 180)

However, disability sport is also saturated with individualistic, heroic, ableist and often hypermasculine, heteronormative, and misogynistic discourses. For some SCI-injured athletes, both male and female, these discourses contribute to the (re)creation of risky and instrumental rationalities towards the body and exposure to further traumatising experiences in seeking enhanced sporting performance (e.g., Brighton, 2014; Sparkes & Brighton, 2020). The impact of these discourses can be demonstrated by drawing on the experiences of 'Stefan' who purposefully induces a state of Autonomic Dysreflexia (AD). AD is a typically traumatic and risky experience for people with SCI above the sixth thoracic spinal level (T6), resulting in elevated blood pressure for the purpose of 'boosting' performance in wheelchair rugby:

> I was literally a year post-injury. I knew the importance of hydrating, and so during rugby matches I would probably drink more water than what I would do in a normal timeframe in between cathing. I just noticed that there were certain times in the game when my bladder would fill and maybe initially it would give me a really nice little energy boost …
>
> (Sparkes & Brighton, 2020, p. 419)

By purposefully distending the bladder by drinking too much and not emptying his catheter (cathing), in the above example, Stefan hints at the risks he is willing to take to enhance his performance. Such research has helped to highlight how disability sport should not be seen as less competitive or in some way 'purer' than able-bodied sport, but rather should be better understood as a contested phenomenon with a dark side and potential for ongoing traumatising experiences. As shown below through my ethnographic explorations and making many mistakes and reflecting on them, I have also highlighted how research with disabled people in sport and PA settings *itself* can be traumatic (e.g., Brighton, 2015; Brighton & Williams, 2018). Having outlined our research in the field, we now address the methodologies and methods we employed which hold potential to assist researchers in this area, and suggest how certain approaches can assist participants who are experiencing trauma.

Methodology and Method

We have both employed different methodological approaches (e.g., narrative, ethnography) and a number of methods of data generation (e.g., participant observation, life history interviews, and timelining) and analysis (e.g., thematic and narrative analyses) to explore the lived experiences of SCI within PA and sport. It is important to recognise that the choice of qualitative approach should be guided by specific objectives of the study, ontological and epistemological assumptions, the phenomena explored, the positionality of the researcher, and evidence-based procedures to avoid further traumatising participants throughout the research process (Brighton & Williams, 2018; McMahon et al., 2022). Fostering a critical ideological positioning is especially meaningful when undertaking research into disability which has been built upon political and activist underpinnings and the historical exploitation of disabled research participants (see Brighton, 2015; Macbeth & Powis, 2022).

While we do not have room to cover each one of the approaches we employed, we selected one methodological aspect each to provide a flavour of the considerations of exploring SCI, trauma, PA, and sport. First, Toni reflects on taking a longitudinal integrated methods approach to exploring the storied experiences of activity-based rehabilitation (ABR) for people with SCI and James reflects on his experiences of undertaking ethnography in disability sport. Both approaches place the researcher in naturalistic terrain, where social behaviour is produced. Given this, analyses of methodology should include the presence of the researcher themselves as well as participants, so we also provide brief considerations of how the research impacted us.

Toni: Longitudinal Integrated Methods

In a narrative study I drew upon an integrated methods approach to explore the storied experiences of ABR for people with SCI (see Williams, 2018). Narrative inquiry is often drawn on in sport and trauma research (Massey & Williams, 2020), and was chosen as the underpinning methodology. Narrative inquiry is largely underpinned and informed by interpretivism and framed by ontological relativism (which assumes reality to be multiple, malleable, and subjective) and epistemological constructionism (which assumes knowledge is socially constructed through relational interactions) (Papathomas, 2016). From this perspective, storytelling is considered a key means by which people make sense of their lives following serious injury such as SCI (Frank, 2013). An integrated methods approach is one type of *pluralism*, whereby multiple qualitative methods are drawn upon throughout the research process to address the complexities of experience (Chamberlain et al., 2011). This 'fusion' of qualitative methods has much to offer trauma-related research by:

- Providing pluralistic data sets that offer 'different takes' on a topic and insights that would not be realised through a single method (Chamberlain et al., 2011).
- Affording opportunities to incorporate chronological, spatial, and corporeal understandings of participants' lifeworld (Papaloukas et al., 2017).
- Capturing multi-dimensional and embodied understandings that are unlikely to be accessed through verbal means alone (Williams, 2018).

Drawing on a longitudinal integrated methods approach allowed me to highlight a more comprehensive understanding of ABR experiences that

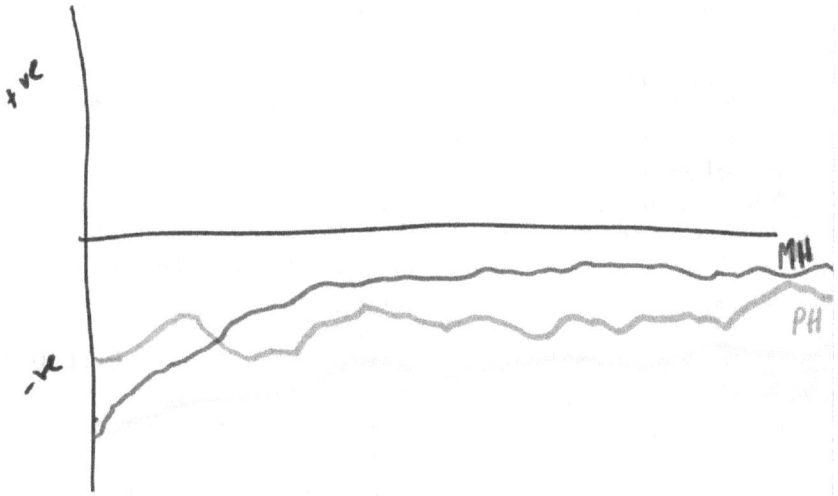

Figure 10.1 Robert's timeline from Williams (2018, p. 231) (note: MH = perceived mental health, PH = perceived physical health, H&E = hope and expectation).

would not have been realised through one method alone. Spending time immersed in the field developing trust and rapport with participants facilitated the telling of personal stories in interviews that went beyond the stories observed on the gym floor. Timelining is a visual representation illustrating how participants made sense of their experiences of health, well-being, and hope since acquiring their SCI (Sheridan et al., 2011). Timelining facilitated a deeper reflection of experiences over time, which was not achieved through questions and interactions during interviews and observations. Longitudinal data collection also highlighted the temporal dynamics of storytelling by providing a more nuanced understanding of how narratives change over time.

A longitudinal multiple methods approach also holds benefits and practical value for people with SCI. By drawing on interviews, timelining and participant observation, participants were able to express themselves in a variety of complementary and congruent ways. For example, reflecting on participants' experiences of health and hope overtime through creating timelines, facilitated difficult conversations about ongoing trauma following SCI that may not be touched upon without this visual representation. This is illustrated in the following quote from 'Robert' and accompanying timeline in Figure 10.1 (see above):

Robert: It (mental health) started really low (on the timeline), and it got a bit better, but it's still not on the positive.

Toni: Why is that?

Robert: Psychologically I can't accept that this has happened to me and I'm in a wheelchair. I don't think I will ever accept it, I just can't. I can't relate and talk to other people in wheelchairs ... Being here I've seen more people who are more severely injured than me, and can do a lot less than me, and that makes me feel guilty the way I feel because, you know. They've even said to me I do brilliant, I motorbike still and it makes me feel quite bad like, when I feel down sometimes I think "oh I can do quite a lot of stuff." It's just I don't think I ever will accept it. But I've seen a psychiatrist and a psychologist and what not, and I've got a bit of an understanding, and they say I don't ever have to accept it as long as I make the most of my life what I can.

(2nd interview, Williams, 2018, p. 231)

That said, there are practical and ethical issues to be considered with multiple methods research and the use of visual methods, in particular to ensure projects are as inclusive, but do not cause further trauma to participants through sharing intimate aspects of their lives and visually representing their experiences (Papaloukas et al., 2017; Sheridan et al., 2011). For example, to avoid causing further trauma to participants through my research, participants were able to choose how they took part in the study by opting in and out of being observed on the gym floor (e.g., if they were having a bad day and wanted to be left alone to exercise) and saying when conversations were not to be included as data. To be as inclusive as possible without highlighting the limitations brought about by SCI (Day, 2013), I also had to consider how participants were going to take part in the timelining to ensure it was a valuable tool to enrich my understanding of participants' experiences. Those with SCI injuries which impacted their hand function asked me to draw their timeline for them based on a timeframe that was meaningful to them, and their detailed descriptions of their health, well-being, and hope over time. Overall, it was important that participants had choice and power (both of which are evidence-based trauma-informed principles) over *how* they took part in the research to minimise any potential traumatising experiences from taking part (Angelo, 2015).

As well as minimising trauma for research participants, I also found I needed to take care of myself as a researcher when listening to participants' traumatic stories to limit the possibility of vicarious trauma resulting:

Today was a fairly emotional day. I interviewed Gareth for the first time and I was shocked and saddened by the stories he told me. Gareth is such a typical Jack-the-lad on the gym floor. He is constantly making jokes, teasing me and having a laugh with everyone. There is never a serious moment with Gareth around. But this all changed when Gareth agreed to be interviewed today. Gone was the comical lad. Instead, I was privileged to listen to some of Gareth's most heart wrenching moments following his SCI. He openly talked to me about his experiences in hospital, problems within the care home, and issues of inaccessibility in his own home and some of his most distressing times. Gareth said that if he didn't have that hope that he will get better, than he wouldn't want to carry on. I actually had a tear in my eye when I reflected on this interview.

(Reflexive journal entry from Williams, 2018, p. 229)

I sometimes found myself distressed after interviews, on more challenging days on the gym floor, or during analysis when re-visiting difficult traumatic moments from participants' stories. Given the relational nature of storytelling (Frank, 2013), I built relationships with participants which led to these emotional experiences as I engaged with their traumatic experiences with empathy (Andersen & Ivarsson, 2015; Smith et al., 2021). To cope with my emotional responses of listening to participants' traumatic stories, I used my reflexive journal to impart my thoughts and emotions. I also confided in my supervisor who offered compassion, support, and strategies for dealing with my own experiences in the field (Sanders et al., 2017). Becoming distressed can be indicative of vicarious trauma which arises from listening to participants' stories of traumatic experiences and can lead to feeling overwhelmed and hopeless, nightmares, intrusive thoughts and images, anxiety, and depression (Smith et al., 2021).

Recommendations to manage and mitigate vicarious trauma include regular debriefing opportunities with other researchers working with traumatised populations and pathways to referral services such as the university counselling service (Sanders et al., 2017; Smith et al., 2021). That said, McMahon et al. (2022) propose that a 'community of care' should be created from the outset of a research project to protect those affected by trauma. For McMahon et al. (2022), a 'community of care' represents the "mutual goal of providing evidence-based strategies to ensure the safety (i.e., physical, social mental) and care of all parties involved … This means strategies and care occur in a reciprocal way, so no further harm results for the entire community" (p. 7). Further examples of promoting physical and psychological safety are included in the final section of this book chapter on trauma-informed approaches to SCI research.

James: Ethnography

O'Reilly (2012, p. 3) outlines ethnography as an umbrella term that "draws on a family of methods, usually including participant observation and conversation" that represents the complexity of the social world and the phenomena under study through developing "rich, sensitive and credible stories".

Employing ethnography is instrumental in revealing powerful insights into the ongoing trauma experienced by SCI athletes in the following ways:

i Traumatic experiences are observed as *they happen* in naturalistic settings. Due to the participatory role of the researcher, some traumatic episodes were experienced jointly with participants. Not only were some traumas experienced by participants interpreted as they occurred, but the *dynamics of how trauma stories are told* in interviews and the 'truths' that are constructed within them can be nuanced with how they were experienced.

ii Traumatic experiences are revealed, contextualised, and analysed *across various social spheres* including in sporting, social, and private fields. For example, the 'psycho-emotional' (Thomas, 2007) trauma experienced by multiple transitions between every day and sport specific wheelchairs and training equipment were exposed (see Brighton, 2015, 2020). Trauma resulting from the unpredictability and uncontrollability of bladder and bowel movements in public and private spaces was also exposed (Moreno-Fergusson & Grace, 2016).

iii The *spontaneity and serendipity* offered by ethnography allowed trauma to be explored in alternative and unanticipated ways, challenging preconceptions and changing the focus of the investigation. For example, in previous work I discussed how SCI athletes have felt compelled to mark experiences of trauma through tattooing and other modificatory practices (see Sparkes et al., 2021) in order to help make sense of new identities embodied post-SCI.

iv Traumatic experience can be *analysed over time*, helping to show: (1) affective responses of trauma of acquiring SCI at differing moments in a lifetime; (2) the multiple, overlapping, and ongoing traumatic experiences; and (3) and the interrelation of past and present experiences of trauma. Prolonged engagement in the field allows for a deeper appreciation of trauma stories and is important in examining performative aspects of identity in response to different traumatic episodes and changes and fluctuations in narrative course.

v Ethnography facilitates *close relationships with participants* and *the generation of collaborative knowledge* (O'Reilly, 2012). Stories of trauma are highly personal and sensitive and lay bare deep-seated fears, anxieties, vulnerabilities, and desires. As Wolcott (2005, p. 60) indicates "intimate, long-term acquaintance" is central in ethnography in order to achieve "some depth of human understanding". Building emotional and affective bonds assist with the richness of interpretations of trauma.

vi Ethnography helps to *reveal experiences of trauma-related oppression* in ways neither participants nor researcher were conscious of. For example, I had not imagined the phenomenon of 'boosting' and the structural oppression present in wheelchair rugby for SCI athletes or other harmful embodied practices present in disability sport (see Sparkes & Brighton, 2020).

Above anything else, however, when undertaking trauma-related research of any sort (e.g., with people with acquired SCI), it is important to recognise that uncritical, un-reflexive research risks reproducing ableist research practices, relationships, and understandings. Careful critical reflection should therefore be given to the researcher's own underlying knowledge of the world and their subjectivities, socialisations, embodiment, and politics. To provide one example of this in research into SCI and trauma, given the unescapable differences between the often able-bodied researcher and participants bodies, there exists an implicit impulse to ask, 'What happened?' Not only can asking such a question cause trauma consciously or subconsciously in the re-telling, it is also politically and ethically dangerous. While the researchers' intentions might be well intended and this line of questioning deemed inexorable in exploring experiences of trauma and any other aspect of people's lives who have acquired SCI, asking "What happened?" defines people primarily by their disability and evokes sympathy. This is offensive as it perpetuates medicalising and tragic understandings of disability (Thomas, 2007) and serves to distinguish, omit, and dismiss people with SCI lives by positioning them as inferior.

To expand this point further, in her work exploring the non-disabled stare, Garland-Thomson (2006) elucidates how staring is followed by asking 'what happened to you?' in a 'stare-and-tell ritual' which is the "social enactment of exclusion from an imagined community of the fully human" (p. 188). For people who have acquired SCI, this ritual places life post-SCI as an 'aftermath' (read: afterthought) further restricting more empowering narrative storylines as individuals attempt to piece together a body and sense of self in an ableist neoliberal capitalist society which already positions them as a 'problem' and burdensome. So, while many (e.g., Moreno-Fergusson & Grace, 2016) argue that gaining in-depth understandings of traumatic life events are important in building effective interventions to trauma, asking 'What happened?' should be avoided. Instead, as discussed below, research strategies should be engendered that prioritise participants' voices and agency, providing them with the power to talk about trauma if they wish, how they wish. Doing so helps position participants at the centre of knowledge construction, all of which requires the researcher to be reflexive.

Trauma-Informed Approach to SCI Research

In the following section, we build on the examples above and outline additional trauma-informed approaches that can be applied to research with people with SCI to minimise further trauma. The Substance Abuse and Mental

Health Services Administration (SAMHSA, 2014) has outlined six evidence-based key principles which are fundamental to trauma-informed approaches. We focus upon three key principles and provide an example of how these principles could be used to guide qualitative research with spinal cord injured people in PA and sport settings who may be negotiating ongoing trauma.

Physical and Psychology Safety

The first principle of trauma-informed approaches that can be applied to research with people with SCI outlines the importance of promoting *physical and psychological safety*. This principle relates to ensuring that the physical setting of any research participation (e.g., location of interviews) and interpersonal interactions (e.g., with researchers and other participations [in focus groups, etc.]) promotes a sense of safety. In our research, a number of steps were taken to promote safety and manage any distress arising from participants' involvement in our projects. For example, from the outset of our interactions with people with SCI, we purposely avoided using problematic – and potentially traumatic – terms such as 'acceptance' or 'recovery' unless participants broached the subject themselves. These terms represent a psychological end point in neurological rehabilitation whereby a patient has accepted their current situation and has realistic hopes and expectations for the future (Soundy et al., 2014). Discussing acceptance and recovery can be problematic because there is often a delicate balance in SCI rehabilitation between managing realistic expectations following SCI and not promoting false hope of recovery (Williams et al., 2018b).

One way we strove to create a safe environment in which participants *could* share their traumatic stories with us, if they chose to, was through building rapport and trusting, reciprocal and open research relationships (McMahon et al., 2022). Although rapport is a unique, context specific, and highly embodied process, time in the field provides opportunities to demonstrate intent, empathy, and compassion for participants and their agendas. These practices facilitated sharing one's own trauma stories and vulnerabilities and affords researchers' own relationships to disability (Brighton, 2015). Another advantage here is that we were both able to demonstrate our commitment to participants through *action* by undertaking a number of assistive roles including being a fitness trainer, carer, mechanic, taxi driver, and personal assistant. Thus, rapport was extended with participants in interactions in the field beyond the basketball court and ABR centre to demonstrate care and empathy (Andersen & Ivarsson, 2015; Angelo, 2015). Our prior experiences (e.g., Toni had worked as a care assistant; James' Dad is disabled) and relationships built with participants and others (e.g., coaches, parents, etc.) meant that we were trusted to carry out such roles. During this time in the field, we took a genuine interest in our participants' lives, as they did with our lives, through the sharing of intimate stories which further enhanced rapport.

As Andersen and Ivarsson (2015) explain, it is paramount that as researchers we are open, accepting, non-judgemental, and curious when responding to participants' stories to avoid causing further trauma. We would therefore recommend that researchers foster safety and rapport with participants with SCI through prolonged ethnographic methods (e.g., observation and participation rather than dropping in, taking data from participants, then leaving) while demonstrating empathy and showing genuine non-judgemental care in participants' lived experiences. Furthermore, we call on researchers of trauma to not just claim, but explicitly address, how rapport was addressed and reflected upon, and how different relationships and selves were managed and negotiated in the field. Attempting and claiming rapport should be approached with caution due to the dangers of navigating human relationships under the pretence of research and the careful management of the presentation of different selves in the field. These practices fundamentally impact on inclusivity and interpretations made of the other (see Brighton, 2015).

Collaboration, Mutuality, Empowerment, Voice, and Choice

The fourth principle highlights *collaboration and mutuality* in relation to the levelling of power differences and the fifth principle emphasises *empowerment, voice, and choice*. A way to empower people with SCI brining these two principles together in future projects is to collaborate *with* them throughout the research process through methods of co-production. There are many different definitions and practices of co-production across the sport, exercise, PA, and health literature. One type of co-production that positions people with SCI at the centre of the research process is *equitable and experientially informed co-produced research*. As Smith et al. (2023) highlight, this type of co-production positions people with lived experience and experiential knowledge as *essential* to the research process. Equitable and experientially informed co-produced research also seeks to form *equitable partnerships* with community and citizen partners by addressing inequalities in power. This process includes addressing oppressive structures, systems, and hierarchies in power to illustrate how they have marginalised or excluded certain people and forms of knowledge. Forming such equitable partnerships is important as they enable communities, citizens, and/or service users to initiate, contribute, influence, and even direct the research process.

This type of co-production can lead to collaborative and equitable research that is not only transformative and impactful, but addresses the needs, concerns, and preferences of people with lived experience (Smith et al., 2023). Following this guiding principle, equitable and experientially informed co-produced research on PA, sport, and SCI could involve sport and exercise practitioners, people working in health promotion or rehabilitation, family, and carers, but must include or be led by people with SCI. What this means in practice is that power is shared so that people with SCI play an active role in driving the research throughout the entire project, and focuses on issues important to the SCI community from the outset. This process can include researchers joining SCI partners in the project they are already leading, or researchers working *with* people with SCI as equitable partners from the beginning of a project. Smith and colleagues (2023) warn that sharing power and forming equitable partnerships may be challenging and uncomfortable in co-produced research. They therefore advise that issues of power and authority can be explicitly addressed by valuing what each member of the partnership can bring to the collaboration and discussing how everyone can influence decision making.

The working principles for equitable and experimentally informed co-produced research highlighted by Smith et al. (2023) are not explicitly stated as trauma-informed. However, many of their recommendations for ensuring equitable partnerships do align with the trauma-informed literature in preventing further emotional and psychological harm. For example, further recommendations for equitable and experimentally informed co-produced research include valuing all knowledge and expertise, embracing conflict and diverse views and genuinely investing in equitable partnerships. These complement the recommendations of trauma-informed co-production proposed by Lonbay et al. (2021) such as creating space for openness and honesty; ensuring time to share experiences during meetings and time to reflect and debrief at the end; asking people how they work; providing inclusive access to the academic world; and identifying pathways to support both during the project and after it ends.

Conclusion

In this chapter, we have reflected upon our empirical research with people who have acquired SCI and their experiences of PA and sport over time following this traumatic life event. Drawing upon the conceptual and methodological considerations discussed, we proposed future directions for trauma-informed research with spinal cord injured people in PA and sport contexts. For instance, we recommend integrating multiple methods with ethnographic approaches to capture multi-dimensional communication, experiences, and embodied understandings of PA and sport following traumatic experiences of SCI. We also advocate for the use of equitable and experientially informed co-produced research which positions people with SCI as essential to the research process to address their needs, concerns, and preferences in relation to PA and sport.

In addition to the points already discussed, we close this book chapter by also encouraging researchers to take an intersectional approach (Crenshaw, 1989) to explore how multiple axes of oppression (e.g., disablism, sexism, racism, etc.) shape people's PA and sport experiences. This is important to recognise as disability represents only one dimension of an individual's identity and their experiences of trauma and how they articulate it will depend on many other embodied identities including race, gender identity, sexual orientation, etc. (see Brighton & Williams, 2018). Examining the intersectional experiences of people with SCI has the potential to challenge the heteronormative and ableist discourses described above and support alternative more inclusive research and representations of disability sport and PA (Irish et al., 2022; Wheeler & Peers, 2022). Taken together, these recommendations foster a critical and reflexive trauma-informed approach to research, challenge ableist research practices, and give participants voice and agency in the research process.

References

Ahuja, C. S., Wilson, J. R., Nori, S., Kotter, M. R. N., Druschel, C., Curt, A., & Fehlings, M. G. (2017). Traumatic spinal cord injury. *Nature Reviews Disease Primers*, *3*, 17018. https://doi.org/10.1038/nrdp.2017.18

Andersen, M. B., & Ivarsson, A. (2015). A methodology of loving kindness: How interpersonal neurobiology, compassion and transference can inform researcher–participant encounters and storytelling. *Qualitative Research in Sport, Exercise and Health*, *8*(1), 1–20. https://doi-org.ezphost.dur.ac.uk/10.1080/2159676X.2015.1056827

Angelo, G. (2015). *Rapport: The art of connecting with people and building relationships*. SN & NS Publications.

Brighton, J. (2014). *Narratives of spinal cord injury and the sporting body: An ethnographic study*. Unpublished PhD Thesis, Leeds Beckett University.

Brighton, J. (2015). Researching disabled sporting bodies: Reflections from an 'able'-bodied ethnographer. In I. Wellard (Ed.), *Researching embodied sport* (pp. 163–177). Routledge.

Brighton, J. (2020). Posttraumatic growth in disability sport following spinal cord injury: A narrative approach. In R. Wadey, M. Day, & K. Howells (Eds.), *Growth following adversity in sport* (pp. 174–188). Routledge.

Brighton, J., & Williams, T. L. (2018). Using interviews to explore experiences of disability in sport and physical activity. In R. Medcalf & C. Mackintosh (Eds.), *Researching difference in sport and physical activity* (pp. 25–40). Routledge. https://doi.org/10.4324/9781315266749-3

Brighton, J., Townsend, R. C., Campbell, N., & Williams, T. L. (2021). Moving beyond models: Theorizing physical disability in the sociology of sport. *Sociology of Sport Journal*, *38*(4), 386–398. https://doi.org/10.1123/ssj.2020-0012

Cairney, J., McGannon, K. R., & Atkinson, M. (2018). Exercise is medicine: Critical considerations in the qualitative research landscape. *Qualitative Research in Sport, Exercise and Health*, *10*(4), 391–399. https://doi.org/10.1080/2159676X.2018.1476010

Canning, K. L., & Hicks, A. L. (2014). Secondary health conditions associated with spinal cord injury. *Critical Reviews in Physical and Rehabilitation Medicine*, *26*, 181–191. https://doi.org/10.1615/CritRevPhysRehabilMed.2014011067

Chamberlain, K., Cain, T., Sheridan, J., & Dupuis, A. (2011). Pluralisms in qualitative research: From multiple methods to integrated methods. *Qualitative Research in Psychology*, *8*, 151–169. https://doi.org/10.1080/14780887.2011.572730

Crenshaw, K. W. (1989). Demarginalizing the intersection of race and sex: A black feminist critique of antidiscrimination doctrine, feminist theory and antiracist politics. *The University of Chicago Legal Forum, 140*, 139–167.

Day, M. C. (2013). The role of initial physical activity experiences in promoting post-traumatic growth in Paralympic athletes with an acquired disability. *Disability and Rehabilitation, 35*, 2064–2072. https://doi.org/10.3109/09638288.2013.805822

Frank, A. W. (2013). *The wounded storyteller* (2nd ed.). University of Chicago Press.

Garland-Thomson, R. (2006). Ways of staring. *Journal of Visual Culture, 5*(2), 173–192. https://doi.org/10.1177/1470412906066907

Irish, T., McDonald, K., & Cavallerio, F. (2022). Race, disability and sport: The experience of black deaf individuals. In B. Powis, J. Brighton, & P. D. Howe (Eds.), *Researching disability sport* (pp. 112–123). Routledge.

Krause, K. S., & Saunders, L. L. (2011). Health, secondary conditions, and life expectancy after spinal cord injury. *Archives of Physical Medicine and Rehabilitation, 92*, 1770–1775. https://doi.org/10.1016/j.apmr.2011.05.024

Lonbay, S., Pearson, A., Hamilton, E., Higgins, Pa., Foulkes, E., & Glascott, M. (2021). Trauma-informed participatory research: Reflections on co-producing a research proposal. *Gateways: International Journal of Community Research and Engagement, 14*(1), 1–8. http://dx.doi.org/10.5130/ijcre.v14i1.7728

Macbeth, J., & Powis, B. (2022). What are we doing here?: Confessional tales of non-disabled researchers in disability sport. In B. Powis, J. Brighton, & P. D. Howe (Eds.), *Researching disability sport* (pp. 55–69). Routledge.

Massey, W. V., & Williams, T. L. (2020). Sporting activities for individuals who experienced trauma during their youth: A meta-study. *Qualitative Health Research, 30*(1), 73–87. http://doi.org/10.1177/1049732319849563

McMahon, J., McGannon, K. R., Zehntner, C., Werbicki, L., Stephenson, E., & Martine, K. (2022). Trauma-informed abuse education in sport: Engaging athlete abuse survivors as educators and facilitating a community of care. *Sport, Education and Society*. https://doi.org/10.1080/13573322.2022.2096586

Moreno-Fergusson, M. E., & Grace, P. J. (2016). Ethical analysis of a qualitative researcher's unease in encountering a participant's existential ambivalence. *Annual Review of Nursing Research, 34*(1), 51–65. https://doi.org/10.1891/0739-6686.34.51

O'Reilly, K. (2012). *Ethnographic method*. Routledge.

Papaloukas, P., Quincey, K., & Williamson, I. R. (2017). Venturing into the visual voice: Combining photos and interviews in phenomenological inquiry around marginalisation and chronic illness. *Qualitative Research in Psychology, 14*(4), 415–441. https://doi.org/10.1080/14780887.2017.1329364

Papathomas, A. (2016). Narrative inquiry: From cardinal to marginal … and back? In B. Smith & A.C. Sparkes (Eds.), *International handbook of qualitative methods in sport and exercise* (pp. 37–48). Routledge.

Papathomas, A., Williams, T. L., & Smith, B. (2015). Understanding physical activity participation in spinal cord injured populations: Three narrative types for consideration. *International Journal of Qualitative Studies on Health and Well-Being, 14*(10), 27295. https://doi.org/10.3402/qhw.v10.27295

Pollard, C., & Kennedy, P. (2007). A longitudinal analysis of emotional impact, coping strategies and post-traumatic psychological growth following spinal cord injury: A 10-year review. *British Journal of Health Psychology, 12*(3), 347–362. https://doi.org/10.1348/135910707X197046

Richardson, E. V., Smith, B., & Papathomas, A. (2017). Disability and the gym: Experiences, barriers and facilitators of gym use for individuals with physical disabilities. *Disability and Rehabilitation, 39*(19), 1950–1957. https://doi.org/10.1080/09638288.2016.1213893

Sanders, P., Wadey, R., Day, M., & Winter, S. (2017). Qualitative fieldwork in medical contexts: Confessions of a neophyte researcher. *Qualitative Research in Sport, Exercise and Health, 11*(1), 106–118. https://doi.org/10.1080/2159676X.2017.1351390

Sheridan, J., Chamberlain, K., & Dupuis, A. (2011). Timelining: Visualizing experience. *Qualitative Research, 11*(5), 552–569. https://doi.org/10.1177/1468794111413235

Singh, A., Tetreault, L., Kalsi-Ryan, S., Nouri, A., & Fehlings, M. G. (2014). Global prevalence and incidence of traumatic spinal cord injury. *Clinical Epidemiology, 6*, 309–311. https://doi.org/10.2147/CLEP.S68889

Smith, B. (2013). Sporting spinal cord injuries, social relations, and rehabilitation narratives: An ethnographic creative non-fiction of becoming disabled through sport. *Sociology of Sport Journal, 30*(2), 132–152. https://doi.org/10.1123/ssj.30.2.132

Smith, E., Pooley, J.-A., Holmes, L., Gebbie, K., & Gershon, R. (2021). Vicarious trauma: Exploring the experiences of qualitative researchers who study traumatized populations. *Disaster Medicine and Public Health Preparedness, 17*, 1–6. https://doi.org/10.1017/dmp.2021.333

Smith, B., Williams, O., Bone, L., & the Moving Social Work Co-production Collective (2023). Co-production: A resource to guide co-producing research in the sport, exercise, and health sciences. *Qualitative Research in Sport, Exercise and Health, 15*(2), 159–187. https://doi.org/10.1080/2159676X.2022.2052946

Soundy, A., Stubbs, B., Freeman, P., Coffee, P., & Roskell, C. (2014). Factors influencing patients' hope in stroke and spinal cord injury: A narrative review. *International Journal of Therapy and Rehabilitation, 21*(5), 210–218. https://doi.org/10.12968/ijtr.2014.21.5.210

Sparkes, A. C., & Brighton, J. (2020). Autonomic dysreflexia and boosting in disability sport: Exploring the subjective meanings, management strategies, moral justifications, and perceptions of risk among male, spinal cord injured, wheelchair athletes. *Qualitative Research in Sport, Exercise and Health, 12*(3), 414–430. https://doi.org/10.1080/2159676X.2019.1623298

Sparkes, A. C., Brighton, J., & Inckle, K. (2018). 'It's a part of me': An ethnographic exploration of becoming a disabled sporting cyborg following spinal cord injury. *Qualitative Research in Sport, Exercise and Health, 10*(2), 151–166. https://doi.org/10.1080/2159676X.2017.1389768

Sparkes, A. C., Brighton, J., & Inckle, K. (2021). 'I am proud of my back': An ethnographic study of the motivations and meanings of body modification as identity work among athletes with spinal cord injury. *Qualitative Research in Sport, Exercise and Health, 13*(3), 407–425. https://doi.org/10.1080/2159676X.2020.1756393

Substance Abuse and Mental Health Services Administration (SAMHSA). (2014). *SAMHSA's concept of trauma and guidance for a trauma-informed approach.* https://ncsacw.samhsa.gov/userfiles/files/SAMHSA_Trauma.pdf.

Thomas, C. (2007). *Sociologies of disability, 'Impairment', and chronic illness: Ideas in disability studies and medical sociology.* Palgrave MacMillan.

van Der Scheer, J. W., Martin Ginis, K. A., Ditor, D. S., Goosey-Tolfrey, V. L., Hicks, A. L., West, C. R., & Wolfe, D. L. (2017). Effects of exercise on fitness and health of adults with spinal cord injury: A systematic review. *Neurology, 89*. https://doi.org/10.1212/WNL.0000000000004224

Wheeler, D., & Peers, D. (2022). Playing, passing, and pageantry: A collaborative autoethnography on sport, disability, sexuality, and belonging. In B. Powis, J. Brighton, & P. D. Howe (Eds.), *Researching disability sport* (pp. 98–111). Routledge.

Williams, T. L. (2018). Exploring narratives of physical activity and disability over time: A novel integrated qualitative methods approach. *Psychology of Sport and Exercise, 37*, 224–234. https://doi.org/10.1016/j.psychsport.2017.09.004

Williams, T. L., Hunt, E. R., Papathomas, A., & Smith, B. (2018a). Exercise is medicine? Most of the time for most; But not always for all. *Qualitative Research in Sport, Exercise and Health, 10*, 441–456. https://doi.org/10.1080/2159676X.2017.1405363

Williams, T. L., Smith, B., & Papathomas, A. (2014). The barriers, benefits and facilitators of leisure time physical activity among people with spinal cord injury: A meta-synthesis of qualitative findings. *Health Psychology Review, 8*, 404–425. https://doi.org/10.1080/17437199.2014.898406

Williams, T. L., Smith, B., & Papathomas, A. (2018b). Physical activity promotion for people with spinal cord injury: Physiotherapists' beliefs and actions. *Disability and Rehabilitation, 40*, 52–61. https://doi.org/10.1080/09638288.2016.1242176

Wolcott, H. (2005). *The art of fieldwork* (2nd ed.). Alta Mira Press.

World Health Organization. (2020). *Spinal cord injury*. https://www.who.int/newsroom/fact-sheets/detail/spinal-cord-injury

Chapter 11

Interview and Arts-Based Approaches for Research with Autistic Adults

Patrick Jachyra, James McLeod, and Simon Rosenbaum

Introduction

Emerging research suggests that autistic people[1] experience high levels of trauma throughout the life course and commonly experience symptoms of post-traumatic stress disorder (PTSD) (Peterson et al., 2019). In childhood, autistic people experience high levels of bullying (Cappadocia et al., 2011), victimization among peers (Gibbs & Pellicano, 2023) and adverse childhood experiences (Rigles, 2021) both within, and beyond, school-based settings. The high levels of trauma noted in childhood extends to adulthood, with researchers highlighting that autistic people experience high levels of victimization through interpersonal violence from a friend or a family member (Pearson et al., 2022), experiences of othering (Pearson et al., 2022), and experiencing significant structural inequalities living in a world that was not designed with their diverse needs, interests, and abilities. Documented traumatic experiences among autistic people include social difficulties and confusion, sensory experiences that are overwhelming, loss of a loved one and/or abandonment, transitions, and change, and/or events related to mental health (Kerns et al., 2022; Rumball et al., 2021). Global events such as the COVID-19 pandemic (Lake et al., 2021) and recruitment into extremist groups (Welch et al., 2022) have also been identified to potentially negatively impact autistic people. Recognizing the high rates of trauma experienced by autistic people, they are more likely to report symptoms of PTSD. In this vein, Rumball et al. (2021) suggest that rates of probable PTSD are between 32% and 45% for autistic people, compared to 4–4.5% observed in the general population. Despite these high rates of PTSD and trauma experienced by autistic people, exposure to potentially traumatic events and traumatic related diagnoses remain poorly understood among autistic people (Hoch & Youssef, 2020). This lack of understanding prompts a clear need to conduct research to better understand how to prevent and support traumatic experiences among autistic people across the life course.

Despite a nascent corpus of research examining trauma experienced by autistic people across the field of autism research illustrated above, there is

DOI: 10.4324/9781003332909-14

little research that has examined traumatic experiences with autistic people in sport and physical activity (PA) spaces. To date, only two studies have described autistic children and young people's experiences of bullying in sport, physical education, and PA environments (see Healy et al., 2013;Jachyra,, 2020; Jachyra, Renwick, et al., 2021). This dearth of research is amplified with autistic adults where there is no previous research that has examined the impact of trauma on sport, PA, and exercise participation. The lack of research in sport and PA spaces with autistic people is problematic given research suggesting that athletes are more likely to experience psychological abuse, and also experience non-contact physical abuse (Mountjoy et al., 2016). The rates of abuse and trauma among disabled people is also grim, with the International Olympic Committee Consensus statement demonstrating that disabled athletes are more likely to be abused (Mountjoy et al., 2016). The paucity of research examining the impact of trauma on PA participation with autistic people is a glaring absence with numerous barriers to sport and PA participation, and lower levels of participation (Gregor et al., 2018; Jachyra, Lai, et al., 2021; Jachyra, Renwick, et al., 2021). Given these knowledge gaps, there is a clear need for research to examine the interconnections between sport, PA, abuse, and trauma among autistic people in an effort to better support their PA participation and prevent (re)traumatization.

In addition to the substantive knowledge gaps described above, there is a paucity of methodological discussion and developments guiding how to conduct qualitative research about PA, sport, and health with autistic people. There is even less research guiding how to conduct trauma-related research in these spaces. To this end, there is no methodological guidance on how to conduct qualitative research with autistic people who have experienced trauma and/or how to conduct trauma-informed research. Yet, given the high rates of trauma experienced by autistic people, there is a heeding need for methodological developments in this domain to ensure that there are trauma-informed research practices reflective of their diverse needs, abilities, and life experiences. In light of this methodological gap, there is a need for researchers to reflect on and share experiences conducting trauma sensitive qualitative research with autistic people to facilitate the deployment of methodologies and study designs that support their diverse needs, interests, abilities, and trauma experiences.

To work towards addressing the methodological gaps described above, this chapter draws on a qualitative research study conducted with autistic women regarding their experiences with sport and PA to reflect on the methodological considerations and adaptions that were associated with the study to limit the possibility of re-traumatization occurring. In this chapter, we reflect specifically on the use of semi-structured interviews and photo-elicitation in the study and discuss the strengths and limitations of these approaches. We also highlight how trauma-informed approaches were used to conduct this research with autistic women, and the importance of their utility in research conducted with autistic people. Towards the end of the chapter, we delve into the impacts of conducting trauma-related research on the researcher and discuss the emergence and impact of vicarious trauma, mitigation strategies, and the importance of temporality, which heretofore has not received extensive attention in the literature. We conclude the chapter by outlining three future directions when conducting qualitative and trauma-related research in the areas of sport, exercise, and health with autistic people to inform future research endeavours.

Methods and Methodology

To begin, we outline the methods and methodology that were deployed in a study examining the PA participation of autistic women. Autistic women between the ages of 18 and 65 years were recruited across the United Kingdom (see Table 11.1).

Table 11.1 Participant Demographic Information

Participant pseudonym	Age	Gender
Barbra	48	Female
Haley	50	Female
Georgia	52	Female
Jude	48	Female
Sarah	46	Female
Ellen	53	Female
Mary	45	Female
Anna	36	Female
Cassie	47	Female
Kathleen	49	Female
Lindsey	53	Female
Valerie	51	Female
Stacey	54	Female
Margaret	29	Female
Georgie	51	Female
Jo	37	Female
Dizzy	47	Female
Samantha	35	Female
Amanda	42	Female
Romelle	21	Female
Veronica	25	Female
Monika	31	Female
Titchy	57	Female
Katie	34	Non-binary
Valerie	40	Non-binary
Kristina	36	Female
Katherine	36	Female
Joanne	51	Female
Melissa	40	Female
Catherine	48	Non-binary

The study was conducted with autistic women, as their perspectives have historically been excluded from previous PA research (Jachyra, 2020; Jachyra, Renwick, et al., 2021). Supporting PA for women has also been identified as a strategic priority area in the new Women's Health Strategy for England. A qualitative study design was selected as this was the first study to solely include the perspectives of autistic women about PA participation. As such, a qualitative design was amenable in an effort to generate an in-depth examination of their perspectives and experiences with PA participation. The use of qualitative approaches was critical to include their voices in research as historically, their voices have been absent. As a result, including their voices was a priority in an effort to learn more about their lives, daily lived contingencies and PA participation. Including a qualitative approach also provided an opportunity to challenge stigma, misunderstandings and gendered assumptions about autistic women given that their perspectives have been excluded from PA research. The use of a qualitative design builds on a larger research programme using qualitative methods (see Campos et al., 2019; Jachyra, Renwick., 2021; Wright Stein et al., 2021) to explore how to optimally support the PA participation and everyday lives of autistic people across the lifespan.

To conduct the research, photo-elicitation and semi-structured interviews were selected to generate data. Photo-elicitation is a research technique that includes photographs as part of a research interview (Harper, 2002) in an effort to generate reflection and further discussion about a particular image (Harrison, 2002). Photo-elicitation was specifically selected to provide multiple opportunities for participants to share their lives using different modes of communication which might be more amenable to their needs and abilities. Finding ways to include the perspectives of autistic people directly was critical as historically, autism research has drawn on the perspectives of parents, caregivers, healthcare professionals, and proxy stakeholders (Fletcher-Watson et al., 2018). Photo-elicitation was also strategically selected to provide participants with opportunities for creativity, as a research tool to promote participant autonomy. The use of photos has also been noted to be a potential vehicle to move towards inclusive research by directly including their perspectives (Courcy & Koniou, 2022). This, in turn, was an important methodological consideration. Finally, photo-elicitation was selected to stimulate discussion in the second interview between the participant and researcher about the perspectives, meanings and experiences with sport and PA. By using photos, the intent was to provide participants with a potential means to highlight the multiple manifestations and modes of trauma that they have experienced, which might not have been captured using only the spoken word through an interview. The combination of photo-elicitation and interviews in this context was an original and important contribution to the literature and knowledge base which heretofore has been absent.

In addition to photo-elicitation, two semi-structured interviews were conducted virtually (i.e., Zoom or MS-Teams) with 30 autistic women, drawn across two studies. While the research team initially sought to conduct interviews in-person, discussions with a group of autistic women advising on the project suggested that participants might feel safer and more comfortable conducting interviews remotely. All participants had access to a computer and online spaces in this study. Also referred to as "anytime anyplace learning" (Veletsianos & Houlden, 2019, p. 455), online or remote interviews were offered to the participants because researchers have shown that people may experience less anxiety in an online environment because their physical space is more predictable (Veletsianos & Houlden, 2019). Given the social pressures of in-person conversations and social conventions which some autistic people may find traumatic (Fuld, 2018), having a safe and predictable physical environment was fundamentally important. Conducting virtual interviews therefore provided a space for participants to share potentially vulnerable experiences, which was important to understand more about, given the high levels of trauma experienced by autistic people in sport, PA, and exercise spaces (Healy, 2013; Jachyra, 2020; Jachyra, Renwick, et al., 2021).

As part of the study, two interviews were conducted and were designed this way to build rapport with the participants over time. The first interview sought to learn about the preferences, habits, and activities of their daily lives, and to build rapport. Building rapport was critical given the high rates of trauma experienced by autistic people and to prevent re-traumatization. This was an important element to build trust with participants and is described further in the Trauma-Informed practices section below. The interviews lasted between 45 and 60 minutes with each participant. All participants communicated verbally during the interviews. At the end of the first interview, participants were provided with the option to take five to ten photographs which reminded them of PA participation, engagement, conceptualizations, and experiences. Participants were asked to email the photos to the first author prior to the scheduling of the second interview. This varied however for each participant and was contingent on their availability and life circumstances at the time of conducting the research. As general guidance, participants were advised to email the photos within two weeks of the first interview in an effort to build on the discussions that developed during the first interview. Through the combination of two interviews and photo-elicitation, the research sought to develop nuanced, detailed, and multifaceted data that likely would not have emerged if the methods were deployed in isolation. This, in turn, is a novel and original contribution to the literature on trauma, sport, and PA participation with autistic people.

Experiences of Trauma among Autistic Women

Across the data with autistic women, there were several and very prominent accounts which highlighted how participants felt misunderstood, misdiagnosed, and misbelieved throughout their lives both within and beyond PA settings. When probing deeper with individual participants, it became clear that these feelings and experiences were connected to various forms of overt and covert traumatic experiences. Traumatic experiences occurred both within and beyond sport and PA arenas and had manifold impacts. For some participants recounting their experiences with physical education class (PE), they highlighted how PE was met with sleeplessness, trepidation and anxiety leading up to, during and after the weekly PE class. One participant noted that she felt "frozen with anxiety" and would "stay up all night" before PE class, as she loathed PE. Other traumatic PE experiences described by participants included wearing uncomfortable kit, the hyper focus on completing drills, and completing the same activities annually with little variety, which predominantly was netball or field hockey.

Some participants highlighted how PE and PA environments themselves were traumatic given their sensory sensitivities. For some autistic women, PA environments such as the gymnasium, swimming pool, and/or outdoor spaces often were overwhelming, given their hyper or hypo sensitives to noise, lights, reverberations, touch, smells, and textures of the floors. Participants described merely entering and being present in these spaces was overwhelming and vividly recalled how this sensory overload at times triggered a complete shutdown. For participants experiencing the traumatic nature of sensory overload, these traumatic experiences were exacerbated by teachers and caregivers who had difficulty relating to what they were experiencing. For some autistic women, they recalled feeling as if they were "irrelevant" and/or were "minimized" when they tried to explain how these spaces made them feel, and how the spaces were not psychologically safe for them. In recounting these experiences, Titchy remarked that she remembered a teacher who told her "to stop being difficult and get in the gym" when she sat curled up in a ball in front of the gymnasium doors and did everything possible to avoid going into a space which typically culminated with a stress response because of the sensory overload. The minimization of sensory experiences was highlighted by Katie who remarked that her father questioned her for "always having a problem with everything" after she was dismissed from her local swimming team for refusing to shower before entering the pool, because the texture of the floor and cold water of the showers triggered a stress response. Without an autism diagnosis for these women (as women have historically been underdiagnosed) teachers, coaches and parents did not understand that their level and type of PA participation in these spaces was not a conscious choice. But rather dovetailed with their sensitivities to the environment. These experiences described above not only created an aversion towards PE and PA, but also afflicted trauma as autistic women described camouflaging in social spaces as a self-preservation strategy.

Camouflaging involves the process of deliberately altering and/or concealing one's dispositions, personality, behaviours, and/or tendencies to try and fit in, within social norms and contexts. Similar to Goffman's concept of passing (Goffman, 1963), autistic women reported camouflaging as a learned self-preservation tactic and habit to compensate, assimilate or mask their differences to minimize trauma. As one participant poignantly put it, "to pretend to be less autistic". For some women, camouflaging included mimicking body language, deliberately maintaining eye contact or employing learned social cues even if not enjoyable, feeling the need to put on an act, and/or rehearsing common phrases or sayings in both sport and PA spaces. These passing techniques were deployed to fit in, but also came at a cost where participants noted that camouflaging was usually met with physical, mental, and emotional exhaustion/burnout, and further trauma to avoid engaging with the social world. The cost of camouflaging not only negatively impacted their mental health, but also negatively impacted their affinity towards PA where they described they felt the need to deploy self-preservation strategies to avoid further traumatization both within and beyond sport and PA spaces. For the participants in the study, trauma was multifaceted in nature and impacted their lives in myriad ways. The trauma shared by autistic women not only shaped the lives of study participants, but also impacted the first author of this chapter (PJ) who conducted some of the interviews. It is to this discussion of these trauma impacts on the researcher that we now turn.

Impacts of Trauma on the Researcher

While the sensitives and mitigations put in place to do no harm to participants is well documented in research (Alessi & Kahn, 2023), one area that has received less attention in qualitative autism research is the impact of vicarious or secondary traumatic stress (STS) experienced by researchers. Vicarious trauma is a process of change resulting from empathetic engagement with trauma survivors (British Medical Association, 2022). Vicarious trauma has also been described as: STS, compassion fatigue, burnout (BO), countertransference, traumatic countertransference, PTSD, emotional contagion, and shared trauma (Branson, 2019). Whereas vicarious trauma can be a "normal reaction to the stressful and sometimes traumatizing work with victims" (McCann & Pearlman, 1990, p. 145), our experience conducting trauma-related research has shown us that vicarious trauma can manifest itself differently across participants, across studies, and importantly, across time. The manifestation of vicarious trauma across time was particularly the case in this study. During the interviews with autistic women, trauma, coping, and mitigation strategies were put in place immediately following the interviews. These coping mechanisms included emotional support from others (i.e., colleagues engaged in a similar line of research), personal counselling, and journal writing (van der Merwe & Hunt, 2019). Despite having these mechanisms in place, one important learning that emerged was the *temporal* nature of vicarious trauma. While vicarious trauma may have immediate onset following a research engagement (such as a research interview), our experience has taught us that, at times, there may be a delayed response in processing the trauma shared by participants. This delay in processing, in turn, can also be presented with a delay in the impact of the trauma on researchers.

In the case of conducting research with autistic women, the impact of this trauma on the interviewer (PJ) was most pronounced when listening back to the interview, reading interview transcripts, and/or when conducting the analysis of the data. When conducting the analysis, PJ noted that he was increasingly fatigued with feelings of lethargy and exhaustion to engage in other activities following analysis work of re-listening, conceptualizing, and trying to make sense of the trauma described by participants. The fatigue that emerged during the analytic process at first was thought to be the result of vigorous physical exertion in sporting contexts. However, as the fatigue, reduced motivation, and reduced productivity to engage with other work-related tasks emerged as a consistent pattern when conducting analysis of the data, the thought of temporal nature of vicarious trauma first emerged through discussions with a friend, colleague, and fellow trauma researcher. From our discussions, engaging with analysis served as a trigger to recall some of the trauma experienced by participants described above. As attention to this recurring temporal trauma was identified, a debriefing plan that was put in place. The plan included engagement with emotional support from others, resting, socializing with others, and engaging in building communities (Saakvitne et al., 2000) with others to work through the (re)emergence of vicarious trauma. This experience highlighted the importance of planning for the temporal nature of STS and BO (Whitt-Woosley & Sprang, 2017) when engaging in this line of research.

Considering the temporality associated with conducting this line of research, it is important for future researchers to think about how trauma can manifest for researchers in manifold ways not only during the data generation where mitigations are commonly put it place. This is new learning that has not received extensive attention in the literature. From our experiences conducting trauma research (see Jachyra, Lai, et al., 2021; Rosenbaum et al., 2022), trauma management strategies and follow-up plans not only need to be in place during data generation phases, but also require careful thinking and planning throughout other phases of the research to manage the (re)emergence of trauma and distress when it might be least expected.

Trauma-Informed Practices

Conducting trauma-related research necessitates thoughtful, preventative, sensitive, and adverse event planning. This is particularly important when working with autistic people given the high levels of trauma that was shared earlier in the chapter. To guide future qualitative trauma research in sport, PA, and health, we draw on two trauma-informed principles and share our experiences of implementing these principles in practice.

Safety

Within trauma-informed practices, safety is a key principle and refers to ensuring practices and interpersonal interactions promote a sense of physical and psychological safety (Edelman, 2022). To support the physical and psychological safety of autistic people, a number of strategies were employed throughout the study. When conducting semi-structured interviews with the autistic women described above, PJ used a series of well-being questions to query their emotional and physical safety throughout the interviews and were informed by the Trauma and Resilience Informed Research Principles and Practice (see Edelman, 2022). For example, a question that was asked at the start of the interview was: Do you feel like you are in a safe space and place to share your life experiences with me today? The well-being questions were especially important to be asked immediately after participants described traumatic details, events, or experiences. For example, after a participant shared her experiences of sensory overload and the traumatic impacts it had on her, PJ asked: "How are you feeling after sharing that experience". Depending on the response of the participant, a series of follow-up questions were asked if there was evidence that the participant may be experiencing any degree of distress. Follow-up questions drew on an active consent approach asking questions such as: "Do you need a break from the interview?", "Would you like to end the interview?", and "Is there anyone you would like to speak to for support?" Asking well-being questions was critical before moving to other aspects of the interview to ensure participant safety remained paramount. Although follow-up questions were not extensively used with participants in the study, these questions were prepared in advance of the interviews in the event that there was a need to use them, as part of the semi-structured interview guide.

In addition to asking well-being questions, the interviewer was attuned to monitoring any potential changes in body language when discussing life experiences. The importance of assessing body language as a form of nonverbal communication to ensure that the participant is emotionally safe is of upmost importance throughout the interview. Informed by Katz et al. (2012), the interviewer paid attention to changes in non-verbal communication such as: change in body language; pitch of voice; pulling on hair, tapping; and selfsoothing movements. If non-verbal changes were observed, the interviewer planned to ask the participant whether they needed to take a break from the interview and any changes to the ways they were feeling. From the participant responses, possible courses of action would have been determined. In addition to these well-being questions, participants were encouraged to have their mobile phone in proximity during the interview in case there was someone they could text or call for support, in the event of any distress. Having a support person at hand may be beneficial to promote social support and safety as research in the general population suggests that a lack of social support can increase the risk of PTSD (Brewin et al., 2000). As a result, mechanisms of social support were included in this study to promote participant safety. Additionally, participants were encouraged to follow-up with their local health practitioner or to access other support mechanisms if needed as part of safety planning. Finally, safety considerations included the physical safety of the interview space which has been identified to be a critical consideration in trauma-informed research. The interview procedures used in this study were informed by Bath (2008) who highlighted that safe environments are created by consistency, reliability, predictability, availability, honesty, and transparency. Safety can also be created by the inclusion of choice and control, as well as cultural and gender awareness (Bath, 2008) in an effort to prevent harm and re-traumatization. To create a safe physical space, the interviews were conducted online and in a location of the participants' choosing. The use of virtual interviews was a strategy to promote physical safety in an effort to shift power imbalances between the interviewer and participants. This was critical, as working at a university is imbued with manifold forms of power and privilege. With a history of distrust of scientific researchers from the autism community (Botha & Cage, 2022), conducting the interviews virtually sought to build trust with participants by recognizing and shifting these power balances. In an effort to build trust, and safety with participants, a social story was used. Social stories combine images and written communication about what to expect during a particular social interaction such as an interview (Gray, 2015a, 2015b) by limiting the ambiguity of the events that will transpire during the research process. Further to outlining the details of what will transpire during each part of the research process, there was information included about the interviewer such as hobbies, interests, and what his role is by conducting research interviews. This was considered to be important to help establish safety as the interviewer PJ was not autistic and a male researcher who conformed to stereotypical notions of masculinity (Jachyra et al., 2015). While it is difficult to ascertain exactly how PJ's gender would impact the data generated (see Jachyra et al., 2014 for a more expansive discussion) thinking these elements through as part of the study design and conduct of the study were critical to ensure participants felt safe, comfortable, and secure as a result of the many different forms of privilege that were accorded to the interviewer. The use of the social stories were critical to build trust with autistic women given a history of institutional trauma and distrust among the autistic community with research initially focused on eugenics (Botha & Cage, 2022). An example of this distrust occurred during participant recruitment where numerous participants initially expressed interest but declined to participate in the study as the interviewer (PJ) was a university researcher. As a result of these considerations, the use of a social story was an important tool to potentially build initial trust and safety with participants, prior to the interviews commencing as participants were fully aware of the nature of activities and interactions that were to take place in the interview space. Further to these safety considerations, the emphasis of choice and the online context sought to create a safe physical space by supporting participant autonomy and avoiding potential physical spaces that may have been triggering as they related to sport, PA, and exercise. Prior to starting the interviews, PJ asked participants' whether they felt they were in a safe physical space, and also suggested participants blur their virtual background if they wished, as a strategy to support the predictability and safety of the space. In addition to these considerations, PJ also asked whether there was anyone else in the immediate vicinity of the online interview space, and to consider selecting a space that was private and away from other people potentially overhearing the conversations if there were other people around. This was critical to a strategy to promote a consistent and reliable space which sought to promote safety. Finally, PJ suggested that participants used headphones during the interviews as a strategy to not only maximize confidentiality, but also promote physical safety. The combination of these safety elements sought to create an honest, transparent, inclusive, and welcoming space for the interviews to learn about difficult aspects of their lives.

Empowerment, Voice, and Choice

Empowerment, voice, and choice are critical aspects to conducting research with autistic people as the perspectives (i.e., voices) of autistic women about PA have been excluded from research (; Jachyra, Renwick, et al., 2021, Jachyra, 2020.). In the research described above, the study methodology sought to promote voice and choice through the use of photo-elicitation where participants represented their lives from their perspective. As suggested by Sinko and Saint Arnault (2021), "photography is an underutilized research method that can allow health researchers to see the world through the eyes of the study participants" (p. 661). The use of photos generated by participants has the potential to provide a deeper understanding of human consciousness than words alone (Glaw et al., 2017). This, in turn, promotes voice and choice by recognizing them as active participants (Sinko & Saint Arnault, 2021) and promotes autonomy of thought. This is particularly crucial for research participants that have experienced trauma or abuse (Pichon et al., 2022) as traumatic experiences can be associated with a loss of choice and control. The use of photo-elicitation aims to restore these potentially lost elements (Chozinki & Gonzalez, 2020) associated with trauma experiences. Providing participants with the choice to use photo-elicitation may be particularly beneficial as it enables autistic people other ways of communicating than relying solely on oral speech. This practice would support multiple communication preferences, but also promotes voice and choice by enabling the participant to become actively engaged in the research process by communicating their experience of the world through their eyes. The use of this approach was a particularly valuable resource for autistic women who identified that they felt genuinely included in the research process as they had the choice to include photos about their lives. Their inclusion in the study was reflected by a participant Veronica who noted:

> Finally, I feel seen and heard. My whole life, people spoke for me and when I spoke up, I was shut down. Nobody believed me. My thoughts didn't matter. This is my experience of exercise through my eyes using photos and nobody can take that away from me.

Given the potential value of photo-elicitation in our study, we recommend it to other researchers conducting studies with autistic people to not only generate rich, in-depth, and insightful data. But mostly importantly, as a trauma-informed tool to promote voice and choice given the long-standing history of autistic voices being excluded from research.

Conclusions

Given the high prevalence of trauma reported in autistic people (Pearson et al., 2022), this chapter drew on a qualitative research study with autistic women in the United Kingdom to highlight the impacts of trauma, impacts of trauma on the researcher, and demonstrated how trauma-informed principles were used to guide this work. This was the first study to solely examine the perspectives of PA participation with autistic women. We conclude this chapter by outlining three future directions for other researchers wishing to conduct studies with autistic people who may be invariably experiencing trauma.

The first relates to qualitative methods where our experience suggests that arts-based approaches may have particular value for individuals who have experienced trauma and abuse. Arts-based approaches refer to "research that uses the arts, in the broadest sense, to explore, understand and represented and even challenge human action and experience" Baden & Wimpenny, 2014, p. 1). The use of arts-based approaches such as photo-elicitation or digital storytelling may be a fruitful avenue where the participant has increased choice and autonomy on how they wish to convey their story (Jachyra, 2020). For children and adolescents exposed to traumatic events, a recent systematic review of evidence highlights that arts-based interventions may have the potential to also reduce symptoms of trauma and negative mood (Morison et al., 2021). Drawing on arts-based methods has the potential to provide much more depth, breadth and nuance to our current understandings of sport, PA, and exercise to reflect the intricacies, complexities, and contradictions of the lives of human beings. We suggest that this may be a very valuable avenue for future research.

The second consideration for researchers wishing to conduct studies with autistic people relates to the use of well-being plans, especially when conducting research in virtual contexts. In a study examining suicidal thoughts and behaviours with autistic adults (see Jachyra, Lai, et al., 2021), the first author of this chapter used a well-being plan to prepare for, direct and respond to potentially difficult situations as they arose during the interviews. The use of the well-being plan was co-created with each participant to help respond, support, and direct a participant during a distressing or a crisis situation until they sought further professional support with a healthcare professional. Preparing for potentially difficult situations in this study was important given that autistic people are at higher risks for premature mortality(see Lunsky et al., 2022). Although the well-being plan was not utilized in this study with autistic women described in this chapter, we believe that a well-being plan may be amenable and an important tool to consider when planning to conduct research on trauma in sport, PA, and exercise given the high rates of trauma experienced by autistic people, and the potential for discussions of trauma to emerge when recounting experiences with PA, sport, and exercise. The use of well-being plans in a virtual context may be of particular relevance where it may be difficult to ascertain and provide support to a participant who may be experiencing distress or a crisis, especially if conducting international or cross-national research where there are different types of supports available, and routes of access to support. As a preventative and supportive tool to promote participant safety, especially when explicitly studying traumatic PA experiences, our experience conducting research in this area reinforces the potential value of using a well-being plan. Elements that have been previously used in our experience creating well-being plans are included below, and might be of potential use to other researchers:

- Names and contact information for family, friends, and next of kin contact.
- Contact information for healthcare professional if consented to disclose.
- Location of nearest accident and emergency room for support.
- Warning signs of what distress may look like.
- Strategies on how to support participant if they are feeling distressed.
- What supports are currently in place, and plans on how to mobilize support if needed.
- Plans for rest of day after partaking in the study.
- Sources of rest, repose, and relaxation.

The third and final direction relates to moving towards co-producing research, policy, and practice. With increasing calls for co-production in sport, health, and PA research (Smith et al., 2022), co-producing research is of utmost importance to ensure that policies, practices, and activities are reflective of the diverse needs, abilities, and sensibilities of autistic people. With a history of doing research on, rather than with autistic people, there is a clear need to change this trajectory. Although co-production is a highly contested term, by co-production, we refer to the potential value in building "equitable partnerships between different contributors … and maintained throughout the research process" (Smith et al., 2022, p. 164). Rather than simply seeking the input of autistic people at the beginning or the end of a research study, we believe it is critical to partner with autistic people from the outset of research and to conduct co-produced research that meets the PA, sport, and exercise priorities of autistic people. Co-producing research increases the possibility of ensuring research, policy and practice to be reflective of their everyday lives, needs, and experiences. This is importance given that there has been little co-produced research in this area to date. Furthermore, by initiating co-production in research, it enables participants to have power in research decision making (McMahon et al., 2022), while having control or power over the process they are involved with (Angelo, 2015). This levelling of power is important within a trauma-informed approach because, as Delker et al. (2019) explain, those who have experienced trauma have often had individual agency, choice, and control taken from them. Co-producing research therefore not only emphasizes agency and choice in an effort to limit the potential or re-traumatization through research but is imperative to ensure that research generated is reflective of their everyday lives, abilities, and circumstances which heretofore has predominantly been absent with autistic people.

Note

1 In this chapter, we use the term autistic people as this has been the expressed preference of the autistic community in the United Kingdom. Importantly, we recognize the diversity of preferences and perspectives within the autism community regarding the use of terminology.

References

Alessi, E. J., & Kahn, S. (2023). Toward a trauma-informed qualitative research approach: Guidelines for ensuring the safety and promoting the resilience of research participants. *Qualitative Research in Psychology*, *20*(1), 121–154. https://doi.org/10.1080/14780887.2022.2107967

Angelo, G. (2015). *Rapport: The art of connecting with people and building relationships*. Seisnama.

Baden, M. S., & Wimpenny, K. (2014). *A practical guide to arts-related research*. SpringerLink. https://link.springer.com/book/10.1007/978-94-6209-815-2

Bath, H. (2008). *The three pillars of trauma-informed care*. https://elevhalsan.uppsala.se/globalassets/elevhalsan/dokument/psykologhandlingar/trauma-informed-care.pdf

Botha, M., & Cage, E. (2022). *"Autism Research Is in Crisis"*: A mixed method study of researcher's constructions of autistic people and autism research. https://doi.org/10.31219/osf.io/w4389

Branson, D. C. (2019). Vicarious trauma, themes in research, and terminology: A review of literature. *Traumatology*, *25*(1), 2–10. https://doi.org/10.1037/trm0000161

Brewin, C. R., Andrews, B., & Valentine, J. D. (2000). Meta-analysis of risk factors for posttraumatic stress disorder in trauma-exposed adults. *Journal of Consulting and Clinical Psychology, 68*(5), 748–766. https://doi.org/10.1037/0022-006x.68.5.748

British Medical Association. (2022). *Vicarious trauma: Signs and strategies for coping.* https://www.bma.org.uk/advice-and-support/your-wellbeing/vicarious-trauma/vicarious-trauma-signs-and-strategies-for-coping#:~:text=Vicarious%20trauma%20is%20a%20process,doctors%20and%20other%20health%20professionals

Campos, C., Duck, M., McQuillan, R., Brazill, L., Malik, S., Hartman, L., McPherson, A. C., Gibson, B. E., & Jachyra, P. (2019). Exploring the role of physiotherapists in the care of children with autism spectrum disorder. *Physical & Occupational Therapy in Pediatrics, 39*(6), 614–628. https://doi.org/10.1080/01942638.2019.1585405

Cappadocia, M. C., Weiss, J. A., & Pepler, D. (2011). Bullying experiences among children and youth with autism spectrum disorders. *Journal of Autism and Developmental Disorders, 42*(2), 266–277. https://doi.org/10.1007/s10803-011-1241-x

Chozinki, B. A., & Gonzalez, A. (2020). Using georeferenced photo-elicitation projects to understand survivor resources: A method for trauma-informed practice in higher education. *Journal of American College Health, 70*(7), 2070–2078. https://doi.org/10.1080/07448481.2020.1842423

Courcy, I., & Koniou, I. (2022). A scoping review of the use of photo-elicitation and photovoice with autistic and neurodiverse people. Moving towards more inclusive research? *Disability & Society.* https://doi.org/10.1080/09687599.2022.2137391

Delker, B. C., Salton, R., & McLean, K. C. (2019). Giving voice to silence: Empowerment and disempowerment in the developmental shift from trauma 'victim' to 'survivor-advocate. *Journal of Trauma & Dissociation, 21*(2), 242–263. https://doi.org/10.1080/15299732.2019.1678212

Edelman, N. L. (2022). Trauma and resilience informed research principles and practice: A framework to improve the inclusion and experience of disadvantaged populations in health and social care research. *Journal of Health Services Research & Policy, 28*(1), 66–75. https://doi.org/10.1177/13558196221124740

Fletcher-Watson, S., Adams, J., Brook, K., Charman, T., Crane, L., Cusack, J., Leekam, S., Milton, D., Parr, J. R., & Pellicano, E. (2018). Making the future together: Shaping autism research through meaningful participation. *Autism, 23*(4), 943–953. https://doi.org/10.1177/1362361318786721

Fuld, S. (2018). Autism spectrum disorder: The impact of stressful and traumatic life events and implications for clinical practice. *Clinical Social Work Journal, 46*(3), 210–219. https://doi.org/10.1007/s10615-018-0649-6

Gibbs, V., & Pellicano, E. (2023). 'Maybe we just seem like easy targets': A qualitative analysis of autistic adults' experiences of interpersonal violence. *Autism,* 136236132211503. https://doi.org/10.1177/13623613221150375

Glaw, X., Inder, K., Kable, A., & Hazelton, M. (2017). Visual methodologies in qualitative research. *International Journal of Qualitative Methods, 16*(1), 160940691774821. https://doi.org/10.1177/1609406917748215

Goffman, E. (1963). *Stigma: Notes on the management of spoiled identity.* Simon & Schuster. https://www.simonandschuster.com/books/Stigma/Erving-Goffman/9780671622442

Gray, C. (2015a). *The new social story book, revised & expanded 15th anniversary edition. Future horizons incorporated.* https://openlibrary.org.books/OL27193688M/The_new_social_story?book

Gray, C. (2015b). *The new social story book*. Future Horizons.

Gregor, S., Bruni, N., Grkinic, P., Schwartz, L., McDonald, A., Thille, P., Gabison, S., Gibson, B. E., & Jachyra, P. (2018). Parents' perspectives of physical activity participation among Canadian adolescents with autism spectrum disorder. *Research in Autism Spectrum Disorders, 48*, 53–62. https://doi.org/10.1016/j.rasd.2018.01.007

Harrison, B. (2002). Photographic visions and narrative inquiry. *Narrative Inquiry, 12*(1), 87–111. https://doi.org/10.1075/ni.12.1.14har

Harper, D. (2002). Talking about pictures: A case for photo elicitation. *Visual Studies, 17*(1), 13–26. https://doi.org/10.1080/14725860220137345

Healy, S., Msetfi, R., & Gallagher, S. (2013). 'Happy and a bit nervous': The experiences of children with autism in physical education. *British Journal of Learning Disabilities, 41*(3), 222–228. https://doi.org/10.1111/bld.12053

Hoch, J. D., & Youssef, A. M. (2020). Predictors of trauma exposure and trauma diagnoses for children with autism and developmental disorders served in a Community Mental Health Clinic. *Journal of Autism and Developmental Disorders, 50*(2), 634–649. https://doi.org/10.1007/s10803-019-04331-3

Jachyra, P. (2020) *Physical activity participation among adolescent boys with autism spectrum disorder*. TSpace. https://tspace.library.utoronto.ca/handle/1807/101004

Jachyra, P., Atkinson, M., & Gibson, B. E. (2014). Gender performativity during interviews with adolescent boys. *Qualitative Research in Sport, Exercise and Health, 6*(4), 568–582. https://doi.org/10.1080/2159676x.2013.877960

Jachyra, P., Atkinson, M., & Washiya, Y. (2015). 'Who are you, and what are you doing here': Methodological considerations in Ethnographic Health and Physical Education research. *Ethnography and Education, 10*(2), 242–261. https://doi.org/10.1080/17457823.2015.1018290

Jachyra, P., Lai, M.-C., Zaheer, J., Fernandes, N., Dale, M., Sawyer, A., & Lunsky, Y. (2021). Suicidal thoughts and behaviours among autistic adults presenting to the Psychiatric Emergency Department: An exploratory chart review. *Journal of Autism and Developmental Disorders, 52*(5), 2367–2375. https://doi.org/10.1007/s10803-021-05102-9

Jachyra, P., Renwick, R., Gladstone, B., Anagnostou, E., & Gibson, B. E. (2021). Physical activity participation among adolescents with autism spectrum disorder. *Autism, 25*(3), 613–626. https://doi.org/10.1177/1362361320949344

Katz, C., Hershkowitz, I., Malloy, L. C., Lamb, M. E., Atabaki, A., & Spindler, S. (2012). Non-verbal behavior of children who disclose or do not disclose child abuse in investigative interviews. *Child Abuse & Neglect, 36*(1), 12–20. https://doi.org/10.1016/j.chiabu.2011.08.006

Kerns, C. M., Lankenau, S., Shattuck, P. T., Robins, D. L., Newschaffer, C. J., & Berkowitz, S. J. (2022). Exploring potential sources of childhood trauma: A qualitative study with autistic adults and caregivers. *Autism, 26*(8), 1987–1998. https://doi.org/10.1177/13623613211070637

Lake, J. K., Jachyra, P., Volpe, T., Lunsky, Y., Magnacca, C., Marcinkiewicz, A., & Hamdani, Y. (2021). The wellbeing and mental health care experiences of adults with intellectual and developmental disabilities during COVID-19. *Journal of Mental Health Research in Intellectual Disabilities, 14*(3), 285–300. https://doi.org/10.1080/19315864.2021.1892890

Lunsky, Y., Lai, M., Balogh, R., Chung, H., Durbin, A., Jachyra, P., Tint, A., Weiss, J., & Lin, E. (2022). Premature mortality in a population-based cohort of autistic adults in Canada. *Autism Research, 15*(8), 1550–1559. https://doi.org/10.1002/aur.2741

McCann, I. L., & Pearlman, L. A. (1990). Vicarious traumatization: A framework for understanding the psychological effects of working with victims. *Journal of Traumatic Stress, 3*(1), 131–149.

McMahon, J., McGannon, K. R., Zehntner, C., Werbicki, L., Stephenson, E., & Martin, K. (2022). Trauma-informed abuse education in sport: Engaging athlete abuse survivors as educators and facilitating a community of care. *Sport, Education and Society, 28*(8), 958–971. https://doi.org/10.1080/13573322.2022.2096586

Morison, L., Simonds, L., & Stewart, S. J. F. (2021). Effectiveness of creative arts-based interventions for treating children and adolescents exposed to traumatic events: A systematic review of the quantitative evidence and meta-analysis. *Arts & Health, 14*(3), 237–262. https://doi.org/10.1080/17533015.2021.2009529

Mountjoy, M., Brackenridge, C., Arrington, M., Blauwet, C., Carska-Sheppard, A., Fasting, K., Kirby, S., Leahy, T., Marks, S., Martin, K., Starr, K., Tiivas, A., & Budgett, R. (2016). International Olympic Committee consensus statement: Harassment and abuse (non-accidental violence) in sport. *British Journal of Sports Medicine, 50*(17), 1019–1029.

Pearson, A., Rees, J., & Forster, S. (2022). "This was just how this friendship worked": Experiences of interpersonal victimization among autistic adults. *Autism in Adulthood, 4*(2), 141–150. https://doi.org/10.1089/aut.2021.0035

Peterson, J. L., Earl, R. K., Fox, E. A., Ma, R., Haidar, G., Pepper, M., Berliner, L., Wallace, A. S., & Bernier, R. A. (2019). Trauma and autism spectrum disorder: Review, proposed treatment adaptations and future directions. *Journal of Child & Adolescent Trauma, 12*(4), 529–547. https://doi.org/10.1007/s40653-019-00253-5

Pichon, L. C., Teti, M., & Brown, L. L. (2022). Triggers or prompts? When methods resurface unsafe memories and the value of trauma-informed photovoice research practices. *International Journal of Qualitative Methods, 21*, 160940692211139. https://doi.org/10.1177/16094069221113979

Rigles, B. (2021). Trajectories of adverse childhood experiences among children with autism. *Research in Autism Spectrum Disorders, 89*, 101876. https://doi.org/10.1016/j.rasd.2021.101876

Rosenbaum, S., Stierli, M., McCullagh, S., Newby, J., Ward, P. B., Harvey, S., & Steel, Z. (2022). An open trial of the RECONNECT exercise program for NSW Police Officers with posttraumatic stress disorder or psychological injury. *Health Promotion Journal of Australia: Official Journal of Australian Association of Health Promotion Professionals, 33*(1), 28–33. https://doi.org/10.1002/hpja.406

Rumball, F., Antal, K., Happé, F., & Grey, N. (2021). Co-occurring mental health symptoms and cognitive processes in trauma-exposed ASD adults. *Research in Developmental Disabilities, 110*, 103836. https://doi.org/10.1016/j.ridd.2020.103836

Saakvitne, K. W., Gamble, S., Pearlman, L. A., & Lev, B. T. (2000). *Risking connection: A training curriculum for working with survivors of childhood abuse.* Sidran Press. https://psycnet.apa.org/record/2000-08464-000

Sinko, L., & Saint Arnault, D. (2021). Photo-experiencing and reflective listening: A trauma-informed photo-elicitation method to explore day-to-day health experiences. *Public Health Nursing, 38*(4), 661–670. https://doi.org/10.1111/phn.12904

Smith, B., Williams, O., Bone, L., & the Moving Social Work Co-production Collective. (2022). Co-production: A resource to guide co-producing research in the sport, exercise, and health sciences. *Qualitative Research in Sport, Exercise and Health*, 1–29. https://doi.org/10.1080/2159676x.2022.2052946

Veletsianos, G., & Houlden, S. (2019). An analysis of flexible learning and flexibility over the last 40 years of *distance education. Distance Education, 40*(4), 454–468. https://doi.org/10.1080/01587919.2019.1681893

van der Merwe, A., & Hunt, X. (2019). Secondary trauma among trauma researchers: Lessons from the field. *Psychological Trauma: Theory, Research, Practice, and Policy, 11*(1), 10–18. https://doi.org/10.1037/tra0000414

Welch, C., Senman, L., Loftin, R., Picciolini, C., Robison, J., Westphal, A., Perry, B., Nguyen, J., Jachyra, P., Stevenson, S., Aggarwal, J., Wijekoon, S., Baron-Cohen, S., & Penner, M. (2022). Understanding the use of the term "Weaponized autism" in an alt-right social media platform. *Journal of Autism and Developmental Disorders.* https://doi.org/10.1007/s10803-022-05701-0

Whitt-Woosley, A., & Sprang, G. (2017). Secondary traumatic stress in social science researchers of trauma-exposed populations. *Journal of Aggression, Maltreatment & Trauma, 27*(5), 475–486. https://doi.org/10.1080/10926771.2017.1342109

Wright Stein, S., Alexander, R., Mann, J., Schneider, C., Zhang, S., Gibson, B. E., Gabison, S., Jachyra, P., & Mosleh, D. (2021). Understanding disability in healthcare: Exploring the perceptions of parents of young people with autism spectrum disorder. *Disability and Rehabilitation, 44*(19), 5623–5630. https://doi.org/10.1080/09638288.2021.1948114

Part IV

Developmental Trauma and Youth Trauma

Chapter 12

Researching *with* Care-Experienced Young People in Sport and Physical Activity

Methodological Reflections and the Need for a Trauma-Aware Lens

Thomas Quarmby, Rachel Sandford, and Oliver Hooper

Introduction

Any individual, of any age, from any neighbourhood or background, and from any social or cultural group can be impacted by trauma (Felitti et al., 1998; Howard, 2021). However, some are more susceptible than others, and this is particularly the case for marginalised young people. Indeed, refugees, asylum seekers, care-experienced young people, children in youth justice services, gender non-binary youth, and young people with disabilities have been shown to be more vulnerable to adverse childhood experiences (ACEs), toxic stress and, thus, trauma (Avery et al., 2022; UNESCO, 2019). ACEs include a range of stressful events that children and young people (up to the age of 18 years) have been exposed to while growing up (Felitti et al., 1998; Smith, 2018). Typically, these events included three specific kinds of adversity (1) abuse – e.g., physical, emotional, and sexual abuse, (2) neglect – e.g., physical and emotional neglect, and (3) household dysfunction – e.g., parental separation, domestic violence, substance misuse, mental illness, and incarceration of a family member. Experiencing any individual ACE may trigger a young person's stress response. However, if a child experiences multiple ACEs over time, those exposures can result in toxic stress, which is the prolonged activation of the stress response system, whereby the body fails to fully recover (Franke, 2014). This stress ultimately results in complex trauma – repeated relational harm that overwhelms a person's capacity to cope (Courtois & Ford, 2009). It is important to note, however, that not all children and young people who have adverse experiences will be traumatised, since how they respond to the same adversity will differ depending on the contexts in which they find themselves and the support that is available to them therein. Individuals respond to trauma in different ways and at different times, and there is therefore an element of flexibility needed with regard to working with/alongside individuals who have experienced trauma.

DOI: 10.4324/9781003332909-16

There are a range of factors that can protect children and young people from the psychological distress that may accompany traumatic experiences. These factors include having nurturing parents, stable family relationships, adequate housing, basic needs being satisfied (e.g., accessing suitable food and water), and caring adults outside of the home who act as mentors (Turner et al., 2012). When these factors are present, they buffer the effects of toxic stress and return the body to its baseline function, allowing an individual to cope despite adversity (Franke, 2014). However, some factors – particularly those associated with stable family relationships and social connections – are not necessarily present for care-experienced young people. This means that their experiences regarding trauma are somewhat different to their (non-cared for) peers (Simkiss, 2018). Broadly speaking, care-experienced youth include those children and young people who have spent a period of time under the care of the state. Care-experienced young people are defined by a variety of terms internationally. For instance, in England, the term 'looked-after children' is used, in Australia, 'children in out-of-home care' is employed and, in the United States, the term 'foster care' is more prevalent. However, throughout this chapter, we use the term 'care-experienced' to capture the transient nature and experiences of those children and young people who have, at some point in their lives, been removed from their family and placed in the care of the state, in foster care, a children's home or in an adoptive placement (Quarmby et al., 2022).

Numbers of care-experienced young people are growing internationally. This growth is partly due to factors such as increased forced migration, international conflict, and the COVID-19 pandemic (UNESCO, 2019). In England, as of March 2022, there were 82,170 children and young people living in care – an increase of 2% from the previous year (Department for Education [DfE], 2022). These trends are reflected in broader international contexts, for instance, in Australia, between 2017 and 2020, the number of young people in out-of-home care rose by 7% (Australian Institute of Health and Welfare, 2021). There is international consensus that this population are among the most vulnerable and marginalised, with widespread evidence suggesting they experience poor physical and mental health, have difficulties with their social and emotional well-being and have poorer educational outcomes than their non-care-experienced peers (O'Higgins et al., 2015; Sebba et al., 2015).

The range of ACEs are disproportionately associated with care-experienced young people, since they are more likely to be exposed to family breakdown, deprivation, and family mental illness (Simkiss, 2018). For instance, in England specifically, 66% of children and young people were reported to enter care in 2020 because of abuse and/or neglect, while 14% entered care because of family dysfunction (DfE, 2022); both specific markers of adversity that may lead to trauma (Felitti et al., 1998). Simkiss (2018, p. 26) has argued that those who enter care because of abuse and/or neglect are likely to have 'experienced the "toxic trio" of parental domestic violence, substance misuse and mental illness', which would inevitably lead to higher ACE scores. In extending the original list of ACEs outlined by Felitti and colleagues (1998), Smith (2018) suggested that being bullied and being placed in foster care are both ACEs that may have detrimental impacts on young people. Such things are pertinent when we consider that care-experienced young people have been identified as a group particularly vulnerable to being bullied (Gallagher & Green, 2012). Moreover, being placed in foster care is also associated with the increased likelihood of placement instability (moving between foster homes and residential homes) and the associated challenges of building meaningful, sustained relationships with peers and adults – key factors that would normally help individuals recover from adversity. This is exemplified in the following research quotes from Matt, a care-experienced young person, and Sam, a care-leaver who had spent time in care but now lives independently:

> I remember, like, I moved primary school about eleven times, not even within the same area, like I've been out of the county a few times. I didn't have many friends at school because of all the moves and I used to get bullied quite a lot.
>
> (Matt, aged 16)

> From a very, very early age, the age of three, I remember episodes of domestic violence. My father wasn't a particularly nice man. He was a fisherman, but he was also incredibly tight … I moved to England from Ireland at the age of nine but the six-year window from the age of three to nine is a bit of a blur. I have some recollections of not particularly happy or joyous years. The best way to describe it was that we were on the move regularly. We were in and out of different types of accommodation, from hostels, flats, houses – what I now know as squatting – to living on the street because we had no place to go. We had no fixed abode. The age of three to nine was about avoiding my father really.
>
> (Sam, aged 32)

The above voices highlight how care-experienced young people may be exposed to a range of prolonged traumatic events in their early development. Importantly, the impact of prolonged exposure to multiple ACEs is associated with poorer outcomes in adulthood in comparison to exposure to just one traumatic event (Simkiss, 2018).

Complex childhood trauma – that which results from repeated exposure to ACEs – can affect young people's development in a number of different ways. For care-experienced young people, Simkiss (2018) identified specific impacts of the increased exposure to ACEs on incidents of mental illness, sexual health, risk taking behaviour, criminality, and mortality. For instance, Simkiss (2018) suggests that there is a four-to-five-fold increase in mental disorder among care-experienced youth, with evidence from the United States, Australia, and Denmark identifying increased mental illness prevalence rates for individuals who have experienced care at some point. In the English context, too, it has been estimated that nearly half of children in care have a diagnosable mental health issue and two-thirds have special educational needs (Oakley et al., 2018).

Notably, such issues are increasingly being discussed in relation to research in sport and physical activity, signifying something of the potential of such activities to ameliorate the detrimental impacts of trauma on young people's development. For instance, physical activity and sport can foster positive emotional climates, facilitate learner-focused activities, and help young people to develop resilience-related skills such as emotional regulation and decision making (D'Andrea et al., 2013; Whitley et al., 2018). Moreover, formal sport and physical activity programmes that are sensitive to the needs of trauma-affected youth can support their development by helping to facilitate psychological escape, enabling them to reconnect and restore feelings of embodiment, and building confidence and competence (Massey & Williams, 2020; Whitley et al., 2018). Hence, participation in physical activity and sport may offer a means of mitigating some of the challenges care-experienced youth encounter.

Reflections on Working with Care-experienced Young People

While our research with care-experienced young people focused primarily on their experiences of and engagement with sport and physical activity (as explained further below), as a research team we were very conscious of the adversity and trauma that they may have experienced in the past. We were, therefore, particularly cognisant of the need to be sensitive to this in our approach to researching with these young people and recognised that we may face challenges in this regard. For instance, we were heavily reliant on gatekeepers (e.g., youth workers) for advice and guidance. From a practical (ethical) perspective we had to penetrate the different layers of the care 'system' in order to even meet with young people – reflecting what Hood et al. (1996, p. 120) refer to as 'a hierarchy of gatekeeping' running from the organisational level to the 'parents' (or, in this case, corporate parents) and finally the child. Moreover, this process also meant that consent to conduct the research was negotiated first through key gatekeepers (e.g., local authorities) and provided in loco parentis by an adult advocate who worked with the young people on a regular basis (e.g., as part of a local authority children in care council). As Kendrick et al. (2008, p. 88) suggest, 'there is the possibility that they [care-experienced young people] have been placed there because of abuse by their parents, or because there has been a breakdown in relationships in the family'. Therefore, it is not always appropriate, nor in the best interests of the young person, to approach their parent(s) for consent (Kendrick et al., 2008).

As noted above, care-experienced young people enter care for a variety of reasons but, more often than not, this is on account of being 'let down' by an adult or adults in their immediate environment. This impact can mean that those who are care-experienced come to be distrustful of 'official adults' (Gooch et al., 2022). Children in care are often surrounded by an array of adults (e.g., social workers, key workers, designated teachers) with whom they are required to meet regularly, as they have a formal role in monitoring (and documenting) their progress and development (Sandford et al., 2021). Therefore, a key priority for us as a research team was to develop positive relationships with the young people we were working with and position ourselves as outside of this 'official' role. To do this, we purposefully explained expectations, established routines in focus group interviews, were responsive to young people and attempted to offer them choice in the activities they engaged in. In this respect, we also looked to avoid being adults who 'parachute' in and 'take data' and worked with young people throughout the process and in producing a young person friendly report that shared the project findings with those involved. This process was incredibly encouraging in that it enabled us to speak with care-experienced young people, listen to their voices, and hear their careful considerations for what might enhance practice.

Right to Be Active (R2BA) Project

Below, we draw on research which we conducted as part of a British Academy-funded project (i.e., Right to Be Active – R2BA) that explored the role and value of sport and physical activity within the day-to-day lives of care-experienced young people in England (see Sandford et al., 2021). The main aim of the project was to examine the strategies in place to support care-experienced young people's engagement with sport and physical activity and, importantly, to explore their lived experiences of these. This research was particularly significant since physical activity has been considered to enhance care-experienced youths' physical and psychological well-being, as well as support their development of social capital, resilience, and identity (O'Donnell et al., 2020). However, concerns remain about the piecemeal nature of physical activity opportunities provided for care-experience youth and their capacity to access these. The broader project therefore consisted of four distinct phases. Within this chapter, we consider how phases three and four were sensitive to the needs of young people who may have been impacted by a range of ACEs, and thus complex childhood trauma. These latter phases explicitly considered care-experienced young people's needs and adopted a qualitative methodology drawing on participatory methods.

Methodology

The methodology that we employed in phases three and four was under-pinned by a youth voice perspective (Hooper, 2018; Sandford et al., 2010) that helped to generate data via a number of participatory methods, which fed into semi-structured focus groups. Montreuil et al. (2021) suggest that 'partici-patory research' is a broad umbrella term that 'covers both the collection of data with children and children's participation in making decisions related to the research process' (p. 2). Hence, they suggest that children and young peo-ple's participation as 'subjects' or co-constructors of research is often blurred and that there is a need to distinguish between participatory methods and a participatory research approach (Montreuil et al., 2021). While a participa-tory research design would have allowed young people in our study to be actively involved in key research decisions (e.g., what questions to ask, how to ask those questions and with whom), Montreuil and colleagues (2021) note that in some contexts the benefits of larger group discussions around key research design and decisions might be outweighed by the need for privacy and confidentiality of participants. We would argue that working with young people who have experienced trauma might be such a context.

As such, in our R2BA study, we employed participatory *methods* rather than a participatory research *approach*. In this respect, we employed differ-ent methods to engage with young people to collect the research data, since we felt this might support them to build rapport with us as researchers and empower them to share their lived experiences. Building rapport and facili-tating voice is essential for care-experienced young people who, as noted, may have difficulty trusting adults, and especially adults they do not know and so these participatory methods enabled the young people to 'take the lead' in engaging with us. Specifically, the participatory methods employed included mind-mapping perceptions of sport and physical activity (e.g., list-ing keywords associated with sport/physical activity), drawing maps of where individuals engaged in sport and physical activity, ranking and debating quotes drawn from the open-ended survey questions, and creating pictorial representations of 'positive' and 'negative' experiences of accessing sport/physical activity as a care-experienced young person ('character creation' – see Sandford et al., 2021).

Importantly, each young person was given the choice over which methods they would like to use and the freedom to be creative within the bounds of the activity (e.g., drawing in particular styles or combining words and pictures in their activity maps), and we were cognisant at all times of the need to ensure that the methods were fun and engaging, yet not perceived as childish (Lundy et al., 2011). In total, 63 care-experienced young people aged 8–21 years (26 males and 37 females), from six different geographical contexts across England, took part in the focus group discussions. These were used as the young people knew each other, were somewhat wary of individual 'official' meetings and were already familiar with taking part in group-based discussions within their contexts. Montreuil et al.'s (2021) review of participatory approaches highlighted the importance of providing young people with an environment that is inclusive and makes them feel safe to express themselves. As such, our research took place in spaces familiar to the young people (e.g., at youth clubs or children in care councils) to ensure that they felt as comfortable as possible during the focus groups and that usual routines were not disrupted.

The use of participatory methods allowed for conversation to build slowly and for individuals to work independently while engaging in informal conversation. Hence, the methods helped us to develop some form of rapport with young people; countering, to some extent, the acknowledged challenge of researchers 'parachuting' in to generate data with young people (e.g., Alderson et al., 2019). As such, this approach aligns with the Substance Abuse and Mental Health Services Administration's (SAMHSA) principles for a trauma-informed approach, namely, (i) safety and (ii) empowerment, voice, and choice (SAMHSA, 2014). For instance, conducting the activity-based focus groups in a space that was convenient and comfortable allowed young people to feel physically (in relation to the setting) and emotionally (in the presence of a trusted adult alongside the research team) safe, while the participatory methods used attempted to purposefully explore, recognise, and value young people's strengths and experiences (SAMHSA, 2014).

In addition to the participatory methods used to support the focus groups with care-experienced young people, we also conducted narrative interviews with four care-leavers (i.e., those who experienced care at some point in their lives but formally left the care system). These participants, consisting of two males and two females, aged 23–32 years, were invited to share stories of being in care and their engagement with sport and physical activity through unstructured interviews. This practice provided participants a degree of control over the stories shared and offered opportunities for them to expand as needed on areas of perceived significance (see Quarmby et al., 2021). SAMHSA (2014) notes that providing choice, in this case which stories and details to share, is particularly important for those who may have previously experienced trauma. Unlike the focus groups with care-experienced youth, the locations of the interviews with care-leavers were negotiated, to maintain a feeling of safety and additional control with the process.

Importantly, the activity-based focus groups and the care-leaver interviews conducted in phase three resulted in the generation of rich, qualitative data. Moreover, it became evident that stories were an important way for individuals to articulate their engagements with sport and physical activity. This phase led to the fourth phase of the project, which was the co-creation of a series of 'concept cartoons' with a graphic designer (Hooper, 2018; Hooper et al., 2021). Following the interviews, we employed the process of creative non-fiction and created multiple stories that showcased different narratives of sport and physical activity. In doing so, we followed a process outlined by Blodgett et al. (2011). We conducted an inductive thematic analysis whereby transcripts were read and re-read before keywords, quotes and ideas that represented individual characters and their stories were highlighted. These key features were transferred to a new document that formed the foundation for the initial skeletons of the different narratives (Blodgett et al., 2011).

Creative non-fiction is the generation of stories that are fictional in form but factual in content grounded in real events and lived experiences of participants (Smith et al., 2015). This approach was considered particularly beneficial since creative non-fiction helps to protect anonymity, while still preserving the integrity of participants' words (Sparkes, 2002). The intention with creative non-fiction is to show, not just tell, complex lived experiences, and layered theoretical aspects of stories (Smith et al., 2015). We used portrait (i.e., individual character's experiences) and composite (i.e., where multiple individuals' experiences are combined into one) vignettes to represent the various sport and physical activity stories of care-experienced youth and care-leavers (Ely et al., 1997). Once the different narratives had been crafted, they were turned into comic strips in the form of a series of four images to reflect the overall story. We considered narratives as social constructions that framed particular stories told and represented through images and text. Therefore, comic strips, as a visual, storied, and narrative medium, were well suited to portray/capture the complexity of lived experiences in both form and content. Following this process, draft comic strips were shared with the care-experienced young people to help refine the images and intended meanings. According to Prosser and Burke (2008), visual stories and narratives serve as a tool to help the researcher and participants co-construct new meaning of their lived experiences. This process helped us (the research team) to engage in further dialogue with participants in the form of repeated focus groups with the young people to share these images and check/refine our interpretations of the stories and how they resonated with their peers. We sought input on the initial draft images created by the graphic designer with the goal of empowering young people in the research by encouraging them to suggest changes to the images that would better (re)present their lived experiences (Sandford et al., 2024). Repeated focus groups took place in four of the six contexts (again, based on a convenience sample) and involved most of those young people who participated in phase three ($n = 40$, 8–21 years of age, 16 male and 24 female). The draft comic strips or 'visual narratives' intensify reflection, whereby the comic strips invited viewers to reflect and 'reimagine' which stimulated further dialogue and the sharing of additional stories with us and each other. Hence, the draft comic strips acted as provocation for further inquiry.

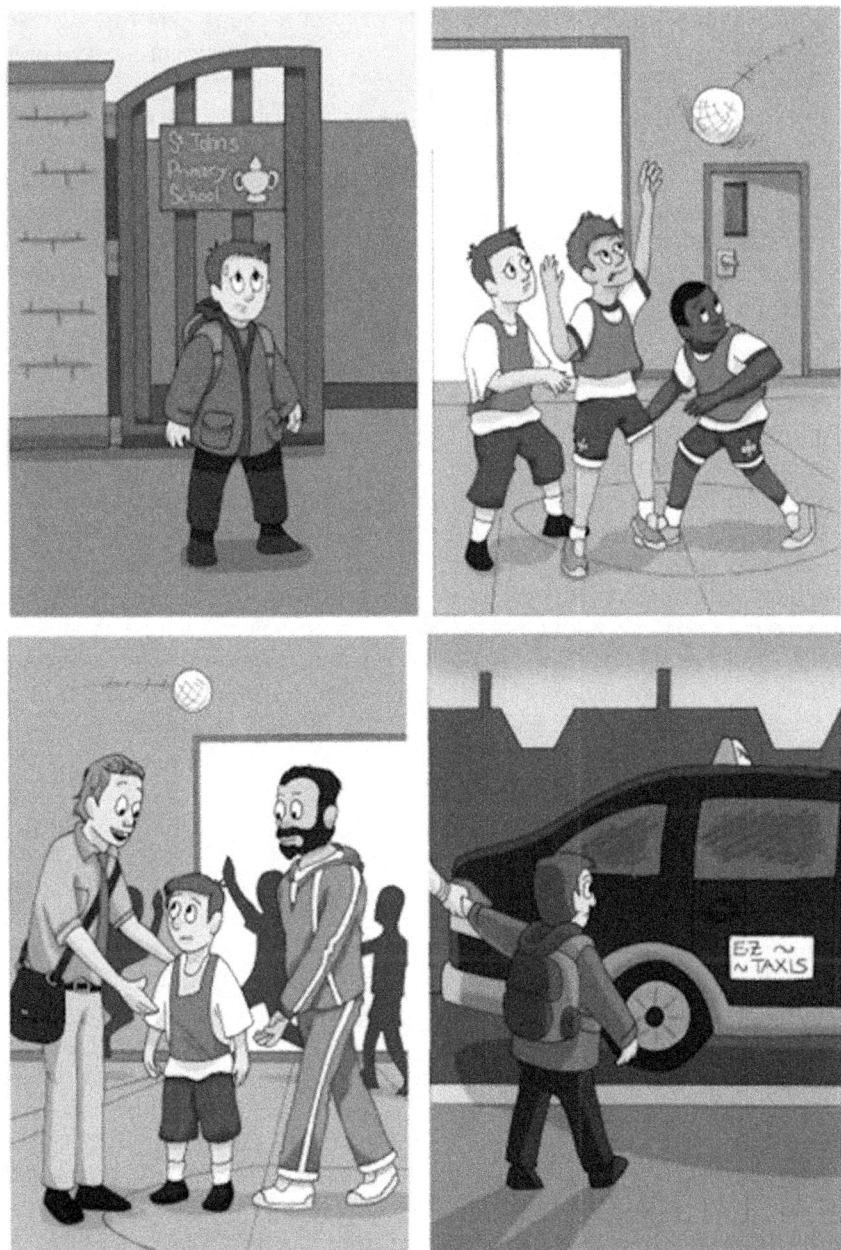

Figure 12.1 'New boy' comic strip.

This cartoon was intended to tell the story of a young care-experienced boy who was starting a new school following a placement move. He is nervous when he is dropped off because he doesn't know anybody there. While he is at school, the boy takes part in a PE lesson but feels a bit left out because the other children all know each other. He is also wearing the wrong PE kit because he hasn't got his new uniform yet, so this makes him feel different. During the PE lesson, the boy needs to go and meet his social worker, which means that he misses out on the rest of the lesson. At the end of the day, the boy doesn't have someone to collect him but is picked up in a taxi to go back to his care home.

Following feedback from the phase four focus groups, the comic strips (see Figure 12.1 example) were finalised and used in additional dissemination events to showcase care-experienced young people's stories about sport and physical activity (Hooper et al., 2021). The fourth phase also reflected SAMHSA's (2014) principle of 'trustworthiness and transparency' for a trauma-informed approach by openly sharing the process of creating the stories and crafting the comic strips with participants which inadvertently helped to build, maintain, and reinforce trust between participants and researchers. Moreover, in sharing the stories with others (both care-experienced young people and adults working with/for them), we enabled them to tell/inspire different stories. We were clear that it was ok to have different interpretations of the stories, and this led to new/alternative conversations about issues of importance.

Protections During the Research Process

There were several protections in place during the research process, both for the care-experienced young people and the researchers. For the care-experienced young people, as part of the ethical process, standard procedures were in place around safeguarding and referral. For instance, we recognised we had a responsibility to support young people and that while the research did not ask questions that would directly elicit difficulties, there could have been situations where we had a duty of care to reveal information that had been provided in confidence, or which we had discovered through inter-actions with the participants. In line with the British Educational Research Association's (BERA) Ethical Guidelines for Educational Research (2018), if it was judged that the effect of the agreements made with participants on confidentiality would allow the continuation of illegal behaviour (this coming to light during the course of the research), then we would have to carefully consider making disclosure to the appropriate authorities. This was in place to support both the young people and us as a research team, as well as to ensure that gatekeepers were able to follow the policies and procedures in their own organisation. As noted earlier in this chapter, we also conducted the research in-situ, in familiar contexts, with trusted adults (e.g., youth workers and social workers) present to support the initial introductions with young people and help with discussions around ethics (e.g., re-checking consent). We feel this helped to access insider knowledge and allowed us to avoid potentially sensitive issues that might be re-traumatising for young people. Finally, adopting a strengths-based approach within the research itself (i.e., ensuring a focus on 'what works' and identifying good practice to support future developments) may have helped to mitigate many of the risks around participants becoming distressed (Enright et al., 2014). For instance, while we explored negative experiences, it was often with a view as to how these might be improved (e.g., considering how teachers might better respond to emotional outbursts, or how social workers might better manage transitions between different care contexts).

In relation to the protections in place for us as a research team, the first thing we identified was the need to conduct the research as a team wherever possible. Aside from it being a pragmatic decision to support the data collection (i.e., allowing for smaller group work within larger focus group sessions), this practice also served to facilitate researcher well-being (Sandford et al., 2024). As an example, we reflected on the participants' conversations following the focus group sessions and talked through difficult or challenging aspects of these. This safeguarded against compassion fatigue (Ashley-Binge & Cousins, 2020). At times, decisions about who would undertake research activities were also made in relation to questions of gender. The BERA Ethical Guidelines for Educational Research (2018) suggests safeguarding the physical and psychological well-being of researchers is part of 'good' ethical practice and hence the team approach helped to mitigate potential issues of a lone researcher working with unknown young people. In addition, after each focus group and interaction with young people we employed team debriefs as part of the research process, sharing experiences within these contexts either via face-to-face discussions or via a WhatsApp group chat.

Trauma-Informed Practices Applied to Research

While the R2BA project was geared towards examining the strategies in place to support care-experienced young people's engagements with sport and physical activity, the research highlighted the need to consider how such contexts could be more sensitive to the needs of young people impacted by trauma. As such, we identified evidence-based trauma-aware pedagogical (TAP) principles grounded in the voices of co-participants that would support those working with/for trauma-affected young people in a physical education (PE) space. We use the term trauma-aware to reflect the start of a transformational journey that involves changes in knowledge, practice, culture and systems that ultimately leads to becoming trauma-informed. We have also argued in subsequent work that as these principles reflect core aspects of 'good' pedagogical practice, they are relevant for broader youth sport and coaching contexts too (Quarmby et al., 2023). These TAP principles are

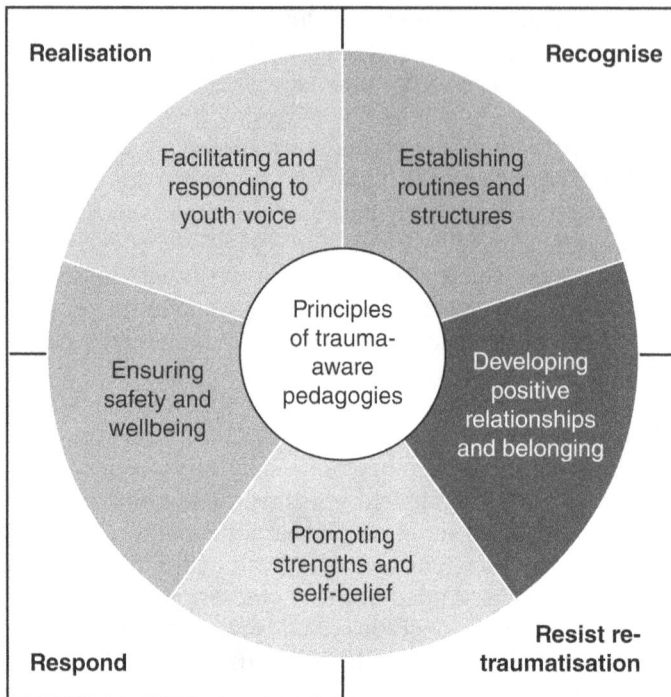

Figure 12.2 Principles for trauma-aware pedagogies (created by Quarmby et al., 2022).

(1) ensuring safety and well-being, (2) establishing routines and structures, (3) developing and sustaining positive relationships that foster a sense of belonging, (4) facilitating and responding to youth voice, and (5) promoting strengths and self-belief.

Importantly, these TAP principles align with, and reinforce SAMHSA's (2014) four key assumptions that underpin a trauma-aware approach – referred to as the four 'Rs' (see Figure 12.2 above).

The first 'R' indicates that people need to have a basic *realisation* about trauma and the adverse effects it can have on an individual. This means viewing people's behaviours in the context of their experiences and realising that behaviours often stem from the traumatised individual developing coping strategies to survive adversity and/or overwhelming situations. The second 'R' is that people are able to recognise the signs of trauma, while the third 'R' assumes that the system (i.e., the school, staff, curriculum PE) responds in a way that embraces our understanding of trauma (i.e., staff are trained in evidence-based trauma practices and schools provide a physically and psychologically safe environment). The final 'R' is used to suggest that practices are put in place to resist re-traumatisation (i.e., practices are considered so they do not interfere with an individual's healing or recovery).

Combined, these four 'Rs' and the TAP principles outlined above provide a foundation for considering research with trauma-affected youth and could be considered as principles that support trauma-aware research. For instance, retrospectively, each of these principles were evident in some shape or form in our R2BA research. Ensuring safety and well-being is important since those who have experienced trauma often perceive the world as 'unsafe'. This practice can then manifest in hypersensitivity to anything that may threaten their sense of physical or psychological safety. As noted above, this was evident in our research when we conducted research in spaces and places that young people felt were familiar and where adults that they had already built relationships with were present. Similarly, establishing clear routines and structures provides young people with a sense of control and helps them to feel like their life can be regulated (Quarmby et al., 2022).

For us, outlining the research process from the start – to avoid any surprises – was a key element of our work with care-experienced youth, ensuring that they knew what to expect and when. Moreover, we sought to demonstrate trust, kindness, empathy, and caring, which have all been shown to help to develop positive relationships (Quarmby et al., 2022). Within the study, we did this through things like actively listening to young people and showing genuine interest in topics that mattered to them – which often extended conversations beyond the immediate context. This is key for young people who have experienced trauma since, as noted earlier, they may have difficulty trusting adults and forming relationships with peers. From a research perspective, we would argue that the choice of approach and methods employed – as detailed above – can help to facilitate this, though there is a need to be aware of how that relationship 'ends' when the research is over. For us, this included creating a specific R2BA 'youth report' – written in plain English – and sharing this with young people via their gatekeepers (Sandford et al., 2020). This enabled us to recognise and acknowledge the contributions that young people had made to the research and to highlight how their involvement was meaningful and would hopefully have impact moving forwards.

Arguably, the principle around facilitating and responding to youth voice was the one we wanted to foreground most in our research. The nature of the participatory, activity-based methods enabled those young people experiencing trauma who may have difficulties communicating via traditional direct means (e.g., face-to-face question and answer interview) the opportunity to share their experiences and foreground their voices (and stories). In this case participants were provided with choice in the focus groups with some opting to take part in certain activities while others chose not to. The co-creation of cartoons further reinforced this principle in our research. Finally, recognising and valuing the strengths that young people bring is a key component of many participatory methods (Coyne & Carter, 2018). These strengths were subsequently captured in the concept cartoons (see Figure 12.1) that reflected young people's stories since we were cognisant of not just depicting the challenges that care-experienced youth encountered, but also the successes they have had.

Conclusions

Moving forward, we propose the following three interconnected considerations when conducting research with youth affected by trauma in sport, exercise, and health contexts.

1 While there is a welcome growth in the number of scholars exploring trauma in sport, physical activity, and health research, there is a tendency to foreground adult voices and perspectives. Although this may reflect the sensitive nature of the work, there is much potential to generate meaningful and relevant insights from trauma-affected youth themselves, if research is conducted sensitively and in line with the trauma-aware research principles we suggest above. We would call for further research engaging with youth voices in the initial conceptualisation and design of research projects. In facilitating youth voices, we suggest that scholars engage with creative, arts-based, participatory methods given the potential of these methods to be used in a way that is sensitive to the histories of youth affected by trauma (Goessling, 2020). Such methods also allow the pedagogical potential of stories to come forward for researchers and co-participants, as part of a shared, and potentially empowering, process for youth. Additionally, recognising that every young person may be affected by trauma differently, with no single uniform approach likely to be sufficient in meeting the needs of all, developing a toolkit of creative, arts-based, participatory methods that young people could draw from would be helpful.

2 Second, more longitudinal research with trauma-affected young people would be beneficial. As used here, longitudinal refers to prolonged engagement with young people. This would help to establish expectations, routines, and structures (ensuring researchers do not simply 'parachute' in) and would likely further facilitate a sense of safety and belonging through the development of relationships with researchers. More longitudinal projects would help to facilitate greater depth and have the potential to engage multiple stakeholders, as well as afford time to initiate changes in practice and determine impact. It would enable a move beyond the 'snapshot' moments so prevalent in short-term-funded research and allow greater recognition of lived experiences of trauma.

3 Finally, it is important to recognise that listening to the stories of those impacted by trauma may result in something akin to compassion fatigue for researchers. Compassion fatigue refers to the negative, though predictable and treatable, psychological consequences of working with, and in

proximity to, suffering people (Ashley-Binge & Cousins, 2020). In short, compassion fatigue relates to the deep emotional exhaustion experienced after repeated exposure to traumatic stories. As such, there is a need to consider the support in place at an individual and institutional level for those researchers working with trauma-affected youth. Such resources may help mitigate any effects of compassion fatigue that may result from the close relationships developed with individuals throughout the course of the research. This practice might also include working with supervisors, mentors, or a research team, and regularly debriefing on the events that have taken place as part of the research.

References

Ashley-Binge, S., & Cousins, C. (2020). Individual and organisational practices addressing social workers' experiences of vicarious trauma. *Social Work in Action*, *32*(3), 191–207.

Alderson, H., Brown, R., Smart, D., Lingam, R., & Dovey-Pearce, G. (2019). You've come to children that are in care and given us the opportunity to get our voices heard': The journey of looked after children and researchers in developing a Patient and Public Involvement group. *Health Expectations*, *22*(4), 657–665. https://doi.org/10.1111/hex.12904

Australian Institute of Health and Welfare. (2021). *Child protection Australia 2019–2020*. Australian Institute of Health and Welfare.

Avery, J., Deppeler, J., Galvin, E., Skouteris, H., Crain de Galarce, P., & Morris, H.. (2022). Changing educational paradigms: Trauma-responsive relational practice, learnings from the USA for Australian schools. *Children and Youth Services Review*. https://doi.org/10.1016/j.childyouth.2022.106506

Blodgett, A., Schinke, R., Smith, B., Peltier, D., & Pheasant, C. (2011). In indigenous words: Exploring vignettes as a narrative strategy for presenting the research voices of aboriginal community members. *Qualitative Inquiry*, *17*(6), 522–533. https://doi.org/10.1177/1077800411409885

British Educational Research Association (BERA). (2018). *BERA Ethical Guidelines for Educational Research*. https://www.bera.ac.uk/publication/ethical-guidelines-for-educational-research-2018-online

Courtois, C., & Ford, J. (2009). *Treating complex traumatic stress disorders: An evidence-based guide*. The Guilford Press.

Coyne, I., & Carter, B. (2018). Participatory research in the past, present and future. In I. Coyne & B. Carter (Eds.), *Being participatory: Researching with children and young people* (pp. 1–13). Springer.

D'Andrea, W., Bergholz, L., Fortunato, A., & Spinazzola, J. (2013). Play to the whistle: A pilot investigation of a sports-based intervention for traumatized girls in residential treatment. *Journal of Family Violence*, *28*(7), 739–749. https://doi.org/10.1007/s10896-013-9533-x

Department for Education (DfE). (2022). *Children looked after in England including adoptions*. https://explore-education-statistics.service.gov.uk/find-statistics/children-looked-after-in-england-including-adoptions

Ely, M., Vinz, R., Downing, M., & Anzul, M. (1997). *On writing qualitative research: Living by words*. Routledge-Falmer.

Enright, E., Hill, J., Sandford, R., & Gard, M. (2014). Looking beyond what's broken: Towards an appreciative research agenda for physical education and sport pedagogy. *Sport, Education and Society, 19*(7), 912–926. https://doi.org/10.1080/13573 322.2013.854764

Felitti, V., Anda, R., Nordenberg, D., Williamson, D., Spitz, A., Edwards, V., Koss, M., & Marks, J. (1998). Relationship of childhood abuse and household dysfunction to many of the leading causes of death in adults: The adverse childhood experiences (ACE) study. *American Journal of Preventative Medicine, 14*(4), 245–258.

Franke, H. (2014). Toxic stress: Effects, prevention and treatment. *Children, 1*, 390–402.

Gallagher, B., & Green, A. (2012). In, out and after care: Young adults' views on their lives, as children, in a therapeutic residential establishment. *Children and Youth Services Review, 34*(2), 437–450.

Goessling, K. P. (2020). Youth participatory action research, trauma, and the arts: Designing youth spaces for equity and healing. *International Journal of Qualitative Studies in Education, 33*(1), 12–31. https://doi.org/10.1080/09518398.2019.1678783

Gooch, K., Masson, I., Owens, A., & Waddington, E. (2022). After care, after thought: The invisibility of care experienced men and women in prison. *Prison Service Journal, 258*(9), 4–12.

Hood, S., Kelley, P., & Mayall, B. (1996). Children as research subjects: A risky enterprise. *Children & Society, 10*(2), 117–128. https://doi.org/10.1111/j.1099-0860.1996.tb00462.x

Hooper, O. (2018). *Healthy talk: Pupils' conceptions of health within physical education*. Unpublished PhD, Loughborough University.

Hooper, O., Sandford, R., Quarmby, T., & Duncombe, R. (2021). Let me tell you a story: Concept cartoons as a tool for representing young people's voices in physical education and youth sport. *Physical Education Matters*. Spring 2021, 56–58.

Howard, J. (2021). *National guidelines for trauma-aware education*. Queensland University of Technology and Australian Childhood Foundation.

Kendrick, A., Steckley, L., & Lerpiniere, J. (2008). Ethical issues, research and vulnerability: Gaining the views of children and young people in residential care. *Children's Geographies, 6*(1), 79–93. https://doi.org/10.1080/14733280701791967

Lundy, L., McEvoy, L., & Byrne, B. (2011). Working with young children as co-researchers: An approach informed by the United Nations Convention on the Rights of the Child. *Early Education & Development, 22*(5), 714–736.

Massey, W., & Williams, T. (2020). Sporting activities for individuals who experienced trauma during their youth: A meta-study. *Qualitative Health Research, 30*(1), 73–87. https://doi.org/10.1177/1049732319849563

Montreuil, M., Bogossian, A., Laberge-Perrault, E., & Racine, E. (2021). A review of approaches, strategies and ethical considerations in participatory research with children. *International Journal of Qualitative Methods, 20*. https://doi.org/10.1177/1609406920987962

Oakley, M., Miscampbell, G., & Gregorian, R. (2018). *Looked-after children: The silent crisis*. Social Market Foundation.

O'Donnell, C., Sandford, R., & Parker, A. (2020). Physical education, school sport and looked-after-children: Health, well-being and educational engagement. *Sport,*

Researching with Care-Experienced Young People   213

Education and Society, *25*(6), 605–617. https://doi.org/10.1080/13573322.2019.1628731

O'Higgins, A., Sebba, J., & Luke, N. (2015). *What is the relationship between being in care and the educational outcomes of children? An international systematic review.* Rees Centre for Research in Fostering and Education.

Prosser, J., & Burke, C. (2008). Image-based educational research: Childlike perspectives. In J. Knowles & A. Cole (Eds.), *Handbook of the arts in qualitative research: Perspectives, methodologies, examples, and issues* (pp. 407–421). Sage Publications.

Quarmby, T., Sandford, R., Green, R., Hooper, O., & Avery, J. (2022). Developing evidence-informed principles for trauma-aware pedagogies in physical education. *Physical Education and Sport Pedagogy*, *27*(4), 440–454. https://doi.org/10.1080/17408989.2021.1891214

Quarmby, T., Sandford, R., & Hooper, O. (2023). Coaching care-experienced children and young people in sport. In M. Toms & R. Jeanes (Eds.), *The Routledge handbook of coaching children in sport* (pp. 204–212). Routledge.

Quarmby, T., Sandford, R., Hooper, O., & Duncombe, R. (2021). Narratives and marginalised voices: Storying the sport and physical activity experiences of care-experienced young people. *Qualitative Research in Sport, Exercise and Health*, *13*(3), 426–437. https://doi.org/10.1080/2159676X.2020.1725099

Sandford, R., Armour, K., & Duncombe, R. (2010). Finding their voice: Disaffected youth insights on sport/physical activity interventions. In M. O'Sullivan & A. MacPhail (Eds.), *Young people's voices in physical education and youth sport* (pp. 65–87). Routledge.

Sandford, R., Hooper, O., & Quarmby, T. (2024). Facilitating conversations and telling stories: Research with and for care-experienced young people. In F. Chambers, R. Sandford, O. Hooper, & L. Schaefer (Eds.), *Research with children and youth in physical education and youth sport (pp. 147-163)*. Routledge.

Sandford, R., Quarmby, T., Hooper, R., & Duncombe, R. (2020). *Right to Be Active: Children and young people's report*. Loughborough University & Leeds Beckett University.

Sandford, R., Quarmby, T., Hooper, O., & Duncombe, R. (2021). Navigating complex social landscapes: Examining care experienced young people's engagements with sport and physical activity. *Sport, Education and Society*, *26*(1), 15–28. https://doi.org/10.1080/13573322.2019.1699523

Sebba, J., Berridge, D., Luke, N., Fletcher, J., Bell, K., Strand, S., Thomas, S., Sinclair, I., & O'Higgins, A. (2015). *The educational progress of looked after children in England: Linking care and educational data*. Rees Centre for Research on Fostering and Education.

Simkiss, D. (2018). The needs of looked after children from an adverse childhood experience perspective. *Paediatrics and Child Health*, *29*(1), 25–33.

Smith, M. (2018). Capability and adversity: Reframing the 'causes of the causes' for mental health. *Palgrave Communications*, *4*(13), 1–5.

Smith, B., McGannon, K., & Williams, T. (2015). Ethnographic creative nonfiction: Exploring the what's, whys and how's. In M. Gyozo & L. Purdy (Eds.), *Ethnographies in sport and exercise research* (pp. 59–73). Routledge.

Sparkes, A. (2002). *Telling tales in sport and physical activity: A qualitative journey*. Human Kinetics.

Substance Abuse and Mental Health Services Administration (SAMHSA). (2014). *SAMHSA's concept of trauma and guidance for a trauma-informed approach*. US Department of Health and Human Services.

Turner, H., Finkelhor, D., Ormrod, R., Hamby, S., Leeb, R., Mercy, J., & Holt, M. (2012). Family context, victimization, and child trauma symptoms: Variations in safe, stable, and nurturing relationships during early and middle childhood. *American Journal of Orthopsychiatry, 82*(2), 209–219.

UNESCO. (2019). *Education as healing: Addressing the trauma of displacement through social and emotional learning (Global Education Monitoring Report No. 38)*. UNESCO. https://data.unicef.org/topic/covid-19-and-children

Whitley, M., Massey, W., & Wilkison, M. (2018). A systems theory of development through sport for traumatized and disadvantaged youth. *Psychology of Sport and Exercise, 38*, 116–125. https://doi.org/10.1016/j.psychsport.2018.06.004

Chapter 13

Using Narrative Inquiry to Understand Street Soccer Players' Experiences of Trauma, Social Exclusion, and Homelessness

Jordan A. Donnelly, Meredith A. Whitley, Daryl T. Cowan, and Sara McLaughlin

Introduction

Exposure to trauma is both an antecedent and an outcome of social exclusion and homelessness (Greenwood et al., 2022). Now a global health crisis (Magruder et al., 2017), complex and developmental trauma is defined as the experience of multiple developmentally adverse events, such as abuse, neglect, and distress (Kemmis-Riggs et al., 2022). Trauma exposure can impede the psychological and social development of young people (Grasser, 2022), acting as an obstacle to integration and functioning in traditional society (i.e., education, employment, housing) (Walsh et al., 2019). Children who experience more than four adverse childhood experiences are at greater risk of lifelong social, psychological, and behavioral health issues, paving the way for future traumas such as alcohol and substance use/addiction, social isolation, and mental health issues (Felitti et al., 1998). For example, a systematic review and meta-analysis of 23 longitudinal cohort studies found that childhood traumas such as bullying, emotional abuse, parental loss, and maltreatment were significantly associated with psychiatric disorders later in life (McKay et al., 2021). In our research project, Makena highlighted her experience of childhood trauma of immigration and social exclusion.

> I get bullied a lot cause I'm from a different country and I came to a new country. I did not know how to speak English and I did not know how to communicate. It's really hard.

For Gary, this trauma manifested in the abuse he was subjected to by his stepfather:

> The physical abuse from my stepdad ... there didn't even need to be a reason for it. It would just happen. And because of this, I was constantly walking on eggshells from a young age.

DOI: 10.4324/9781003332909-17

Complex and developmental trauma exposure is common in those battling social exclusion and homelessness later in life (Ayano et al., 2020), with reports
of intertwined familial trouble, abuse, neglect, bullying, violence, sexual violence, and substance misuse/abuse (Whitley et al., 2022). The compounding
experiences of developmental traumas, and their psychological and social
impact, can force people toward a life of social exclusion and homelessness
(Ayano et al., 2020). There are an estimated 216 million people reported to be
homeless worldwide (Tipple & Speak, 2009), 1.6 billion globally without adequate housing (Habitat for Humanity, 2014), and 113 million people across
Europe at risk of poverty or social exclusion (Eurostat, 2017). This relationship
between trauma, social exclusion, and homelessness has intensified with the
COVID-19 pandemic (Barocas et al., 2021) and the refugee crisis (Strang &
Quinn, 2021), which has had a disproportionate impact on people who have
experienced trauma (Grasser, 2022).

Individuals who experience social exclusion and homelessness are con-
fronted with complex barriers when attempting to access basic healthcare,
rendering them more vulnerable to common communicable and non-
communicable diseases (Malden et al., 2019). Such issues are compounded
by many homeless and socially excluded people being at unequal risk of exposure to violence, sexual abuse, extreme hunger, injectable drugs (increasing the risk of hepatitis and HIV exposure), and damp and cold environments,
resulting in deteriorated health with scarce access to healthcare (Fazel et al.,
2014). In addition, many homeless and socially excluded people carry the
weight of their unresolved childhood trauma (Greenwood et al., 2022), without familial support or access to services (Malden et al., 2019). As a result,
these traumas are often aggravated by their current environments and isolation, which can have a devastating impact on their mental health (Whitley
et al., 2022). Worryingly, experiences of complex and developmental trauma –
coupled with the cumulative effects of social exclusion and homelessness –
may prevent people from ever having fair and equal participation in society.
Indeed, many who are socially excluded and/or homeless find themselves in
an "institutional cycle" of homelessness, hospitals, jails, and prisons (Greenwood et al., 2022). Others face condemnation and stigma, even from social
and health professionals (Chamberlain & Johnson, 2018), which can trigger
re-traumatization or negative coping strategies (i.e., drug use, self-harm) (Fazel et al., 2014). To this end, multidisciplinary services (i.e., housing, psychological, health, social) must understand the challenges and needs of people
battling social exclusion and homelessness (Greenwood et al., 2022).

As the socioeconomic landscape becomes more uncertain, combined with
scarce public resources, those who have experienced trauma are turning to
alternative services (Lima, 2019). This includes the use of creative therapies
such as art and performance-based programming (i.e., music, dance, art),
acting in conjunction with psychotherapy and trauma-informed practices to
promote resilience and healing in trauma survivors (D'Andrea et al., 2013).

Other services embrace sport as a pathway to serving socially excluded and homeless populations given its mass appeal, with many of these Sport for Development interventions using trauma-informed practices (Massey & Whitley, 2020). These interventions can provide access to a supportive climate, caring mentors, meaningful friendships, and new opportunities. Such spaces also provide routes to health and housing services which are seldom available to socially excluded and homeless individuals (Whitley et al., 2022). Moreover, participation in sport-based interventions has been credited with developments in emotional, social, and cognitive skills, which can transfer into other life domains such as education, relationships, and employment (Donnelly et al., 2023). Our research examined two of these Sport for Development interventions: Street Soccer Scotland (SSS) and Street Soccer USA (SSUSA). SSS and SSUSA offer support for people who experience social exclusion, homelessness, and the causal and concurrent traumas associated with these experiences such as substance abuse, mental health issues, isolation, and poverty. As long-standing national partners of the Homeless World Cup (HWC), SSS and SSUSA also select players to attend this annual, week-long soccer tournament, which raises awareness and changes attitudes about homelessness by bringing players together from over 50 nationalities to play soccer and engage in other opportunities (e.g., travel, networking, service support) (Homeless World Cup Foundation, 2021).

Our research was conducted with 16 players (eight from SSS, eight from SSUSA) who embarked on their HWC journey. Over a period of nine months, players took part in interviews with the first two authors (Jordan and Meredith) which explored their life histories and current realities, along with their engagement in the HWC and Street Soccer (SS) programming. The interviewers also spoke with the significant others of some of the participants (e.g., family, friends, and coaches). Within all these interviews, stories of trauma and resilience during childhood emerged, with connections to their experiences of social exclusion and homelessness later in life. These stories are examined in Whitley et al. (2022), Whitley (2022) and Donnelly et al., (2024), however, below is a composite narrative that represents a synthesized experience from SSS and SSUSA players – composed through creative nonfiction (i.e., research findings conveyed in a "fictional" tale that is grounded in authentic empirical data) (Monforte & Smith, 2020).

Looking back at my childhood, I realize that we were desperately poor and how that put so much pressure on my Mum and Dad. In the beginning, we survived, but by the time I went to school, the cracks started to show. Dad was either working or drinking and Mum was too scared to even look him in the eye. She just tried to keep us all together, but she couldn't. I was bullied at school because we didn't have enough money to wash my clothes, so I smelled really bad. Then when I returned home, I would have these moments of peace with Mum before Dad came home from work in a drunken rage. He would beat up me and my Mum, often for no reason. This made my social anxiety skyrocket. I was constantly looking over my shoulder, scared of my own shadow. I was petrified of Dad coming to get me, and that was absolute torture.

When you grow up in a dysfunctional family, you leave home before you are ready, and you don't have the tools to survive on your own. I left just before I was 16 and everything felt hopeless. I was livin' on the streets for a long time. I first turned to weed to block what I was feeling inside – feeling guilty leaving home and feeling shameful leaving Mum with him – but it got to the point where weed no longer soothed what I felt inside. For a while, cocaine helped me check out and numb my feelings, but over time, I started experimenting with amphetamines and heroin. On the streets, I was still looking over my shoulder because I felt like someone was coming to get me. Sometimes I was right. I've been mugged, assaulted, and verbally abused on the streets of my own town. On several occasions, people pulled a gun on me and stole everything I had. When you start again with nothing, it can feel like you are nothing. That's when I used a lot of heroin. I thought about suicide quite a bit, and I even tried it once. I have this vivid memory of standing on top of a chair with a belt tied around my neck, but the belt snapped, and I survived and was rushed to the hospital and referred to a treatment center.

Using drugs was how I coped, letting me escape my feelings of hatred, loneliness, and fear. But in the addiction center, they took away my coping mechanism. This began a cycle … for months, I would be clean and have structure to my days, with a new job and even a new relationship. Eventually though, I'd look for drugs. I'd relapse and lose everything again. It was shameful. A disgrace. I was a disgrace. I'd go back to treatment, where they helped me begin to look at things in a new way. It felt like extra support and more defined boundaries between all the drugs, the feelings, and my experiences with living on the streets. I learned to let my hypervigilance go, as I didn't have to worry about scoring drugs or finding a place to sleep that night. When in treatment, I could think about the good things I had and the support I was receiving. Over time, I realized my whole life had been a trauma, but I also realized that I wasn't tied to this. I could move forward.

Our use of narrative inquiry to explore the experiences of trauma is part of a growing trend using this approach (e.g., McGannon & McMahon, 2022 McMahon et al., 2021, 2022). Qualitative researchers must be cognizant of ethical and optimal approaches to elicit stories from individuals who have experienced complex and developmental trauma. Such sensitivity may be particularly important when engaging people who have experienced social exclusion and/or homelessness, given the challenges cited earlier. In the section below, we describe the methodological approach we used in this project, along with the decisions we made to ensure our methods were both ethical and optimal (i.e., evidence-based, trauma-informed) for the participants, the interventions, and ourselves as researchers.

Methodology and Methods

Philosophy and Methods

Our narrative inquiry was framed within a relativist ontology and a constructionist epistemology (Monforte & Smith, 2020). A relativist ontology stipulates that multiple viewpoints and realities exist, while constructionism acknowledges that both the researcher and the researched create knowledge through a collaborative and subjective process (Smith, 2016). Narrative inquiry is both a theory and methodology that explores stories as a source of meaning, as people construct and use stories to make sense of their identities, experiences, and (inter)actions (McGannon & McMahon, 2022; Smith, 2010). Briefly put, stories are specific tales that people tell. In contrast, narratives are socially and culturally available resources that can shape people's beliefs and influence the construction of the stories they tell (Monforte & Smith, 2020). Within our relativist narrative inquiry, we explored the stories of individuals who experienced social exclusion and/or homelessness, including their experiences of trauma and the impact of SSS, SSUSA, and the HWC on their lives (see Figure 13.1 below for interview timeline and participation). This approach aimed to explore the underlying ideologies and psychological implications of the stories by treating them as co-constructed cultural narratives

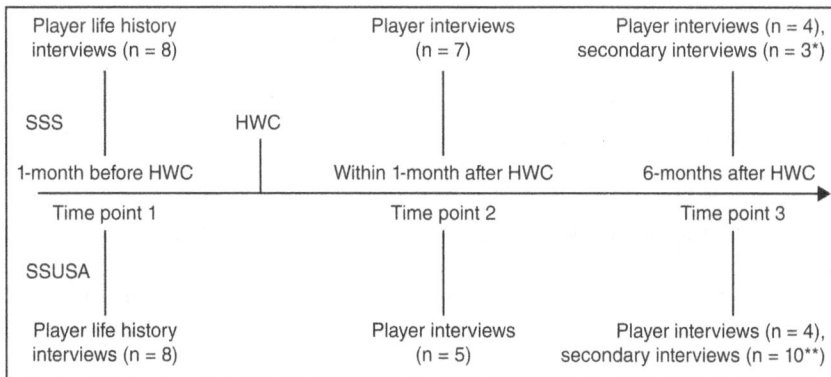

Player life history interviews (n = 8)		Player interviews (n = 7)		Player interviews (n = 4), secondary interviews (n = 3*)
SSS	HWC			
1-month before HWC		Within 1-month after HWC		6-months after HWC
Time point 1		Time point 2		Time point 3
SSUSA				
Player life history interviews (n = 8)		Player interviews (n = 5)		Player interviews (n = 4), secondary interviews (n = 10**)

*SS coach (n = 2), sister (n = 1).   **SS coach (n = 6), sister (n = 1), friend (n = 1), (step) parents (n = 2).

Figure 13.1 Interview timeline and participation.

that can *do things* to humans by altering views of and interactions with the world (McGannon & McMahon, 2022; Smith, 2013).

Narrative inquiry was used to create space for players to share stories and feel heard, which can help promote catharsis and healing among socially excluded populations (McGannon & McMahon, 2021; McMahon et al., 2021). However, it is important to consider that eliciting stories can also cause distress and even additional trauma. Stories can *move us* by shaping our emotions and how we interpret future worlds, whether in a positive or a negative direction (Smith, 2016). To combat this issue, we adopted an open-ended, flexible, and conversational approach to narrative interviewing, as opposed to a more structured interview. Narrative interviewing differs from sequential and mechanical styles of interviewing, and instead actively encourages participants to tell *their* story (Smith, 2010). In our approach, the interviewer relinquishes responsibility to the participants within the interview, with each person deciding how to communicate their story: what information to share, how much information to share, and what direction they want to take the interview (Alessi & Kahn, 2022). This approach may be particularly important when interviewing people who have experienced trauma, as they can share their version of the story, without delving into instances that could be particularly distressing or cause re-traumatization. In our research, narrative interviewing facilitated rich, deep explorations of players' lives and the impact of SS and HWC programming, while prioritizing their comfort and safety.

Another way we were cautious in our approach to this research project was with participant selection, as we knew that some players might not be ready to discuss their life histories. With that in mind, we collaborated with SS staff members to identify players who would feel most comfortable being interviewed, yet we maintained confidentiality in the interview itself. We asked SS staff to identify *more* players than were needed, so staff members did not know who actually took part in the interview process. We also discussed at length the "ins and outs" of the research process with potential participants, ensuring they understood all their rights while discussing how confidentiality and anonymity would be maintained throughout the research process. We made it clear that their decision on whether or not to participate – or if they chose to withdraw later in the study – would not impact their participation in SS programming or the HWC. Finally, we were cognizant that some players were at different stages of recovery and/or had quite a bit of variability in their lives (e.g., multiple moves, new jobs, new services and support). We also recognized the wide range of feelings players held toward significant others in their lives, from feeling incredibly supported or feeling that they were a source of trauma.

This awareness led to a more flexible research design, ensuring players never felt pressured throughout the research process. For example, we were only able to interview 12 of the original 16 players at time point 2 (1 month after the HWC) and just 8 players at time point 3 (6 months after the HWC). While we certainly could have reached out multiple times to the players who did not respond to our initial requests for second and third interviews, we were cautious not to overstep or insert any pressure on players to respond to our requests. Another example comes in our approach to asking players interviewed at time point 3 (6 months after the HWC) if we might speak with one (or more) significant others in their lives, who might be able to provide us with a more holistic understanding of their experiences during childhood and/or more recently. Some players were comfortable identifying individuals for us to speak with, while others were hesitant. Yet again, we did not insist, which is why we did not have secondary participants (e.g., friends, family, and coach) for all of the final 8 players interviewed. These are just some examples of the decisions we made to protect participants during the research process. We explore more of these decisions in the next section. Before we shift to a deeper exploration of the trauma-informed practices used in our research process, we outline the ways that narrative inquiry – along with our analytic approach – might assist the wider audience in learning more about trauma.

Analysis and Representation of Narratives

Narrative inquiry facilitated the exploration and presentation of complex stories in a holistic manner, rather than breaking up the stories into parts (e.g., codes, meaning units). We felt this approach would create a more accessible representation of the players' stories and experiences by helping readers understand more about the complexities and nuances associated with trauma, social exclusion, and homelessness. Through narrative analysis, we embraced both the role of *story analyst* (communicating analytical accounts of narratives) and then *storyteller* (creative practices producing narratives as a story) (Monforte & Smith, 2020). We adopted the role of story analyst in Whitley et al. (2022) to communicate findings as a realist tale represented in themes of trauma experiences, growth, and resilience among SS players. As the term is used here, a "realist tale" reflects a closely disseminated and tightly theorized depiction of participant quotes from stories placed under analysis (Smith, 2010). In this chapter and in Donnelly et al. (2024), we embrace the role of the storyteller, sharing composite vignettes (i.e., short-storied descriptions created from participants' own words) of the central theme – "living through and with trauma" – which were identified in our initial story analyst phase (e.g., approaches outlined by McGannon & McMahon, 2021). The storyteller approach allows the researcher to "produce an analysis *in* storytelling and *show* rather than tell theory *in* and *through* the story" (Smith, 2013, p. 134). A storyteller approach can enhance accessibility to the narrative, with the possibility for interpretation and meaning left in the hands of the reader (Whitley, 2022).

Considering the hidden traumas faced by people around us, the intent is for these stories to resonate with the readers, allowing them to gain insight and empathy toward those who have experienced trauma, social exclusion, and/or homelessness. Such flexibility of moving between storyteller and story analyst positions promotes greater accessibility and appreciation of a particular subject matter (Smith, 2016). However, while recognizing that stories *do things* to humans (Smith, 2013), we must also acknowledge that these stories may resonate in multiple ways and do different things to different humans (e.g., evoke empathy vs. stigma). Ultimately, varying "takes" on stories told within certain narratives may hold significant pedagogical potential by generating critical reflections, challenging assumptions, and encouraging dialogue (McGannon & McMahon, 2022).

Retrospective Reflectivity

We agree with Smith's (2016) arguments that narratives can change humans (e.g., shape our emotions and behaviors), since narratives and the stories told within them are theorized to allocate meaning to personal identities and unfolding storylines within a changing social world (Smith, 2010). We are also acutely and reflexively aware that researchers can be impacted by their research experiences and shaped by their immersion within tales of complex and developmental trauma. Therefore, we must be conscious of *retrospective* reflexivity – which is the impact that research may have on us as researchers (Attia & Edge, 2017). This impact comes to the fore as we dedicate significant time to familiarizing ourselves with traumatic stories (i.e., interviewing, listening, re-reading, transcribing). In Jordan's case (the primary Scottish researcher), the research was emotionally distressing at times and exposed him to the deeply troubling unfairness and inequalities that existed in the town where he grew up. Over a period of four years, he developed strong relationships with the players at SSS, rendering the process of interviewing and analysis for this study as a reminder of the suffering that they faced. To cope with these impacts, Jordan utilized a reflexive diary and consulted with his PhD supervisor (Daryl) for support and guidance. Similarly, Meredith (the primary US researcher) felt strong connections with the SSUSA players during her interviews with them, which led to feelings of being overwhelmed when hearing their stories. She managed her emotions during the interviews, so that players would not feel uncomfortable or feel as though they needed to care for her. After each interview, she felt emotionally exhausted and used reflexive writing to capture insights from the interview as well as to help process the story itself. Ultimately, combining reflexive writing with peer support can help researchers digest and deal with particularly distressing interviews (Qhogwana, 2022). However, both Jordan and Meredith acknowledge that a better plan could have been in place. This is explored in the next section below, along with other trauma-informed practices that were (or should be) applied to research.

Trauma-Informed Practices Applied to Research

Qualitative approaches are often considered the most appropriate method for understanding the lived experiences of trauma (McGannon & McMahon, 2021). However, without an appreciation for how trauma affects humans and their social interactions, qualitative researchers may find themselves unintentionally re-traumatizing participants or misusing their power during the research process (Alessi & Kahn, 2022). We were aware of these concerns and used a set of trauma-informed practices to mitigate the risk of the participants potentially experiencing re-traumatization. Writing this chapter also prompted further reflection on these practices in accordance with these trauma-informed approaches (Alessi & Kahn, 2022; SAMHSA, 2014). Below, we outline our implementation of SAMHSA's (2014) key principles, along with reflections and recommendations for trauma-informed research practice with populations who have experienced trauma, social exclusion, and homelessness.

Safety

Feelings of physical, social, and psychological unsafety are particularly threatening to individuals who have experienced trauma, which can lead them to experience hypersensitivity, extreme anxiety, and re-traumatization (SAMHSA, 2014). Thus, consideration was placed on the potential vulnerability SS players might feel during interviews. We were cognizant that conversations surrounding trauma would be distressing for the SS players and endeavored to ground the research in the "here and now" to establish clear distinctions between *recounting* and *reliving* trauma (Alessi & Kahn, 2022). To achieve this practice, we formulated our questions surrounding trauma in accordance with life history approaches (e.g., "What was your life like for you growing up?"), which emphasize that their experiences of events happened in the past, despite any lingering negative emotions (Alessi & Kahn, 2022). In addition, through narrative interviewing and open-ended questioning, the players could decide what stories to tell and how much of the story we should be privileged to hear. Ultimately, this flexible line of questioning allowed players to delve deeply into their journeys, while ensuring they could set boundaries for their own psychological safety.

To further protect SS players' safety, we believe it would be beneficial to have greater consideration of the physical space in which the research is conducted. We conducted longitudinal research in two nations (Scotland, USA) over three time points, which resulted in a pragmatic approach to gathering data (i.e., at the intervention site, at a national tournament, by telephone; Whitley et al., 2022). In the future, research participants should have a greater degree of ownership over where and how they engage in the research process. While working with SS organizations, it may be possible to use their resources (e.g., laptops, tablets) to conduct online video calls, provided participants feel comfortable with this format. Online video calls enable participants to be interviewed in a familiar and convenient environment (i.e., accommodation, sport setting) while having immediate access to those who might provide support (i.e., family, program staff) during pauses and/or after the interview (Gray et al., 2020). The predictability of a familiar and (potentially) psychologically safe environment in online data gathering is also less intrusive than face-to-face methods, affording participants access to their own space and can be less anxiety-provoking for those who have experienced trauma (McMahon et al., 2022). Despite being less intrusive, video calling still provides the ability to observe the participant's non-verbal communication (Gray et al., 2020), allowing researchers to monitor for signs of distress, while taking action to mitigate feelings of unsafety or anxiety (McMahon et al., 2022).

Trustworthiness and Transparency

The principles of trustworthiness and transparency are outlined by SAMHSA (2014) as "operations and decisions conducted with transparency with the goal of building and maintaining trust with clients and family members" (p. 11). Individuals who are experiencing social exclusion and/or homelessness are often less trusting of others, organizations, or authorities because of abuse, manipulation, or apathy to which they have been subjected to (Barocas et al., 2021). Thus, transparency was a crucial factor for us to gain the trust of the SS players, which then allowed us to gain insight into their lived experiences of trauma through narrative interviewing.

With this in mind, the SS players were made aware of our long-term partnership with the respective SS organizations. SSS and SSUSA had achieved trusted status in the eyes of the players, given their welcoming, non-judgmental approach and commitment to trauma-informed practices (Whitley et al., 2022). At a foundational level, our association and *being seen* with trusted partners was an important aspect of securing trust with SS players (Alessi & Kahn, 2022), while strengthening the notion that our research was not being conducted for exploitive or nefarious reasons (e.g., coercion, control, bullying, legal reasons). Additionally, the interviews conducted before/after SS programming meant players could opt for peer support from trained and trauma-informed staff when reflecting upon and revisiting instances of trauma (McMahon et al., 2022).

Trust and transparency were further achieved by our predictability and the predictable nature of our research. We endeavored to be predictable (i.e., *did what we said we would*), consistent (i.e., *did what we said we would over time*), and accepting (i.e., *did not judge nor shame*) (Alessi & Kahn, 2022). As researchers, we strove to be transparent and unambiguous, mirroring our written participant information sheets and consent forms which players were asked to read and understand prior to the commencement of the study. Though considered as standard ethical practice, SS players were made explicitly and consistently aware of their rights (i.e., right to non-participation, right to withdraw without reason or consequence, right to pause/reschedule) to further foster transparency and our predictability. In addition, we strove to show empathy without trivializing or commodifying participants' experiences of trauma, social exclusion, homelessness, addiction, poverty, and beyond. This process manifested in a non-judgmental approach (e.g., not being reactionary to stories) and being appreciative (e.g., saying thank you for their stories and their time), while highlighting the valuable implications of the stories that the players entrusted us to hear.

Collaboration and Mutuality

SAHMSA's (2014) principle of collaboration and mutuality highlights the need to level power differentials and share decision-making. Through reflexive practices, we can be cognizant that the researcher occupies a position of power while eliciting traumatic stories (Drozdzewski & Dominey-Howes, 2015), particularly when engaging overlooked or marginalized populations (Massey & Whitley, 2020). Attempts were therefore made to redistribute that power in the research process through consideration of researcher reflexivity and the construction of a collaborative research space. In the first instance, our constructionist epistemology positions the researcher and participants as co-constructors of stories and co-creators meaning (Smith, 2016). Shared power manifested in our conversations with SS players, emphasizing that as storytellers, their stories were valuable and meaningful, and that as co-researchers, we were there to listen attentively and to learn, without interruption or judgment (McMahon et al., 2022). Second, we were mindful that our *prospective reflexivity* (e.g., beliefs, biases, lived experiences) influenced our interactions with the players (Attia & Edge, 2017). Thus, we were conscious of our positioning (e.g., class, age, gender, education) and aimed to take subsequent actions (i.e., engaging critical friends, self-reflection) to thwart unintentional power imbalances, while emphasizing the need for collaboration with and empowerment of the participants (Alessi & Kahn, 2022). This process was ultimately achieved by engaging in ongoing collaborative dialogue with our community partners (SSS, SSUSA), so that they could advise on the best approach to interviewing (i.e., location, interview guides), and through sharing control of the interview process with the SS players. Sharing power during interviews was especially valuable for the players, as control was often absent during the times they experienced complex and developmental trauma (Whitley, 2022; Whitley et al., 2022).

Self-reflection and reflexive practice were also critical for Jordan and Meredith as they sought to safeguard the players – and themselves – during and after interviews, as discussed in a previous section. While writing this chapter, Jordan and Meredith considered how researchers tend to engage positionality and *prospective* reflexivity to ensure their research is ethical and aligns with the philosophical roots guiding the study – along with the population and/or context under study. Yet, despite the prevalence of trauma in contemporary sport, exercise, and health research, scarce consideration is directed toward *retrospective* reflexivity or the countertransference of trauma from researcher to the research participants (McMahon & McGannon, 2019). In line with our approaches of engaging in reflexive writing, working collaboratively, and asking for emotional guidance, qualitative researchers must consider care for themselves to ensure the care of others (Drozdzewski & Dominey-Howes, 2015). In the future, we should implement trauma-informed approaches into university ethics applications while creating space and time during the research process to explicitly discuss and reflect upon potential experiences of trauma among research teams (Drozdzewski & Dominey-Howes, 2015). Additionally, qualitative researchers should be explicit in using strategies for reflexive practice throughout the research process, which Jordan and Meredith strived to do. Although the practice of reflexivity in qualitative research is often recommended, this was especially valuable in our project as we endeavored to elicit traumatic accounts without triggering or causing SS players to relive trauma. Reflexive strategies in this case included a proactive approach to self-care involving the organization of time, space, resources, and support to allow for reflection and processing of the participants' traumatic experiences, as well as our own (Qhogwana, 2022).

Empowerment, Voice, and Choice

Once a foundation of safety, trust, and shared decision-making is established, qualitative researchers must be mindful of processes and practices that foster unifying empowerment. SAMHSA's (2014) trauma-informed principle of empowerment, voice, and choice builds on the practices that acknowledge power differentials and the importance of shared decision-making (as outlined above). However, there is also a need to foster belief, resilience, and the future potential of those who have experienced trauma (SAMHSA, 2014). Regarding empowerment and by recognizing that stories *do things*, we started each interview by reminding the SS players about the value of their voice, lived experiences and the stories that *they decide* to communicate:

> In this interview, there are no right or wrong answers. Instead, I'm most interested in hearing about your experiences, your perspectives, your beliefs and your stories.

SS players were also made explicitly aware that we appreciated their time, that we understood sharing stories would be emotionally taxing and that we were committed to their preferences and views on how the research would be conducted. For instance, we engaged in close dialogue with the players and staff to facilitate choice on where (e.g., inside Soccer club-houses vs. outside on pitches) and how (e.g., in person vs. telephone) the interviews would take place when possible. Additionally, given the non-sequential and non-mechanical nature of narrative interviewing, we relinquished *some* power by championing methods which allowed play-ers to tell *their* story (Smith, 2010). To illustrate this and while conceding the principles of constructionism (knowledge is co-constructed), we argue narrative interviewing fosters choice and empowerment by allowing inter-viewees to decide what stories we should be privy to and what plotlines and characters should be omitted/included within each story (Alessi & Kahn, 2022).

When prioritizing participant self-determination and empowerment, it is also important that we do not assume a participant is "too traumatized" or emotionally incapable of answering questions, as this deprives them of the opportunity to tell their story (Alessi & Kahn, 2022). Trauma re-searchers are faced with a tough predicament when engaging in narrative interviews with those who have experienced trauma, as there can be a fine margin between causing undue stress and nullifying someone's voice. Ultimately, we recommend that researchers approach interviewing with careful consideration of how and when to show empathy (e.g., pausing or stopping an interview, providing reassurance) versus when to reinforce empowerment (e.g., letting the interview continue uninterrupted) (Alessi & Kahn, 2022).

Conclusion

An increasing number of researchers are using narrative inquiry approaches to explore experiences of trauma in sport, exercise, and health contexts (e.g., McGannon & McMahon, 2021; McMahon et al., 2021, 2022; Whitley et al., 2022). In line with this growing use of narrative inquiry, there needs to be thoughtful consideration of when and how to use different forms of reflexivity throughout the research process. As discussed earlier, qualitative research-ers must acknowledge their own lived experiences before and during the research process. When conducting trauma-informed work, much more is involved than simply acknowledging one's lived experiences. For example, when conducting an interview that might reference complex and develop-mental trauma, researchers should be mindful of how their own reflexive bag-gage might compound the hardship of the participants. In turn, researchers should also be conscious of *retrospective* reflexivity, which is concerned with the effect that research can have on researchers (Attia & Edge, 2017). Moving forward, it would be advisable that researchers studying trauma share their strategies of how they mitigate the transference of trauma from the researched to the researcher, as well as countertransference.

Eliciting stories from those who have experienced complex and developmental trauma can also be a vehicle for catharsis and healing, given the empowerment that can be associated with feeling valued and being heard (McGannon & McMahon, 2021; McMahon et al., 2021). Furthermore, as stories offer new possibilities to think, feel, and behave (Smith, 2016), qualitative researchers could construct their own retrospectively reflexive stories to challenge their basic assumptions about their narrative view (Smith, 2010), while also endeavoring to make sense of difficult moments within their research. These constructions and the sharing of tales may be of particular significance to those researching populations whose voices may often be overlooked or marginalized (Donnelly, 2024). Yet, researchers should be cognizant that as narratives do different things to different people (e.g., healing vs. re-traumatization), they may have unintended negative outcomes for research participants (Smith, 2013). Indeed, as more researchers use narrative inquiry to explore trauma within sport, exercise, and health contexts, there should be greater awareness of how research participation can promote healing among participants, and not simply as a means for sharing meaningful stories to educate others.

Finally, researchers might consider the use of creative analytical practices grounded in narrative inquiry, such as creative non-fiction and vignettes. Creative non-fiction is a growing creative writing practice (see McGannon & McMahon, 2022; McMahon et al., 2021) that centralizes participants' experiences through fictional storylines grounded in authentic data, often communicated in short-storied vignettes (Smith, 2016). Such approaches allow researchers to synthesize connected and intersecting voices into meaningful, shared accounts that tell co-constructed stories across space and time (McMahon et al., 2021). For many, vignettes and stories are a more accessible and evocative way to convey empirical data (Smith, 2010), which can open a necessary and meaningful dialogue with a wider audience (McGannon & McMahon, 2022). Stories from those who have experienced trauma, social exclusion, and homelessness should also be shared with those who are in the field (e.g., coaches, counselors, therapists) working directly with these populations. In doing so, we recognize that narrative inquiry can engage and change humans by eliciting multiple interpretations of stories that may present new conditions to think and feel about basic narrative assumptions (Smith, 2010, 2016). Ultimately, as socially excluded and homeless people often endure narratives of stigma and apathy from society (Chamberlain & Johnson, 2018), narrative inquiry may yield a pathway to (re)shape perceptions through accessible stories that promote education, compassion, and healing to wider audiences.

References

Alessi, E. J., & Kahn, S. (2022). Toward a trauma-informed qualitative research approach: Guidelines for ensuring the safety and promoting the resilience of research participants. *Qualitative Research in Psychology, 20*(1), 1–34. https://doi.org/10.10 80/14780887.2022.2107967

Attia, M., & Edge, J. (2017). Be(com)ing a reflexive researcher: A developmental approach to research methodology. *Open Review of Educational Research, 4*(1), 33–45. https://doi.org/10.1080/23265507.2017.1300068

Ayano, G., Solomon, M., Tsegay, L., Yohannes, K., & Abraha, M. (2020). A systematic review and meta-analysis of the prevalence of post-traumatic stress disorder among homeless people. *Psychiatric Quarterly, 91*(4), 949–963. https://doi.org/10.1007/s11126-020-09746-1

Barocas, J. A., Jacobson, K. R., & Hamer, D. H. (2021). Addressing the COVID-19 pandemic among persons experiencing homelessness: Steps to protect a vulnerable population. *Journal of General Internal Medicine, 36*(5), 1416–1417. https://doi.org/10.1007/S11606-020-06434-5

Chamberlain, C., & Johnson, G. (2018). From long-term homelessness to stable housing: Investigating 'liminality'. *Housing Studies, 33*(8), 1246–1263. https://doi.org/10.1080/02673037.2018.1424806

D'Andrea, W., Bergholz, L., Fortunato, A., & Spinazzola, J. (2013). Play to the whistle: A pilot investigation of a sports-based intervention for traumatized girls in residential treatment. *Journal of Family Violence, 28*(7), 739–749. https://doi.org/10.1007/s10896-013-9533-x

Donnelly, J., Arthur, R., Arthur, C., & Cowan, D. (2023). The indirect effects of transformational leadership in soccer programmes for socio-economically disadvantaged individuals: Need satisfaction as a mechanism towards personal development. *International Journal of Sports Science & Coaching, 19*(1), 1–11. https://doi.org/10.1177/17479541231158693

Donnelly, J.A., Whitley, M.A., Cowan, D.T., McLaughlin, S. and Arthur, R., (2024). The Homeless World Cup through storytelling: The narratives of Street Soccer players from Scotland and the USA. *Psychology of Sport and Exercise, 70*, 102549. https://doi.org/10.1016/j.psychsport.2023.102549

Drozdzewski, D., & Dominey-Howes, D. (2015). Research and trauma: Understanding the impact of traumatic content and places on the researcher. *Emotion, Space and Society, 17*, 17–21. https://doi.org/10.1016/j.emospa.2015.09.001

Eurostat. (2013). People at risk of poverty or social exclusion. Population and Social Conditions. Publications Office of the European Union.

Fazel, S., Geddes, J. R., & Kushel, M. (2014). The health of homeless people in high-income countries: Descriptive epidemiology, health consequences, and clinical and policy recommendations. *The Lancet, 384*(9953), 1529–1540. https://doi.org/10.1016/S0140-6736(14)61132-6

Felitti, V. J., Anda, R. F., Nordenberg, D., Williamson, D. F., Spitz, A. M., Edwards, V., Koss, M. P., & Marks, J. S. (1998). Relationship of childhood abuse and household dysfunction to many of the leading causes of death in adults: The adverse childhood experiences (ACE) study. *American Journal of Preventive Medicine, 14*(4), 245–258. https://doi.org/10.1016/S0749-3797(98)00017-8

Grasser, L. R. (2022). Addressing mental health concerns in refugees and displaced populations: Is enough being done? *Risk Management and Healthcare Policy, 15,* 909–922. https://doi.org/10.2147/rmhp.s270233

Gray, L. M., Wong-Wylie, G., Rempel, G. R., & Cook, K. (2020). Expanding qualitative research interviewing strategies: Zoom video communications. *The Qualitative Report, 25*(5), 1292–1301. https://doi.org/10.46743/2160-3715/2020.4212

Greenwood, H., Gupta, A., & Sanderson, C. (2022). Distressing unusual experiences and beliefs in the lives of previously homeless individuals: A narrative analysis of the stories of white British men. *Psychosis.* https://doi.org/10.1080/17522439.2022.2068645

Habitat for Humanity. (2014). Shelter finance report 2014. Habitat for humanity international. https://www.habitat.org/sites/default/files/annual-report-2014.pdf

Homeless World Cup Foundation. (2021). *Cardiff 2019 Homeless World Cup.* https://homelessworldcup.org/cardiff-2019-tournament/

Kemmis-Riggs, J., Dickes, A., Rogers, K., Berle, D., & McAloon, J. (2022). Improving parent–child relationships for young parents in the shadow of complex trauma: A single-case experimental design series. *Child Psychiatry and Human Development,* 1–13. https://doi.org/10.1007/s10578-022-01379-8

Lima, V. (2019). Urban austerity and activism: Direct action against neoliberal housing policies. *Housing Studies, 36*(2), 258–277. https://doi.org/10.1080/02673037.2019.1697800

Magruder, K. M., Mclaughlin, K. A., & Borbon, D. L. E. (2017). Trauma is a public health issue. *European Journal of Psychotraumatology, 8*(1), 1375338. https://doi.org/10.1080/20008198.2017.1375338

Malden, S., Jepson, R., Laird, Y., & McAteer, J. (2019). A theory-based evaluation of an intervention to promote positive health behaviors and reduce social isolation in people experiencing homelessness. *Journal of Destress and Homelessness, 28*(2), 158–168. https://doi.org/10.1080/10530789.2019.1623365

Massey, W. V., & Whitley, M. A. (2020). Adverse experiences of children and youth: Can sport play a role in growth following psychologically traumatic events? In R. Wadey, M. Day, & K. Howells (Eds.), *Growth following adversity in sport: A mechanism to positive change* (pp. 204–215). Routledge.

McGannon, K. R., & McMahon, J. (2022). (Re)Storying embodied running and motherhood: A creative non-fiction approach. *Sport, Education and Society, 27*(8), 960–972. https://doi.org/10.1080/13573322.2021.1942821

McKay, M. T., Cannon, M., Chambers, D., Conroy, R. M., Coughlan, H., Dodd, P., Healy, C., O'Donnell, L., & Clarke, M. C. (2021). Childhood trauma and adult mental disorder: A systematic review and meta-analysis of longitudinal cohort studies. *Acta Psychiatrica Scandinavica, 143*(3), 189–205. https://doi.org/10.1111/ACPS.13268

McMahon, J., & McGannon, K. R. (2019). Acting out what is inside of us: Self-management strategies of an abused ex-athlete. *Sport Management Review, 23*(1), 28–38. https://doi.org/10.1016/j.smr.2019.03.008

McMahon, J., McGannon, K. R., & Palmer, C. (2021). Body shaming and associated practices as abuse: Athlete entourage as perpetrators of abuse. *Sport, Education & Society, 27*(5), 578–591. https://doi.org/10.1080/13573322.2021.1890571

McMahon, J., McGannon, K. R., Zehntner, C., Werbicki, L., Stephenson, E., & Martin, K. (2022). Trauma-informed abuse education in sport: Engaging athlete abuse survivors as educators and facilitating a community of care. *Sport, Education and Society,* 1–14. https://doi.org/10.1080/13573322.2022.2096586

Monforte, J., & Smith, B. (2020). Conventional and postqualitative research: An invitation to dialogue. *Qualitative Inquiry*, *27*(6), 650–660. https://doi.org/10.1177/1077800420962469

Qhogwana, S. (2022). Research trauma in incarcerated spaces: Listening to incarcerated women's narratives. *Emotion, Space and Society*, *42*, 100865. https://doi.org/10.1016/j.emospa.2021.100865

Smith, B. (2010). Narrative inquiry: Ongoing conversations and questions for sport and exercise psychology research. *International Review of Sport and Exercise Psychology*, *3*(1), 87–107. https://doi.org/10.1080/17509840903390937

Smith, B. (2013). Sporting spinal cord injuries, social relations, and rehabilitation narratives: An ethnographic creative non-fiction of becoming disabled through sport. *Sociology of Sport Journal*, *30*(2), 132–152. https://doi.org/10.1123/ssj.30.2.132

Smith, B. (2016). Narrative analysis in sport and exercise: How can it be done? In B. Smith & A. C. Sparkes (Eds.), *Routledge handbook of qualitative research in sport and exercise* (pp. 260–273). Routledge. https://doi.org/10.4324/9781315762012-31

Strang, A. B., & Quinn, N. (2021). Integration or isolation? Refugees' social connections and wellbeing. *Journal of Refugee Studies*, *34*(1), 328–353. https://doi.org/10.1093/jrs/fez040

Substance Abuse and Mental Health Services Administration. (2014). A treatment improvement protocol: Trauma-informed care in behavioural health services. U.S. Department of Health and Human Services. TIP 57.

Tipple, G., & Speak, S. (2009). *The hidden millions: Homelessness in developing countries* (1st ed.). Routledge. https://doi.org/10.4324/9780203883341

Walsh, D., McCartney, G., Smith, M., & Armour, G. (2019). Relationship between childhood socioeconomic position and adverse childhood experiences (ACEs): A systematic review. *Journal of Epidemiology & Community Health*, *73*(12), 1087–1093. https://doi.org/10.1136/jech-2019-212738

Whitley, M. A. (2022). In her own words: A refugee's story of forced migration, trauma, resilience, and soccer. *Sport in Society*, *25*(3), 551–565. https://doi.org/10.1080/17430437.2022.2017817

Whitley, M. A., Donnelly, J. A., Cowan, D. T., & McLaughlin, S. (2022). Narratives of trauma and resilience from Street Soccer players. *Qualitative Research in Sport, Exercise and Health*, *14*(1), 101–118. https://doi.org/10.1080/2159676X.2021.1879919

Chapter 14

Development Despite Trauma

Critical Reflections on Our Research Journey with Sport Participants

William V. Massey and Meredith A. Whitley

Introduction

Trauma can be defined as a stressor that overwhelms an individual's stress response capabilities, and as a result changes one's core identity in a negative or maladaptive way (Conti, 2021). In the United States, experiences of childhood trauma or traumatising events have received increasing attention since Felitti et al. (1998) examined adverse childhood experiences (ACEs). Subsequent research has shown trauma prevalence rates higher than 30% in children and adolescents (Fletcher, 2003), yet this research was narrowly focused on ACEs (i.e., individual trauma). Other forms of trauma, such as collective trauma that persists across generations and communities (e.g., natural disasters, war, geocide, terrorism), historical trauma in which emotional and psychological injury accumulates over time and generations (e.g., slavery, colonialism, forced relocation), and intergenerational trauma carried within families (e.g., mistrust of people or systems due to oppression and abuse) (Dekel & Goldblatt, 2008; Hirschberger, 2018), likely account for higher levels of trauma than might be published in the academic literature.

Despite the negative impact of trauma, some sport researchers have suggested that for athletes pursuing peak performance, their *"talent needs trauma"* (Collins & MacNamara, 2012, p. 907), an assertion that is both dangerous and not supported by research. Collectively, researchers have shown, with little to no ambiguity, that the effects of trauma are devastating (D'Andrea et al., 2012), can have generational consequences, and are more severe the earlier and more repeated the exposure (Hambrick et al., 2019; O'Neill et al., 2016). For example, individuals with at least four ACEs are more likely to be depressed, have difficulty controlling their anger, use illicit drugs, engage in domestic violence, and suffer from alcoholism (Anda et al., 2006). Similar findings have been reported for physical health outcomes (Irish et al., 2010; Williamson et al., 2002), psychological health outcomes (Anda et al., 2007; Dube et al., 2001), and behavioural health outcomes (Anda et al., 2002; Chapman et al., 2011).

DOI: 10.4324/9781003332909-18

While researchers have begun to investigate the negative effects of trauma in sport (e.g., D'Andrea et al., 2013; Ley et al., 2021; McMahon et al., 2023; Van Ingen, 2016; Whitley et al., 2022), there is still a long way to go in terms of how trauma, including systematic oppression and inequity, shape sport experiences, and performance. As such, our work described in this chapter was conceptualised at the intersection of the assets required to pursue peak performance in sport and the devastating effects of childhood trauma. Given accounts of successful athletes having endured challenging and traumatic childhoods, and at the time a dearth of research examining the intersection of ACEs and sport, our central research aims were to develop a theory that elucidated how, in the context of experiencing trauma, some athletes went on to experience high levels of performance-related success, and how systemic influences interacted to shape this development. Not surprisingly, the data generated were complex and did not provide a clear and consistent picture of the role sport played in the lives of participants. For example, for some, sport was a powerful antidote to trauma. The participant below represents an individual who reached the highest possible level in his sporting profession:

My father was a major importer of cocaine in the city of [redacted] from a Mexican cartel … So, I remember my mom always had after hours, she was always going to jail. Every weekend she would go to jail, like she go on Friday, wouldn't see her until Monday 'cause she got locked up. And, the weekends she didn't go to jail, she would have after hours and those after hours, she was selling coke to whoever came to the house basically. So, I just remember those memories, those loud nights like where music's blasting, people so loud, and coming downstairs and seeing people that I have never seen in my life in front of my kitchen. Some of them smoking or cooking up coke so they can smoke it. My uncles making lines and shooting in. And I remember vividly sitting at the bottom of the staircase and screaming for my mom, like screaming and they looked at me like, "Who is this kid? Why is he up?" and I'm looking at them like, "Why are you in my house?" But then someone would go get my mom and then she come and yell at me and more often than not whoop me for getting out of bed. So, when my parents would have those after hours and those parties, we would go upstairs and, I remember the police always kicking in our door, house getting raided … Sports was a getaway from reality, it was where I could be a kid. I think that's why going to the gym is much fun too, because when I go to the gym, I don't have no worries. I could have the worst day ever, as soon as I hit that mat, it's gone. I don't even think about any of my fears or anything I'm dealing with when I'm on the mat. It really takes me out of reality.[1]

For others, sport was a reinforcement of the trappings and trauma of other parts of life, as explained by another participant, who had also reached the highest level of his sport:

> Everything was six inches from your face for me growin' up. The first thing we learned to do was fight. Whatever it is, the key is to humiliate the person and so with the threat of humiliation and every relationship that you're in you develop this hard cast that you don't wanna be humiliated. Growin' up in [redacted] it shaped my aggression. It shaped my thought process. I'm not takin' no shit from people ... 'cause it was relentless violence, very psychological, social, it was relentless. I told you Princess, my dog, so she had puppies, so a couple of my crew got the puppies and one of them was Poncho. And Poncho was aggressive, bit the hell out of people. So, we leave to go home one night ... we get back to the neighbourhood someone had got Poncho, set Poncho on fire. They lit the garbage can full of fire and then put Poncho in it. It was constantly violent ... physical, psychological, social, it was just violence.

> Sport helped me magnify [my neighbourhood].

Methodology

In this section, we describe and briefly summarise reflections on our methodological processes in an effort to contextualise recommendations for other qualitative researchers conducting research with athletes who have experienced trauma. Readers interested in this work are also referred to publications associated with our research on sport participants and developmental trauma discussed in this chapter (Massey & Whitley, 2016, 2021; Whitley & Massey, 2018; Whitley et al., 2016, 2018). Collectively, this work examined how sport intersected with the lives of athletes who experienced developmental trauma, to better understand the role of sport in their lives.

At the onset of our work, we planned to conduct a constructionist grounded theory study. In doing so, we used an iterative process of data collection and data analysis. Yet, early into data collection and analysis, we began debating whether we were doing the participants justice by reducing their lives to themes to compare/contrast the data, as this analytical approach was not representing the complexity of the participants' lives. Specifically, complex, and interwoven nature of the data made it impossible (and, in our eyes, unethical) to parse them down into line-by-line codes. For context, the inclusion criteria for participants at the start of our work included having: (a) achieved a high level of athletic success (e.g., collegiate or professional sport); (b) attended college; (c) self-reported to be living a healthy and/or fulfilling life; and (d) experienced at least three ACEs. The criteria for ACEs were based on the United States Centers for Disease Control and Prevention's (2010) classifications, along with research (e.g., Chapman et al., 2004, 2007, 2011; Zolkoski & Bull-ock, 2012) exploring developmental risk factors for youth (e.g., emotional/physical abuse, emotional/physical neglect, sexual abuse, homelessness, community violence, lived below the poverty line, lived with a parent who suffered from mental illness, had a parent incarcerated). As an example, one participant noted as she reflected back on her childhood:

> One day, I think I was 15 … my brother came over to my house and I didn't really see him that much 'cause he lived with my dad and was do-ing drugs … he looked at me and he was like, "We need to go for a walk. Will you go for a walk with me?" … So I'm walking with him, he doesn't say anything, so I don't say anything either. We walk into this field … and he cuts me off and he pulls out a knife and I'm wiggin' out like, "What the hell are you doing? What's the deal?" And he's like, "You need to shut the fuck up, I'm gonna kill you." And so I did, and he throws me on the ground, kind of straddled me with his knees, so sittin' on my stomach, and pressed the knife into my throat and was like, "Fuck mom, fuck [re-dacted], I'll kill them too. I can't stand them …" So I was not doing shit, not moving, and then for whatever reason, he got off me, and left …[1]

In our view, the quote directly above, along with the quotes presented in the introduction section, highlight the challenges mentioned in conducting line-by-line coding that could remove data from its context. We struggled with how to address these (and other) data, as parsing out statements (i.e., coding this as conflict with family; violence) left the data void of context, that ultimately undermined the quality and complexity of the data. As such, with the guidance of outside mentorship and through further study of the research literature on methodological plurality (e.g., Lal et al., 2012), we ultimately decided to "start over" and take on an analytical approach that blended grounded theory and narrative inquiry traditions. Despite utilising multiple qualitative methodologies, we intentionally did not position our re-search within a framework of methodological pluralism, but rather our study purpose and ongoing data collection led to the decision to blend method-ologies that could achieve coherence through an underlying epistemology (see Lal et al., 2012). As the term is used here, "methodological pluralism" refers to using multiple methods or methodologies, each with their own un-derlying epistemological assumptions. Drawing from a non-foundational ontological stance, coupled with the belief that knowledge is socially con-structed, subjective, and relative to time and place, we felt that construction-ist grounded theory allowed us to identify relationships across concepts and themes using a constant comparative analysis, while narrative inquiry (i.e., studying how stories unfold across time and space) (Smith, 2010) allowed us to examine theory within each case, without fragmenting data and thus maintaining the social context of the data. We grounded this approach in symbolic interactionism (i.e., similar events may take on different meanings depending on the context and interactions) (Blumer, 1969) and pragmatism (i.e., the connection between actions, consequences, and beliefs) that shape grounded theory research (Corbin, 2009). We also contextualised the form of various narratives and the interaction between personal and social narratives (Smith, 2010). This was done through an iterative process in which we mapped personal and cultural stories for each participant independently, then in comparison with other participants in a sequential and holistic manner, and finally against the published literature. During these phases we also crafted these narratives into vignettes that explained the data in storied form. Ultimately, we felt that this was the most ethical way to move forward to best represent the stories of our participants and make a meaningful contribution to the academic literature.

In addition to shifting methodological and analytical processes, we also had to rethink and reconfigure our original plan for recruiting participants, as we realised (and will discuss below) we felt our recruitment strategy could be causing residual harm. We began the study with a theoretical orientation that made space for the realities of: (a) the individual's experience of trauma, (b) that trauma is often an interpersonal process, and (c) that system-level factors play a role in trauma exposure and responses. As such, our research took a systems approach, examining both individual development and broader social systems. At an individual level, we drew from Bioecological Systems Theory (Bronfenbrenner, 1995), which posits that individual development occurs through the interaction of interpersonal, contextual, socio-cultural, and chronological factors that influence individual behaviour. However, sitting with and bearing witness to the grotesque atrocities against the participants in our study, as well as the darker side of humanity in general, led to critical reflections on ways our study could cause harm. One such example was that our original design included interviewing family members, friends, coaches, and others who supported their growth and development over time of the athlete participants we were interviewing. The strategy to connect with secondary participants proved difficult for a number of reasons. For some participants, the challenge was benign, such as availability issues (e.g., their most influential person was a high-profile coach who was unavailable for a research interview). Others had parents and siblings who were deceased, in jail, or not in a physical or psychological place for which the primary participant should ethically contact them to take part in the interview process. Perhaps most impactful was the difficulty in separating those in a proximal position to influence development with those who were perpetrators of interpersonal trauma. This led to a change in our recruitment strategy midway through the first wave of data collection, where we stopped asking participants if there were significant others we could contact for the study. Instead, we continued interviewing athlete participants through an iterative process of data collection and analysis, while adding interviews with community experts (i.e., coaches, community organisers, police officers, counsellors, teachers) who worked with populations of youth impacted by trauma.

In making this shift, community expert participants were able to add unique perspectives that allowed us to broaden our understanding of the impacts of trauma, while minimising the risk of harm described above. The following excerpt from an interview with a community expert, in which we were exploring a core concept (i.e., sport as a form of escape) identified through analysis of athlete interviews, demonstrates this point:

> I would say the short answer is yes, I agree, I also think … calling it an escape, it doesn't do justice to what it really is … [we] haven't really deconstructed what works … [sport] needs to be well thought through and it works because it's the interplay: the right coach, with the right culture, with the right people and the right community, all those things. So, in terms of the escape piece, that's a key element in that, but I think there's a lot more to it than that … I think what sport actually does is it creates a special environment … where the expectation is clear, the goal is very explicit, you can measure your progress almost immediately and these tiny little feedback loops … And sport, with enough practices in a week and enough time playing … you actually get this virtuous cycle of development for kids which sport is a phenomenal container for. And I think it's because it's built around really explicit skill building.[1]

While this participant mentioned sport as an escape, he also discussed the environment, the interactions with the coach and culture of sport (which other participants connected to developing social capital), the need for explicit skill building, and how feedback loops can shape development. Importantly, we saw in the data that when these conditions did not occur, real harm could be done. For example, one participant discussed how he became socially and psychologically disabled because he was socialised to be addicted to sport: "I was a human lottery ticket and not knowing I was a human lottery ticket, I was addicted to playing football as a way to demonstrate who I was as a person that didn't know the power of addiction." The participant went on to discuss years of drug abuse, time in jail, and stunted development after being used by those around him as a 'ticket' to cash in. Ultimately, being able to pivot from our original plan mitigated possible issues for participants, and also enhanced our understanding of trauma and development. Notably, we were able to make connections in the data with both the depth of individual narratives of athletes and the breadth of perspectives from those working directly in our populations of interest.

Trauma-Informed Practices Applied to Research

The Substance Abuse and Mental Health Services Administration (SAMHSA, 2014) has listed six evidence-based key principles central to a trauma-informed approach. Below, we focus on three of those approaches: (a) *safety*; (b) *empowerment, voice, and choice*; (c) *trustworthiness and transparency*; and (d) *peer support*. We employed a range of strategies to ensure participants were safe, felt connected through trust and transparency, and felt supported as a function of their participation in our research (Bath, 2015; SAMHSA, 2014). In doing so, we tried to ensure these strategies were part and parcel of our research philosophies, methodologies, and methods. Critical to the success of our work, and perhaps less discussed in the literature, was the need for us to create these structures with one another as co-researchers. Without establishing safety, connection, and support for one another, we would not have been able to successfully and ethically navigate these processes with participants. Below, we provide examples of the trauma-informed strategies we used with participants and with one another, which we encourage researchers to consider when conducting research that engages populations that have experienced trauma.

Safety and Empowerment, Voice, and Choice

In terms of safety and empowerment, voice, and choice (Bath, 2015), we believe it is first critical to note our non-foundational ontological stance, coupled with the belief that knowledge is socially constructed, subjective, and relative to time and place (Smith, 2009). Importantly, taking this approach allowed us to show up as fellow and empathic humans as opposed to 'objective' and distant researchers. Researchers have highlighted how telling one's story can be a painful experience, yet it can also have benefits, with differing research traditions impacting the participant experience (Campbell et al., 2010; Wolgemuth et al., 2015). For example, research interviews conducted within a constructionist (Carter et al., 2008) or feminist (Campbell et al., 2010) lens can produce a therapeutic effect (e.g., acute positive affective responses), despite challenges that might occur during the interview process. From a constructionist point of view, this could be a by-product of shifting the power from the researcher's agenda to a more compassionate approach in which participants direct and lead the interview, thereby increasing participant control (Corbin & Morse, 2003; Råheim et al., 2016). As White university researchers in the United States, we were intentional about normalising experiences (discussed in greater detail below), particularly when narratives were shared at the intersection of race, oppression, poverty, and trauma. Moreover, while the strategies described above are a function of constructionist research, they can conflict with methodological strategies in positivist or post-positivist research traditions. Guided by our philosophical position, and in conjunction with the sensitive nature of the research, we intentionally implemented strategies to minimise hierarchies, normalise experiences, and link participants to mental health resources (Campbell et al., 2010). For example, we purposefully scheduled interviews to increase the comfort and safety of the participants. Participants had the option of taking part in the interview in a setting of their choice whether it be a public setting or in an online space. Online interviews (i.e., Skype, Zoom) or those conducted via telephone have been shown by researchers (McMahon et al., 2023) to be more predictable for the participants (i.e., particularly those who have experienced abuse or trauma), as they experience less anxiety because their environment was more expectable.

As participants had ultimate control over where and when they would like the interview to be conducted, it meant that we travelled to different states and sites, such as participants' homes, sport training facilities, public libraries, restaurants, and business offices. In hindsight, this practice meant taking risks with our own safety at times, such as travelling alone to meet with [then] strangers in their homes. To be transparent, we had not considered how our methodological choices might impact our own safety until Meredith, a female researcher on the team, entered a male participant's home for an interview. While she trusted this participant and nothing untoward happened (nor did anything inappropriate occur in any interview), she realised as he locked the front door behind them that no one knew where she was. Moving forward, we communicated before and after each interview, detailing whether the interview was conducted in a private setting, and sharing the interview location as a precaution (yet still following ethics board procedures to ensure participant protection).

Another strategy we used to mitigate power hierarchies was to begin interviews by asking participants to describe their lives growing up. This often led to unscripted and less structured interviews in which we followed where the participant wanted to take us. Some have suggested that this interview practice could pose the risk of distracting the interview from the intended topic or increasing researcher vulnerability (Råheim et al., 2016), yet this approach has been described as more healing centred for participants (Cutcliffe & Ramcharan, 2002). We also took steps to promote reflection for participants throughout the interview process. First, we did not put any time constraints on the interviews, with some lasting up to three hours. Second, at the end of each interview, we offered space (outside of the recorded research process) for the participant to reflect, to provide feedback, or to discuss anything that had come up (Wolgemuth et al., 2015). Finally, we offered a list of local and national resources (e.g., mental health practitioners, trauma networks) if the participant was interested. Following participation in the study, several participants reached out to us after interviews to thank us for listening. Some participants indicated it was the first time they had told their story (or parts thereof) and were surprised at how much they gained through the conversation.

While it might go without saying, proper training and experience in a range of topics and settings was critical to conducting this work. When we began collecting data in 2013, we both had received PhDs in sport and exercise psychology with training, experience, and publications utilising qualitative methodologies. Yet this knowledge and training was insufficient given the topic we were exploring and the range of participant experiences we encountered. William had also completed 600 supervised hours of clinical training as a trauma therapist for homeless youth and adolescents, was trained in motivational interviewing, and was a licensed foster-care parent in the state he resided. Moreover, he had previous experience as a sport coach, a sport psychology consultant, and served on the board of directors of multiple organisations that worked with inner-city youth. As for Meredith, she had received an earlier degree in counselling with a specialisation in sport psychology, supported athletes, teams, and coaches as a mental skills consultant, and served as a coach at both youth and collegiate levels. Additionally, she had accumulated years of experience working in sport-based settings with individuals who are marginalised, have experienced trauma, and/or reside in under-resourced communities (domestic and abroad), including those experiencing generational poverty, systemic and structural racism, community violence, forced relocation, and beyond. Thus, our training and experiences intersected to provide the necessary skill set to protect the psychological safety of participants and ourselves. At a minimum, we would advise that sport researchers interested in studying the effects of trauma receive supervised training and mentorship prior to, and throughout engagement in this type of research.

Trustworthiness and Transparency

We worked hard to build connections with participants by building trust and maintaining transparency (Bath, 2015). This started in the recruitment process but lasted throughout the duration of study procedures. While we both had experiences with interpersonal trauma inside and outside of sport, as white university researchers, it was unlikely that we would be perceived as having any form of insider status. Yet, Bulk and Collins (2023) argue that insider status is a process in flux, with less to do about shared identities and more to do with shared emotions and experiences. By starting recruitment with known contacts and snowball sampling techniques, individuals could vouch for us as people who 'do the work' and not disconnected academics who were focused only on the data. This initial rapport was then furthered through shared understanding of the issues faced for many participants in the study, with awareness that our goal was to share the knowledge with others who were helping to do the work (Pollock, 2012). Further, by following up as promised after interviews, sharing data with participants, and sharing data with community organisations that participants cared about, we were able to maintain trust and transparency throughout the entire research process.

While we needed to build relationships with participants, the work was also not possible without a strong relationship between us as co-researchers. Our relationship, both professional and personal, was not rushed and we intentionally took steps to invest interpersonally. Roughly two years passed between our first conversations about this research and the commencement of data collection. In hindsight, we needed this time to build the connection that was needed to feel safe, be vulnerable, and critically engage with one another (Curry et al., 2012; Trussell et al., 2017). In essence, we played the long-game, which often seems counter-cultural in a system that prioritises quantity over quality and productivity over relationships. As a result, we learned to respect each other as colleagues, and to use humour (a common coping strategy; Abel, 2002) within our working relationship. Both respect and humour were effective strategies that allowed the creation of a safe, collective learning environment where honest, candid discussions emerged around vulnerabilities, concerns, questions, and new ways of thinking (Curry et al., 2012; Trussell et al., 2017).

Peer Support

A final area was understanding our own capacity, and what it took to conduct this research. In addition to helping participants process their emotions related to the research interviews, we also had to address our own reactions and emotions during the research process. The intense emotionality of narratives shared cultivated a sense of responsibility for us, as the researchers, to communicate these narratives that appropriately honoured the participants' stories. For us, 'deciding what story to tell, how to tell it, and to whom' (Lingard et al., 2007, p. 513) were complex, fraughtful decisions, as we wanted to be true to the participants' experiences (Paulus et al., 2010). Moreover, we knew that the stories shared by the participants were creating a range of emotional reactions within ourselves (e.g., anger, hopelessness, hope, sadness, connection, empathy) (Lalor et al., 2006). Thus, we took the step of creating formal support structures for ourselves and each other. This included a scheduled debriefing session after each interview, in which the interviewer could discuss with the other researchers how they were affected by the interview. We also constructed written memos following each interview to help the interviewer reflect on the interview, similar to the written disclosure paradigm (Sloan & Marx, 2004). Finally, we paced our data collection to ensure we had space to process along the way. These steps allowed us to support one another (i.e., peer support), but they also align with some of the other principles central to a trauma-informed approach (e.g., promoting a sense of safety, building trust between team-members, collaboration, and mutuality; SAMHSA, 2014).

As we reflect on this work, as co-researchers, we were both all in on this project. While we occasionally included students in support roles, this work was our priority for several years. This meant we needed to carve out time for long, intense periods of work. Sometimes, this meant limiting other forms of work (e.g., teaching, advising, other research projects) so we could dive more deeply into data analysis; on other occasions, we chose to work during times we might usually spend with family or away from the office, knowing we would not have work-related distractions vying for attention. That said, analysing the data was intense, not just because of the powerful stories shared with us but also because of our commitment to sharing the stories in the right way. There were times when we had to step away from the project, whether for a few minutes, a few days, or a few weeks, allowing for a 'reset.' So our emphasis in this subsection on capacity refers not only to carving out the time necessary to engage in research activities, but also the mental acuity to invest in the research process.

Conclusion

In conducting the research that informs this chapter, it was necessary to frame the research in a theoretical context that made space for the realities of: (a) the individual's experience of trauma, (b) that trauma is often an interpersonal process, and (c) that system-level factors play a role in trauma exposure and responses. As such, our research took a systems approach, examining both individual development and broader social systems. At an individual level, we drew from Bioecological Systems Theory (Bronfenbrenner, 1995), which posits that individual development occurs through the interaction of interpersonal, contextual, socio-cultural, and chronological factors that influence individual behaviour. Yet, we recognised that systems level factors shaped individual development through sport, and so we also theorised on a macro-level. For this, we drew from social science applications of dynamical systems theory, particularly that posited by Ricigliano (2012). This view accepts that micro- or individual-level change does not automatically lead to macro-level change (Massey et al., 2015). Instead, there is a need to examine the interconnectedness of systematic influences, dynamic causality and feedback loops, delays in the system influences over time, and leverage points that incite ripple effects through a system (Coleman et al., 2007; Massey et al., 2015; Woodrow & Chigas, 2011). Thus, our focus was not merely on the traumas experienced by participants, but also how individual development (including the effects of trauma) takes place within a system of influence. We believe that future researchers working with populations affected by trauma should take a systems approach to their work.

Another consideration for future researchers is a deep commitment to ethical practices, even if that means shifting directions, starting over, or even stopping a research study entirely. Pollock (2012) discussed the need for qualitative researchers to expand beyond ethical compliance and consider micro-ethical decisions that happen outside of the context of administrative ethics review. Notably, Pollock argued for ongoing judgements about ethical dilemmas as they appear in real time for qualitative researchers, who should constantly consider the well-being of the participants and the quality of the research. For us, described earlier in this chapter, we had a significant change in our recruitment strategy midway during the first wave of data collection, which was driven by our commitment to participant safety. Additionally, we recognised challenges with our initial analytical approach, leading us to 'start over' despite the lost time and effort. When conducting research with populations affected by trauma, it is critical to be mindful of ongoing ethical decision-making, which is not possible without researchers engaging in critical and ongoing reflection and reflexivity at all stages of the research process.

A final consideration is one that sits at the intersection of many of the points made above. Namely, we encourage researchers, particularly early career researchers, to strongly consider and assess their own personal and professional capacity to conduct qualitative research in populations affected by trauma. As discussed above, we both had extensive preparation to engage in this study, yet both recognise that it felt insufficient once engaged in the process of doing the work. From an ethical point of view, without the time and personal capacity to engage in the work over a long period of time, we may have made decisions that were more about our own goals (e.g., academic outputs) rather than the needs of participants and the community at large (Pollock, 2012). Thus, assessing and receiving guidance on whether or not research teams have the appropriate training, building strong interpersonal relationships within research teams, and carving out appropriate capacity are all important steps for facilitating successful research projects, productive research teams, and – most importantly – the safety of research participants.

Note

1 **Acknowledgement:** This chapter is derived in part from an article published in *Qualitative Research in Sport, Exercise and Health*, May 14, 2018, copyright Taylor & Francis, available online: https://www.tandfonline.com/doi/abs/10.1080/2159676X.2018.1470559

References

Abel, M. H. (2002). Humor, stress, and coping strategies. *International Journal of Humor Research*, *15*, 365–381.

Anda, R. F., Brown, D. W., Felitti, V. J., Bremner, J. D., Dube, S. R., & Giles, W. H. (2007). Adverse childhood experiences and prescribed psychotropic medications in adults. *American Journal of Preventive Medicine*, *32*, 389–394.

Anda, R. F., Felitti, V. J., Walker, J., Whitfield, C. L., Bremner, J. D., Perry, B. D., Dube, S. R., & Giles, W. H. (2006). The enduring effects of abuse and related adverse experiences in childhood: A convergence of evidence from neurobiology and epidemiology. *European Archives of Psychiatry and Clinical Neuroscience, 56*, 174–186.

Anda, R. F., Whitfield, C. L., Felitti, V. J., Chapman, D., Edwards, V. J., Dube, S. R., & Williamson, D. F. (2002). Adverse childhood experiences, alcoholic parents, and later risk of alcoholism and depression. *Psychiatric Services, 53*, 1001–1009.

Bath, H. (2015). The three pillars of traumawise care: Healing in the other 23 hours. *Reclaiming Children and Youth, 23*(4), 6–11.

Blumer, H. (1969). *Symbolic interactionism: Perspective and method*. University of California Press.

Bronfenbrenner, U. (1995). Developmental ecology through space and time: A future perspective. In P. Moen, G. H. Elder, & K. Luscher (Eds.), *Examining lives in context* (pp. 619–649). APA.

Bulk, Y. L., & Collins, B. (2023). Blurry lines: Reflections on "Insider" research. *Qualitative Inquiry*. https://doi.org/10.1177/10778004231188048

Campbell, R. A., Adams, A. E., Wasco, S. M., Ahrens, C. E., & Sefl, T. (2010). "What has it been like for you to talk with me today?" The impact of participating in interview research of rape survivors. *Violence Against Women, 16*, 60–83. https://doi.org/10.1177/1077801209353576

Carter, S. M., Jordens, C. F. C., McGrath, C., & Little, M. (2008). You have to make something of all that rubbish, do you? An empirical investigation of the social process of qualitative research. *Qualitative Health Research, 18*, 1264–1276.

Centers for Disease Control. (2010). Adverse childhood experiences reported by adults – Five states, 2009. *Morbidity and Mortality Weekly Report, 59*(49), 1609–1613.

Chapman, D. P., Anda, R. F., Felitti, V. J., Dube, S. R., Edwards, V. J., & Whitfield, C. L. (2004). Adverse childhood experiences and the risk of depressive disorders in adulthood. *Journal of Affective Disorders, 82*(2), 217–225. http://dx.doi.org/10.1016/j.jad.2003.12.013

Chapman, D. P., Dube, S. R., & Anda, R. F. (2007). Adverse childhood events as risk factors for negative mental health outcomes. *Psychiatric Annals, 37*, 359–364.

Chapman, D. P., Wheaton, A. G., Anda, R. F., Croft, J. B., Edwards, V. J., Liu, Y., Sturgis, S. L., & Perry, G. S. (2011). Adverse childhood experiences and sleep disturbances in adults. *Sleep Medicine, 12*, 773–779.

Coleman, P. T., Vallacher, R. R., Nowak, A., & Wrzosinka, L. (2007). A dynamical systems approach to conflict escalation and intractability. *American Behavioral Scientist, 50*, 1454–1475.

Collins, D., & MacNamara, A. (2012). The rocky road to the top: Why talent needs trauma. *Sports Medicine, 42*, 907–914. https://doi.org/10.1007/BF03262302

Conti, P. (2021). *Trauma: The invisible epidemic. How trauma works and how we can heal from it*. Sounds True Publishing.

Corbin, J. (2009). Taking an analytic journey. In J. M. Morse, P. N. Stern, J. Corbin, B. Bowers, K. Charmaz, & A. E. Clark (Eds.), *Developing grounded theory: The second generation* (pp. 35–54). Left Coast Press.

Corbin, J., & Morse, J. M. (2003). The unstructured interactive interview: Issues of reciprocity and risks when dealing with sensitive topics. *Qualitative Inquiry, 9*, 335–354.

Curry, L. A., O'Cathain, A., Plano Clark, V. L., Aroni, R., Fetters, M., & Berg, D. (2012). The role of group dynamics in mixed methods health sciences research teams. *Journal of Mixed Methods Research, 6*, 5–20.

Cutcliffe, J. R., & Ramcharan, P. (2002). Leveling the playing field? Exploring the merits of the ethics-as-process approach for judging qualitative research proposals. *Qualitative Health Research, 12*, 1000–1010.

D'Andrea, W., Bergholz, L., Fortunato, A., & Spinazzola, J. (2013). Play to the whistle: A pilot investigation of a sports-based intervention for traumatized girls in residential treatment. *Journal of Family Violence, 28*(7), 739–749. https://doi.org/10.1007/s10896-013-9533-x

D'Andrea, W., Ford, J., Stolbach, B., Spinazzola, J., & van der Kolk, B. A. (2012). Understanding interpersonal trauma in children: Why we need a developmentally appropriate trauma diagnosis. *American Journal of Orthopsychiatry, 82*, 187–200.

Dekel, R., & Goldblatt, H. (2008). Is there intergenerational transmission of trauma? The case of combat veterans' children. *American Journal of Orthopsychiatry, 78*(3), 281–289. https://doi.org/10.1037/a0013955

Dube, S. R., Anda, R. F., Felitti, V. J., Chapman, D., Williamson, D. F., & Giles, W. H. (2001). Childhood abuse, household dysfunction and the risk of attempted suicide throughout the life span: Findings from adverse childhood experiences study. *JAMA, 286*, 3089–3096.

Felitti, V. J., Anda, R. F., Nordenberg, D., Williamson, D. F., Spitz, A. M., Edwards, V., Koss, M. P., & Marks, J. S. (1998). Relationship of childhood abuse and household dysfunction to many of the leading causes of death in adults: The adverse childhood experiences (ACE) study. *American Journal of Preventive Medicine, 14*, 245–258.

Fletcher, K. E. (2003). Childhood posttraumatic stress disorder. In E. J. Mash & R. A. Barkley (Eds.), *Child psychopathology* (pp. 330–371). The Guildford Press.

Hambrick, E. P., Brawner, T. W., Perry, B. D., Brandt, K., Hofmeister, C., & Collins, J. O. (2019). Beyond the ACE score: Examining relationships between the timing of developmental adversity, relational health, and developmental outcomes in children. *Archives in Psychiatric Nursing, 33*, 238–247.

Hirschberger, G. (2018). Collective trauma and the social construction of meaning, *Frontiers in Psychology, 9*, 1441. https://doi.org/10.3389/fpsyg.2018.01441

Irish, L., Kobayashi, I., & Delahanty, D. L. (2010). Long-term physical health consequences of childhood sexual abuse: A meta-analytic review. *Journal of Pediatric Psychology, 35*, 450–461.

Lal, S., Suto, M., & Unger, M. (2012). Examining the potential of combining the methods of grounded theory and narrative inquiry: A comparative analysis. *The Qualitative Report, 14*, 1–22.

Lalor, J. G., Begley, C. M., & Devane, D. (2006). Exploring painful experiences: Impact of emotional narratives on members of a qualitative research team. *Methodological Issues in Nursing Research, 56*, 607–616.

Ley, C., Karus, F., Wiesbauer, L., Barrio, M. R., & Spaaij, R. (2021). Health, integration and agency: Sport participation experiences of asylum seekers. *Journal of Refugee Studies, 34*(4), 4140–4160. https://doi.org/10.1093/jrs/feaa081

Lingard, L., Schryer, C. F., Spafford, M. M., & Campbell, S. L. (2007). Negotiating the politics of identity in an interdisciplinary research team. *Qualitative Research, 7*, 501–519.

Massey, W. V., & Whitley, M. A. (2016). The role of sport for youth amidst trauma and chaos. *Qualitative Research in Sport, Exercise, and Health, 8*, 487–504. https://doi.org/10.1080/2159676X.2016.1204351

Massey, W. V., & Whitley, M. A. (2021). The talent paradox: Disenchantment, disengagement and damage through sport. *Sociology of Sport Journal, 38*(2), 167–177. https://doi.org/10.1123/ssj.2019-0159

Massey, W. V., Whitley, M. A., Blom, L. C., & Gerstein, L. H. (2015). Sport for development and peace: A systems theory perspective on promoting sustainable change. *International Journal of Sport Management and Marketing, 16*, 18–35. http://dx.doi.org/10.1504/IJSMM.2015.074921

McMahon, J., McGannon, K. R., Zehntner, C., Werbicki, L., Stephenson, E., & Martin, K. (2023). Trauma-informed abuse education in sport: Engaging athlete abuse survivors as educators and facilitating a community of care. *Sport, Education and Society, 28*(8), 958–971. https://doi.org/10.1080/13573322.2022.2096586

O'Neill, L., Fraser, T., Kitchenham, A., & McDonald, V. (2016). Hidden burdens: A review of intergenerational, historical and complex trauma, implications for indigenous families. *Journal of Child & Adolescent Trauma, 11*(2), 173–186.

Paulus, T. M., Woodside, M., & Ziegler, M. F. (2010). "I tell you, it's a journey, isn't it?" Understanding collaborative meaning making in qualitative research. *Qualitative Inquiry, 16*, 852–862.

Pollock, K. (2012). Procedure versus process: Ethical paradigms and the conduct of qualitative research. *BMC Medical Ethics, 13*, 25. https://doi.org/10.1186/1472-6939-13-25

Råheim, M., Magnussen, L. H., Sekse, R. J., Lunde, Å, Jacobsen, T., & Blystad, A. (2016). Researcher-researched relationship in qualitative research: Shifts in positions and researcher vulnerability. *International Journal of Qualitative Studies on Health and Well-Being, 11*, 30996. https://doi.org/10.3402/qhw.v11.30996

Ricigliano, R. (2012). *Making peace last: A toolbox for sustainable peacebuilding*. Paradigm Publishers.

Substance Abuse and Mental Health Services Administration (SAMHSA). (2014). *SAMHSA's concept of trauma and guidance for a trauma-informed approach*.

Sloan, D. M., & Marx, B. P. (2004). Taking pen to hand: Evaluating theories underlying the written disclosure paradigm. *Clinical Psychology: Science and Practice, 11*, 121–137.

Smith, B. (2010). Narrative inquiry: Ongoing conversations and questions for sport and exercise psychology research. *International Journal Review of Sport and Exercise Psychology, 3*(1), 87–107. https://doi.org/10.1080/17509840903390937

Smith, J. (2009). Judging research quality: From certainty to contingency. *Qualitative Research in Sport and Exercise, 1*(2), 91–100. http://dx.doi.org/10.1080/19398440902908928

Trussell, D. E., Paterson, S., Hebblethwaite, S., Xing, T. M. K., & Evans, M. (2017). Negotiating the complexities and risks of interdisciplinary qualitative research. *International Journal of Qualitative Methods, 16*, 1–10.

Van Ingen, C. (2016). Getting lost as a way of knowing: The art of boxing within Shape Your Life. *Qualitative Research in Sport, Exercise and Health, 8*, 472–486. https://doi.org/10.1080/2159676X.2016.1211170

Whitley, M. A., Donnelly, J. A., Cowan, D. T., & McLaughlin, S. (2022). Narratives of trauma and resilience from Street Soccer players. *Qualitative Research in*

Sport, Exercise and Health, 14(1), 101–118. https://doi.org/10.1080/2159676X. 2021.1879919

Whitley, M. A., & Massey, W. V. (2018). Navigating tensions in qualitative research: Methodology, geography, personality, and beyond. *Qualitative Research in Sport, Exercise, and Health, 10*, 543–554. https://doi.org/10.1080/2159676X.2018.1470559

Whitley, M. A., Massey, W. V., & Leonetti, N. (2016). 'Greatness (un)Channelled': The role of sport in the life of an elite athlete who overcame multiple developmental risk factors. *Qualitative Research in Sport, Exercise, and Health, 8*, 194–212. https://doi.org/10.1080/2159676X.2015.1121913

Whitley, M. A., Massey, W. V., & Wilkison, M. (2018). A systems theory of development through sport for traumatized and disadvantaged youth. *Psychology of Sport and Exercise, 38*, 116–125. https://doi.org/10.1016/j.psychsport.2018.06.004

Williamson, D. F., Thompson, T. J., Anda, R. F., Dietz, W. H., & Felitti, V. J. (2002). Body weight, obesity, and self-reported abuse in childhood. *International Journal of Obesity, 26*, 1075–1082.

Wolgemuth, J. R., Erdil-Moody, Z., Opsal, T., Cross, J. E., Kaanta, T., Dickmann, E. M., & Colomer, S. (2015). Participants' experiences of the qualitative interview: Considering the importance of research paradigms. *Qualitative Research, 15*(3), 351–372. https://doi.org/10.1177/1468794114524222

Woodrow, P., & Chigas, D. (2011). Connecting the dots: Evaluating whether and how programmes address conflict. In D. Körppen, N. Roper, & H. Giessmann (Eds.), *The non-linearity of peace process: Theory and practice of systemic conflict transformation* (pp. 205–228). Barbara Budrich Publishers.

Zolkoski, S. M., & Bullock, L. M. (2012). Resilience in children and youth: A review. *Children and Youth Services, 34*(12), 2295–2303. http://dx.doi.org/10.1016/j. childyouth.2012.08.009

Chapter 15

Future Directions in Trauma-Informed Research in Sport, Exercise, and Health

Kerry R. McGannon and Jenny McMahon

Modest Reflections and Openings for Future Research

In bringing this edited volume to a close, we reiterate that trauma is an important focus for qualitative researchers. Trauma is now recognized as a global health epidemic with well-established physical, psycho-social, behavioural, and health impacts (Substance Abuse and Mental Health Services Administration [SAMHSA], 2014, 2023). Qualitative researchers in physical activity and sport are advancing discourses of 'trauma-informed practice' (TIP) (e.g., trauma awareness, safety, trust, empowerment) to avoid participants' re-traumatization and build resilience. Such work includes explorations of physical activity programming/services grounded in TIP to mitigate impacts of trauma and gender-based violence for adults (Darroch et al., 2022; van Ingen, 2016; Whitley et al., 2022), traumatized youth in sport (Massey & Williams, 2020) and in physical education (Quarmby et al., 2023). Researchers have also called for TIP in sport cultures concerning abuse and the physical and mental health impacts on athletes, and risk of further harm and re-traumatization (McMahon et al., 2023; Mountjoy et al., 2022). This research call coincides with public discussions of gender-based violence and safeguarding in a 'crisis of trauma in sport' discourse, where TIP is recommended to understand and mitigate the impacts of interpersonal violence in sport (Hayhurst & Darroch, 2023).

In addition to a growing body of trauma research conducted with populations in physical activity and sport, the chapters in this book affirm that an engagement with TIP is timely and important for qualitative researchers. Accordingly, Alessi and Kahn (2023, p. 123) note that:

> Whether or not qualitative researchers specifically aim to target participants who have experienced traumatic events, it is almost certain that they will interact with those who have encountered trauma when considering that trauma exposure is high.

Alessi and Kahn's (2023) assertion is part of an emerging body of work in the social sciences detailing guidelines for trauma-informed qualitative research

DOI: 10.4324/9781003332909-19

methods and why this matters (see Campbell et al., 2009; Edelman, 2023a; Isobel, 2021; McMahon et al., in press). While differing in orientations and trauma-impacted participants, proponents of this work effectively argue that without trauma-informed understanding in the research process, researchers may re-traumatize participants, and potentially themselves, given the emotional and socio-political demands of this work (Edelman, 2023b; Shankley et al., 2023; Tujague & Ryan, 2021). It is also important to affirm a strength-based approach without silencing sensitive questions that centralize participants' voices, when conducting trauma-informed qualitative research (Alessi & Kahn, 2023; Nonomura et al., 2020).

Trauma researchers have established that people affected by trauma differ in their support needs and are at risk of re-traumatization (SAMHSA, 2014, 2023). As result of these points, along with the above discussions and tensions concerning TIP in qualitative research methods, researchers are beginning to implement trauma-informed strategies in research in physical activity (e.g., Palladino et al., 2023) and sport (e.g., McMahon et al., 2023) to prevent inflicting any unintended further harms in the research process. Given that TIP in qualitative methods is still an emerging area, the authors in this book showcase their trauma work as a collection centralizing qualitative research on trauma and outline evidence-based TIP used as its core theme. The chapters also sparked conversations about nuanced understandings, tensions, and ethics in TIP in qualitative research, leaving us wanting more. In this chapter, we use a broad-brush approach to summarize some modest reflections concerning TIP categories, with which the chapters engaged. While presented as distinct, these categories should be viewed as dynamic and interdependent, to form a platform for future trauma-informed qualitative research. These points are not offered as definitive steps or rules, but as openings to build on the emerging area of TIP in qualitative research methods in the social sciences, sport, exercise, and health research.

Honouring Context and Complexity: Reflecting on Trauma Meanings

Although it is beyond our scope to detail the vast amount of research on trauma conceptualizations and meanings, before designing and executing research, the chapters in this book made clear to us that qualitative researchers must seek a *critical* understanding of trauma meanings. Doing so facilitates a contextualization of research themes and participants' lives, so that researchers enter this field with empathy and informed understandings (Alessi & Kahn, 2023; Isobel, 2021; Shankley et al., 2023). SAMHSA (2014, p. 7) outlines a commonly cited conception of 'trauma' in a practice context, as resulting from

... an event, or circumstance resulting in physical harm, emotional harm, and/or life-threatening harm which has a lasting adverse effect on the

individual's mental, physical, and emotional health as well as social and/
or spiritual well-being.

Because trauma comprises an external event and an individual's or community's response, the impact of a given traumatic experience should not be
viewed and/or understood in a 'one size fits all' manner (Nonomura et al.,
2020; SAMHSA, 2023). Further, researchers should be aware that the effects
of trauma can be short- and long-term, occurring immediately following
exposure to adversity, or have a delayed onset, which means that research
participants affected by trauma differ in their support needs (Alessi & Kahn,
2023; Nonomura et al., 2020; SAMHSA, 2014). When conducting research
on trauma, and with survivors, these impacts and meanings are better contextualized when researchers have an awareness of trauma beyond general,
biomedical, and individualized definitions. Expanded trauma meanings include historical, cultural, and structural forms (Alessi & Kahn, 2023; Isobel,
2021; SAMHSA, 2023; Shankley et al., 2023). Such understanding is part of a
critically informed approach that problematizes individualized or superficial
conceptions of TIP as developed in a colonial context, which perpetuates victim blame, shame, structural trauma, and stigmatizing processes (e.g., racism,
sexism, ableism, homophobia, transphobia, and xenophobia) (Alessi & Kahn,
2023; Goodman, 2015; Nonomura et al., 2020). Trauma-informed researchers should thus begin with a sensitivity to the impact of historical and cultural
trauma to centre marginalized populations (e.g., Indigenous peoples, people
of colour, people with disabilities, sexual and gender minority individuals,
girls, and women) and the needs of the communities in which they live (Darroch et al., 2022; Tujague & Ryan, 2021; van Ingen, 2016). Attending to these
trauma meanings and those effected holds value for TIP in qualitative research
in sport, given that sport is predicated on a White, male, hegemonic system,
that perpetuates intergenerational and cultural trauma, inequity, and gender-
based violence (Hayhurst & Darroch, 2023; McMahon et al., 2023).

To cultivate meaningful awareness of trauma in the qualitative research
process that honours the complexity of trauma, it is incumbent upon qualitative researchers to 'do the work' and avoid a 'tick box' or performative
exercise in which multiple trauma meanings are glossed over or simply acknowledged (Alessi & Kahn, 2023; Tujague & Ryan, 2021). Once researchers are aware of trauma meanings and the effects of trauma on people's
lives (SAMHSA, 2023), there should be reflection linked to ethical questions of "why the research is being undertaken, who undertakes it, who
participates, and whom it may benefit" (Isobel, 2021, p. 1461). While qualitative researchers often consider such questions in research design, implementation, and ethics, the additional component of being trauma-informed
entails an awareness where participants are asked to share distressing
experiences, and/or probing hidden/unshared trauma, can be voyeuris-
tic, exploitive, or tokenistic, which can do further harm (Nonomura et al.,

2020). It is recommended that researchers deeply reflect on whether their research aims are legitimate enquiry or in contrast, informed by mere curiosity and/or opportunism to advance their personal careers/educational achievement (Alessi & Kahn, 2023; Isobel, 2021).

Operating with an awareness of the above before entering the field honours the ethical complexity of trauma, along with researchers recognizing that they are not treating trauma, but instead using TIP to co-design and co-conduct qualitative research to avoid causing further harm, while fostering strength and resilience (Alessi & Kahn, 2023; Edelman, 2023a). Embracing this standpoint in research aligns with critically engaged TIP to support the complex ways that trauma is negotiated by participants and researchers (Nonomura et al., 2020). Next, we outline reflections contextualized in trauma-informed principles to offer suggestions for how qualitative researchers might further engage with critically informed TIP in the research process.

Trauma-Informed Principles in Qualitative Research: Reflections and Openings

SAMHSA's (2014, 2023) six trauma-informed principles for a practice/services context, served as an evidence-based resource for authors in their chapters. Social science researchers are also drawing on SAMHSA's principles to make additional recommendations for trauma-informed qualitative research methods (e.g., Alessi & Kahn, 2023; Edelman, 2023a; Isobel, 2021; Shankley et al., 2023). These principles include (1) safety; (2) trustworthiness and transparency; (3) peer support; (4) collaboration and mutuality; (5) empowerment, voice, and choice; and (6) cultural, historical, and gender issues. We outline these principles linked with some recommendations for methods and methodologies, followed by a discussion of researcher reflexivity and vulnerability.

Safety, Trustworthiness, and Transparency

Given that trauma has intersectional meanings and effects, *safety* is a core principle of TIP, since trauma survivors in physical activity and sport contexts may feel unsafe due to past experiences and/or current relationships, living situations, discrimination, and stigmatization (Darroch et al., 2022; McMahon et al., 2023; Quarmby et al., 2023; van Ingen, 2016; Whitley et al., 2023). SAMHSA's (2014) principle of *safety* is conceptualized as multifaceted, in that there are physical, social, cultural, and emotional safety aspects to consider. Future qualitative investigations should carefully consider methods in the research process to address and/or mitigate these multiple forms of safety. The chapters in this book outlined several well-established considerations to address these forms safety. We will not outline these again but repeat the importance of learning participants' trauma histories before entering the field. Additionally, the provision of comfortable/safe spaces for the research, along with restorative routines, and providing culturally sensitive access to care and support throughout the research process are foundational considerations. The principle of *trustworthiness and transparency* whereby "operations and decisions are conducted with transparency with the goal of building and maintaining trust" (SAMHSA, 2014, p. 11) is intertwined with addressing safety in the research process. Each chapter again offers considerations to achieve trust and transparency that readers should consider as foundational (e.g., ensuring informed consent and confidentiality is explained and maintained throughout the research process, following through with protocols, or if necessary, adapting protocols).

The implementation of the above well-established TIPs by chapter authors in their research provides an emerging platform on which to build future qualitative research from a critical perspective. Moving forward, engaging in reflections regarding tensions in the research process that mirror social science researchers' 'confessional tales' of 'behind the scenes challenges' when researching TIPs (Edelman, 2023b; Shankley et al., 2023) would be useful. While researchers cannot plan for everything, reflecting on completed trauma research projects can build on TIP in qualitative research, to inform what worked or fell short, and how to address issues. To assist qualitative researchers with critically informed decisions concerning *safety, trustworthiness*, and *transparency*, an intersectionality lens holds value (Alessi & Kahn, 2023). Intersectionality refers to the critical insight that identities and meanings of race, social class, gender, ethnicity, sexuality, dis/ability, or age are not exclusive from one another, but rather, co-constitute people's lived realities (Crenshaw, 1991). Intersectionality holds value for recognizing enduring historical and cultural traumas, and the structural, systemic discrimination that perpetuate violence (Darroch et al., 2022; Goodman, 2015; Tujague & Ryan, 2021; van Ingen, 2016). This recognition means that qualitative researchers acknowledge that intersectional identities of *all* involved (i.e., researchers, participants), which is infused with systems of oppression and power. While we explore this in greater detail when discussing remaining trauma-informed principles, for now it can be noted that attending to intersectionality and power dynamics is crucial to address physical, social, cultural, and emotional safety (SAMHSA, 2023).

Using an intersectionality lens, researchers might engage with participatory qualitative methodologies to co-create knowledge *with* participants to reimagine who owns the research processes, outcomes, and shift the power (Alessi & Kahn, 2023; Darroch et al., 2022). Researchers may also use other interpretive qualitative methodologies that prolong engagement in exercise/sport cultures, and centralize participants' voices, such as ethnography, autoethnography, narrative inquiry, and phenomenology. While different in orientations, these methodologies enable a 'deep dive' into participants' lives, which may be combined with participatory methods to include cultural insiders (e.g., survivor researchers, people with contextual knowledge) that affirm communities of care, safety, and trust (see McMahon et al., 2023; Mc-Mahon & McGannon, submitted; Darroch et al., 2022; Palladino et al., 2023).

Peer Support, Collaboration, and Mutuality

The principles of *peer support, collaboration, and mutuality*, also intertwine with *safety, trust, and transparency*. SAMHSA (2014, p. 11) outlines 'peers' as individuals who are survivors with lived experience of trauma, who may enhance safety and trust, through sharing their stories to promote a realistic picture, and strength-based approach (McMahon et al., 2023). *Peer support* involves survivor researchers working in *collaboration and mutuality* as co-researchers, to co-design and co-lead the research, which is akin to participatory qualitative research methodologies (Darroch et al., 2022; McMahon et al., 2023; Quarmby et al., 2023; van Ingen, 2016). *Peer support* in a trauma-informed approach grounded in *collaboration and mutuality* may also come from 'practitioner-experts' who are immersed in the community and have insider contextual knowledge (Hira et al., 2023; Palladino et al., 2023). *Peer support* might also be used to facilitate shared understanding of trauma meanings and experiences throughout the research process, to enhance safety and trust with co-researchers (McMahon et al., 2023; Shankley et al., 2023).

Given the collaborative and shared partnership emphasis of these intertwining TIPs, SAMHSA (2014) and social science researchers emphasize the need to attend to the role of power and privilege in the research process (Alessi & Kahn, 2023; Campbell et al., 2009; Shankley et al., 2023). One way to accomplish this is to use an intersectional lens coupled with participatory or co-production methodologies, to identify, address, and reconfigure power relations (Alessi & Kahn, 2023). An important part of this process is researchers' *reflexive acknowledgement* of intersecting identities – including critiquing their own – and the relationship of these with privileges and trauma(s), which can silence stories, create mistrust, stigmatization, and/or re-traumatization (Darroch et al., 2022; Goodman, 2015; Isobel, 2021). Researchers with racialized identities that intersect with historical and cultural traumas, when working with trauma survivors in sport and exercise contexts, may also engage in this reflexive acknowledgement (Moola & Krahn, submitted), with support from the research team. We explore additional future directions related to these points in the next principle of *empowerment, voice, and choice*, due its centrality in *peer support, collaboration, and mutuality*.

Empowerment, Voice, and Choice

The principle of *empowerment, voice, and choice* relates to ensuring that research practices and processes are designed to empower those affected by trauma by addressing power relations and differentials (as outlined above) (SAMHSA, 2014). This principle also emphasizes *peer support and collaborative/shared decision-making*, with *choices* facilitated within a co-participatory framework (Darroch et al., 2022; McMahon et al., 2023; Palladino et al., 2023). Fundamentally, to be trauma-informed, it should be reiterated that researchers need to operate from a strength-based approach, to promote *self-determined* recovery from trauma, even in the research process (Darroch et al., 2022; Edelman, 2023a). From an intersectional lens and critically informed participatory methodology, these points mean that power in the research process is reconfigured not erased, in ways that honour multiple meanings of trauma, grounded in oppressive systems (Goodman, 2015). Lest it be unclear, this TIP principle reminds researchers that they do not 'bestow power', 'give voice', or 'allow for choice', as such language may position researchers as holding *hierarchical power* (Alessi & Kahn, 2023; Edelman, 2023a). Rather, researchers should strive to work *alongside* trauma survivors, to dismantle dominance, and shift power and control, in research practices to benefit their lives (Goodman, 2015).

Several qualitative methods might be used to shift or reconfigure power relationships, to enhance *empowerment, voice, and choice* in the research process, while bolstering participants' coping strengths. In some of the chapters in this book, researchers recommended using narrative inquiry to centre stories as pedagogical and cathartic resources. In TIP, stories can be shared and (re)negotiated by peers/co-participants in ways that are comfortable for them, while providing opportunities for understanding and healing (McMahon et al., 2023). This process might include participants *choosing* arts-based methods (e.g., drawings, comics, poems) to reduce privileging the spoken word, particularly for those whose intersecting identities, trauma history, and experiences are not easily expressed in interviews or through colonized ways of knowing (Forsyth et al., 2023). Participants might share stories rather than answering (semi)structured interview questions, to facilitate *empowerment to choose* what they tell and how they tell it; some may express life histories while others find this difficult and choose to express non-linear or fractured tales. The visual method of mind-mapping (i.e., visual images, and short meaningful words are used to 'sketch' out one's journey) can also be used to facilitate participants' control over how, and what, stories they tell (Zehntner et al., submitted). In the principle of *empowerment, voice, and choice*, all content and storytelling forms should be valued by peer support and collaborative research team.

For those occupying survivor-researcher roles, autoethnography may be used to explore, and share, complex experiences throughout the research process (McMahon & McGannon submitted; McMahon et al., in press; Michell, 2020). As a form of theoretically layered self-storytelling, autoethnography can be a valuable tool for cultural outsiders, to learn more about TIP in research. Such stories also offer researchers insight into their own intersecting identities but should be shared only if they feel safe to do so (McMahon & McGannon, submitted, McMahon et al., in press).

While the above research methods may facilitate *empowerment, voice, and choice*, we caution using arts-based methods, interviews, or story-based methods, without a critical understanding of trauma meanings and TIP. While researchers have shown that survivors' research participation can be beneficial and strengthen resilience (see Jaffe et al., 2015), sharing experiences and stories should not be viewed as a panacea without risks and critical awareness of trauma histories. To avoid stigmatizing 'vulnerability' as weakness (Edelman 2023b), researchers may expand peer support/partnerships to include communities of care, enhanced by 'friendship as method' (McMahon & McGannon, submitted). 'Friendship as method' replaces objectivity and power held by academic researchers who 'know best', with co-researchers whose knowledge is trusted and honoured (Edelman, 2023a; McMahon et al., 2023; Papathomas et al., submitted; Williams & Brighton, submitted). 'Friendship as method' can also be expanded to replace the often-used concept of 'critical friends', which can have connotations of criticism and thus silence *empowerment and voice*, for survivor researchers (McMahon & McGannon, submitted).

Cultural, Historical, and Gender Issues

Within SAMHSA's (2014, 2023) guidelines, the principle of *cultural, historical, and gender issues* circles back to a key point with which we began this chapter: being aware of trauma meanings that include historical, intergenerational, cultural, and structural forms, and centring intersectional identities (e.g., race, ethnicity, social class, gender, sexuality, dis/ability, age). SAMHSA (2023, p. 10) reinforces this point, noting that "there are overarching generational, cultural, and societal issues that have caused trauma in the past and continue to re-traumatize individuals". Applied to sport and exercise research, this principle means that research participants come to these spaces for healing, with historical and complex intersecting traumas (Darroch et al., 2022; van Ingen, 2016; Whitley et al., 2022). Others have complicated, repeated, or triggered traumas linked to sport cultures grounded in a history of gender-based violence, linked with their intersecting identities (Hayhurst & Darroch, 2023; McMahon et al., 2023).

The centring of intersectional identities within the principle of *cultural, historical, and gender issues* remains a cornerstone of culturally informed TIP, which begins with *cultural humility* (SAMHSA, 2023). In the qualitative research process, cultural humility entails opening conversations with participants, to seek genuine understanding of identities related to race and ethnicity, gender, sexual orientation, socioeconomic status, social needs, and others (Goodman, 2015; SAMHSA, 2023). While there is no 'one-size fits all' approach to cultural humility, researcher reflexivity is central in this process, whereby researchers interrogate (not simply acknowledge) their own intersecting identities, privilege, and power (Isobel, 2021). We will discuss researcher reflexivity in the final section. But for now, before entering the field, and throughout the research process, researchers need to 'do the work' to seek deep understanding of historical and generational traumas, to understand the implications (Alessi & Kahn, 2023).

Returning to the five trauma-informed principles outlined, it is useful for qualitative researchers to reflect on how these may intersect with *cultural, historical, and gender issues*. While we will not rehash these points, we reiterate that qualitative researchers have participatory research methodologies, and interpretive methodologies at their disposal, to accomplish deep cultural learning, witnessing experiences/stories of trauma and healing, and prolonged engagement in the field. Each of these methodologies is a research craft with nuances, so understanding epistemological underpinnings and implications for each is also essential. The use of qualitative research methods outlined earlier to enhance *empowerment, voice, and choice* (e.g., arts-based methods, stories, autoethnography, mind-mapping, friendship as method) can also facilitate cultural humility by way of witnessing and shared understanding of *cultural, historical, and gender issues* (Forsyth et al., 2023; Zehntner et al., submitted).

Alessi and Kahn (2023) also suggest using 'anti-oppressive research' frameworks when working with historically marginalized participants/communities to further transform oppressive Euro-centric research methods that undermine self-determined community knowledges, co-produced by, and for, survivor researchers. Decolonizing approaches might also be used to acknowledge the history, legacy of exploitation and oppression of Indigenous peoples and racialized communities (Forsyth et al., 2023). In decolonizing approaches, trauma-informed research in sport and exercise must be led by these communities and/or scholars, not by White mainstream academics (Forsyth et al., 2023). Anti-oppressive and decolonizing approaches can also be useful to bring racialized scholars' historical and cultural traumas to the fore, for self-reflexive learning for all members of the research team (Moola & Krahn, submitted). As a final point, the principle of *cultural, historical, and gender issues* can also be critically explored by understanding how aspects of sport cultures (e.g., normalized maltreatment/abusive practices, win at all costs) intersect with cultural identities and traumas (e.g., McMahon & McGannon, submitted; Papathomas et al., submitted; Williams & Brighton, submitted; Zehntner et al., submitted). All previously outlined trauma-informed principles are relevant here, including allyship with peers/survivors leading the process where possible, supported with *safety, trust, choice, and empowerment* forms of qualitative research methods.

Researcher Reflexivity and Vulnerability: Tensions in a Protectionist Ethos

Throughout this chapter, we touched on researcher reflexivity in various ways, across TIP in qualitative research methods. Although it is beyond our scope to detail reflexivity origins and iterations, in trauma-informed qualitative research, reflexivity is regarded as essential to honour intersecting meanings of trauma and effects, to avoid re-traumatization (Alessi & Kahn, 2023; Isobel, 2021). In a general sense, reflexivity in qualitative research means questioning the notion that data are collected and evaluated with detachment/ objectivity, and that researchers act and speak for others, from power and omnipotence. Reflexive researchers acknowledge their own intersecting identities and privilege, as co-constructed in and through the research process, with psychological, emotional, and material consequences for all involved (Alessi & Kahn, 2023).

As noted, researcher reflexivity is an essential practice for engaging with *cultural humility*, through a critical look at one's intersecting identities and power, without marginalizing, stigmatizing, and re-traumatizing co-participants (Isobel, 2021; Shankley et al., 2023). Power dynamics are further intensified when researchers are cultural outsiders, even when using co-participatory frameworks and partnerships to dismantle oppressive research practices (Alessi & Kahn, 2023). Researcher reflexivity runs the risk of becoming another 'tick box' or performative activity, when researchers simply acknowledge and/or state their intersecting identities, without action and/or follow-through (Isobel, 2021). Engaging thoughtfully, honestly, and collaboratively with participants' backgrounds by openly stating one's own using the principles of *peer support, collaboration, and mutuality,* can be useful towards practising meaningful reflexivity (Alessi & Kahn, 2023). Affirming support by following through in the process, along with advocacy, while working with co-participants, community partners, or being a cultural insider (e.g., survivor researcher), can also be a meaningful way to show, not just 'tell', researcher reflexivity.

Alessi and Kahn (2023) recommend that trauma-informed researchers expand reflexivity practices beyond identity positioning and power, to attend critically to emotions experienced before, during, and after research planning and implementation phases of a study. Forms of writing such as 'confessional tales' and 'autoethnography' are useful qualitative methods to assist with this self-reflexive knowledge, shared learning, and critical reflection. The chapters in the book engaged with these forms of writing, in some cases briefly, and in others, more deeply, to outline the impacts of trauma-informed research on themselves. The recommendation for this expanded reflexivity brings forward another aspect of trauma-informed research outlined by researchers in this book: the vulnerability of the researcher in relation to emotional transference, psychological fatigue and distress when hearing difficult stories, and providing support to co-researchers and the research team (Berger, 2020; Edelman, 2023b). The concept of the 'vulnerable researcher' is an important, and complex one in self-reflexive work moving forward, particularly given that TIP in qualitative research emphasizes avoiding re-traumatization, while bolstering resilience (Edelman, 2023b).

Recommendations to assist with transference and psychological impacts of trauma research on researchers relate to enhancing well-being and psychological safety of the researcher. Examples might include forms of self-care (e.g., exercise, mindfulness), supportive members within and outside the research team, journaling/diary methods (Berger, 2020), and as noted earlier, 'friendship as method' (McMahon & McGannon, submitted; Papathomas et al., submitted). It is also important to support and avoid stigmatizing vulnerable researchers, if/when vulnerability is expressed. Contemporary discussions concerning 'vulnerable researchers' and care practices also centre on empathic researchers and/or those holding positions of survivor researchers. Practices include avoiding media stories related to the trauma context that may re-traumatize some (McMahon et al., in press), and journal/diary writing to process deeper feelings and reactions (Alessi & Kahn, 2023; Michell, 2020). These individuals may need additional support and consideration from colleagues, formal institutional support, or qualified health professionals, who can assist with their unique needs. The provision and availability of culturally relevant support and care is underscored by the need for sensitivity and awareness of all co-researchers' intersecting identities, and their link to historical and cultural traumas (Forsyth et al., 2023; McMahon & McGannon, submitted; Moola & Krahn, submitted).

Concluding Reflections

This book had three central aims, the first of which was to showcase the trauma research of a collection of world-leading and early career scholars who have conducted qualitative studies in sport, exercise, and/or health contexts. A second aim was to have chapter authors outline evidence-based TIPs they used, or recommended, for qualitative trauma-informed research work. Finally, based on these two aims, this novel book provides researchers interested in working with populations affected by trauma with a qualitative research resource to build on, and spark new directions in, trauma research in sport, exercise, and health.

We are indebted to these scholars who gave their time to contribute insightful and novel qualitative research that centralizes TIP, in this emerging area of research in sport, exercise, and health, and in the social sciences. We are also indebted to the sport and exercise participants whose stories and lives featured in each chapter's insightful and thought provoking research. Their stories and experiences profoundly matter. Moreover, their voices contribute towards witness, shared understanding of trauma, and the value of trauma-informed research.

As we reflect on our journey of putting together this edited collection, in conjunction with our backgrounds and experiences, it is our hope that the chapters in this book, and our introduction and closing chapters, expands dialogues and sparks additional research. We recognize that the topics, populations featured, sport/exercise contexts, and qualitative research methods utilized only begin to scratch the surface of TIP, and it's potential, in qualitative research. The evidence-based trauma-informed qualitative methods and methodologies featured in each chapter have brought tensions to the fore, but also exciting questions for us to pose, ponder, and explore. We hope that the book has a similar impact for readers interested in the emerging area of trauma-informed qualitative research methods, in sport and exercise research.

References

Alessi, E. J., & Kahn, S. (2023). Toward a trauma-informed qualitative research approach: Guidelines for ensuring the safety and promoting the resilience of research participants. *Qualitative Research in Psychology, 20*(1), 121–154. https://doi.org/10.1080/14780887.2022.2107967

Berger, R. (2020). Studying trauma: Indirect effects on researchers and self – and strategies for addressing them. *Dissociation, 5*(1), 100149. https://doi.org/10.1016/j.ejtd.2020.100149

Campbell, R., Adams, A. E., Wasco, S. M., Ahrens, C. E., & Sefl, T. (2009). Training interviewers for research on sexual violence: A qualitative study of rape survivors' recommendations for interview practice. *Violence Against Women, 15*(5), 595–617. https://doi.org/10.1177/1077801208331248

Crenshaw, K. (1991). Mapping the margins: Intersectionality, identity politics, and violence against women of color. *Stanford Law Review, 43*, 1241–1299. https://doi.org/10.2307/1229039

Darroch, F. E., Varcoe, C., Montaner, G. G., Webb, J., & Paquette, M. (2022). Taking practical steps: A feminist participatory approach to cocreating a trauma-and violence-informed physical activity program for women. *Violence Against Women*. https://doi.org/10.1177/10778012221134821

Edelman, N. (2023a). Trauma and resilience informed research principles and practice: A framework to improve the inclusion and experience of disadvantaged populations in health and social care research. *Journal of Health Services Research & Policy, 28*(1), 66–75. https://doi.org/10.1177/13558196221124740

Edelman, N. (2023b). Addressing researcher vulnerability with the trauma resilience informed research principles and practices framework. In B. C. Clift, I. Costas Batlle, S. Bekker, & K. Chudzikowski (Eds.), *Qualitative researcher vulnerability: Negotiating, experiencing and embracing* (pp. 94–120). Routledge.

Forsyth, J., O'Bonsawin, C., Field, R., & Pillips, M. G., (2023). Ways of knowing: Sport, colonialism and decolonization. In J. Forsyth, C. O'Bonsawin, R. Field, & M.G. Phillips (Eds.), *Decolonizing sport* (pp. 12–30). Fernwood Publishing.

Goodman, R. (2015). A liberatory approach to trauma counseling: Decolonizing our trauma-informed practices. In R. Goodman & P. Gorski (Eds.), *Decolonizing "multicultural" counseling through social justice* (pp. 55–72). Springer.

Hayhurst, L. M. C., & Darroch, F. (2023). Why taking a trauma-and-violence-informed approach can make sport safer and more equitable. *The Conversation*. https://theconversation.com/why-taking-a-trauma-and-violence-informed-approach-can-make-sport-safer-and-more-equitable-213349

Hira, S., Sheppard-Perkins, M., & Darroch, F. (2023). The facilitator is not a bystander: Exploring the perspectives of interdisciplinary experts on trauma research. *Frontiers in Psychology, 14*, 1225789. https://doi.org/10.3389/fpsyg.2023.1225789

Isobel, S. (2021). Trauma-informed qualitative research: Some methodological and practical considerations. *International Journal of Mental Health Nursing, 30* (Suppl. 1), 1456–1469. https://doi.org/10.1111/inm.12914

Jaffe, A. E., DiLillo, D., Hoffman, L., Haikalis, M., & Dykstra, R. E. (2015). Does it hurt to ask? A meta-analysis of participant reactions to trauma research. *Clinical Psychology Review, 40*, 40–56. https://doi.org/10.1016/j.cpr.2015.05.004

Massey, W. V., & Williams, T. L. (2020). Sporting activities for individuals who experienced trauma during their youth: A meta-study. *Qualitative Health Research, 30*(1), 73–87. https://doi.org/10.1177/1049732319849563

McMahon, J., & McGannon, K. R. (submitted). Abstracting the legacy of abuse in post-sport: Using arts-based methods and friendship as method to limit re-traumatisation in abuse and trauma research. In J. McMahon & K.R. McGannon (Eds.), *Trauma-informed research in sport, exercise, and health: Qualitative methods*. Routledge

McMahon, J., McGannon, K. R., & Zehntner, C. (under review). Arts-based methods as a trauma-informed approach to research: Enabling survivors and victims' experiences to be visible and limiting the risk of re-traumatisation. *Methods in Psychology*.

McMahon, J., McGannon, K. R., Zehntner, C., Werbicki, L., Stephenson, E., & Martin, K. (2023). Trauma-informed abuse education in sport: Engaging athlete abuse survivors as educators and facilitating a community of care. *Sport, Education and Society, 28*(8), 958–971. https://doi.org/10.1080/13573322.2022.2096586

Michell, D. E. (2020). Recovering from doing research as a survivor-researcher. *The Qualitative Report, 25*(5), 1377–1392. https://doi.org/10.46743/2160-3715/2020.4048

Moola, F. J., & Krahn, A. (submitted). On breasts and blood: Exploring the contours of forms of trauma for one professional female ballet dancer using a trauma-informed lens. In J. McMahon & K.R. McGannon (Eds.), *Trauma-informed research in sport, exercise, and health: Qualitative methods*. Routledge, Taylor & Francis.

Mountjoy, M., Vertommen, T., Denhollander, R., Kennedy, S., & Majoor, R. (2022). Effective engagement of survivors of harassment and abuse in sport in athlete safeguarding initiatives: A review and A conceptual framework. *British Journal of Sports Medicine, 56*, 232–238.

Nonomura, R., Giesbrecht, C., Jivraj, T., Lapp, A., Bax, K., Jenney, A., Scott, K., Straatman, A.-L., & Baker, L. (2020). *Toward a trauma-and violence-informed research ethics module: Considerations and recommendations*. Centre for Research & Education on Violence Against Women & Children, Western University.

Palladino, E., Darroch, F., Jean-Pierre, L., Kelly, M., Roberts, C., & Hayhurst, L. (2023). Landscape of practice: A participatory approach to creating a trauma- and violence-informed physical activity social learning space. *Qualitative Research in Sport, Exercise and Health, 15*(2), 297–312. https://doi.org/10.1080/2159676X.2022.2146163

Papathomas, A., Pereira Vargas, M. L., & Prior, E. (submitted). Embracing trauma informed practices in athlete disordered eating research. In J. McMahon & K.R. McGannon (Eds.), *Trauma-informed research in sport, exercise, and health: Qualitative methods*. Routledge.

Quarmby, T., Sandford, R., Hooper, O., & Gray, S. (2023). Co-creating strategies for enacting trauma-aware pedagogies with pre-service physical education teachers. *Physical Education and Sport Pedagogy*. https://doi.org/10.1080/17408989.2023.2194905

Shankley, W., Stalford, H., Chase, E., Iusmen, I., & Kreppner, J. (2023). What does it mean to adopt a trauma-informed approach to research?: Reflections on a participatory project with young people seeking asylum in the UK. *International Journal of Qualitative Methods, 22*, 1–12. https://doi.org/10.1177/1609406923118360

Substance Abuse and Mental Health Services Administration (SAMHSA). (2023). *Practical guide for implementing a trauma-informed approach*. https://store.samhsa.gov/sites/default/files/pep23-06-05-005.pdf

Substance Abuse and Mental Health Services Administration (SAMHSA). (2014). *SAMHSA's concept of trauma and guidance for a trauma-informed approach*. https://ncsacw.samhsa.gov/userfiles/files/SAMHSA_Trauma.pdf

Tujague, N. A., & Ryan, K. L. (2021). Ticking the box of 'cultural safety' is not enough: Why trauma-informed practice is critical in indigenous healing. *Rural and Remote Health, 21*, 1–5. https://doi.org/10.22605/RRH6411

van Ingen, C. (2016). Getting lost as a way of knowing: The art of boxing within shape your life. *Qualitative Research in Sport, Exercise and Health, 8*(5), 472–486. https://doi.org/10.1080/2159676X.2016.1211170

Whitley, M. A., Donnelly, J. A., Cowan, D. T., & McLaughlin, S. (2022). Narratives of trauma and resilience from Street Soccer players. *Qualitative Research in Sport, Exercise and Health, 14*(1), 101–118. https://doi.org/10.1080/2159676X.2021.1879919

Williams, T. L., & Brighton, J. (submitted). Trauma and spinal cord injury: Reflections from research into physical activity and sport. In J. McMahon & K.R. McGannon (Eds.), *Trauma-informed research in sport, exercise, and health: Qualitative methods*. Routledge.

Zehntner, C., McMahon, J., & McGannon, K. R. (submitted). Investigating gender-based violence experienced by female coaches and how trauma-informed research approaches can be used to prevent further harm. In J. McMahon & K.R. McGannon (Eds.), *Trauma-informed research in sport, exercise, and health: Qualitative methods*. Routledge.

Index

For Product Safety Concerns and Information please contact our EU
representative GPSR@taylorandfrancis.com
Taylor & Francis Verlag GmbH, Kaufingerstraße 24, 80331 München, Germany

www.ingramcontent.com/pod-product-compliance
Lightning Source LLC
Chambersburg PA
CBHW060237220326
41598CB00027B/3959

* 9 7 8 1 0 3 2 3 6 6 1 3 5 *